Poverty and Neglected Tropical Diseases in the American Rural South

Poverty and Neglected Tropical Diseases in the American Rural South

Christine Crudo Blackburn and Macey Lively

LEXINGTON BOOKS
Lanham • Boulder • New York • London

Published by Lexington Books
An imprint of The Rowman & Littlefield Publishing Group, Inc.
4501 Forbes Boulevard, Suite 200, Lanham, Maryland 20706
www.rowman.com

6 Tinworth Street, London SE11 5AL, United Kingdom

British Library Cataloguing in Publication Information Available

Library of Congress Cataloging-in-Publication Data Available

ISBN 978-1-4985-9386-1 (cloth)
ISBN 978-1-4985-9387-8 (electronic)

Contents

Preface

The idea for this project came about several years ago as I sat in an auditorium on the Texas A&M University campus listening to a presentation by Dr. Peter Hotez from Baylor College of Medicine. I had just moved from the small town of Pullman, Washington, located 8 miles from the Idaho border, to the "college town" (it has the same population as the largest city in Eastern Washington) of College Station. I had come from the College of Veterinary Medicine, where I had spent my time walking calf hutches at 4 a.m. and analyzing samples in a microbiology lab in the afternoon. I was now adjusting to the 8–5 office routine in a public policy school and trying to determine what direction to take my research.

As Dr. Hotez discussed Neglected Tropical Diseases (NTDs) that day, diseases which I admittedly had not thought much about, I found myself fascinated. Following the presentation, I began months of investigation into what work had been done on NTDs here in the United States. What I found was shocking. Despite Dr. Hotez's estimation that there are approximately 12 million Americans living with at least one NTD, the narrative that I kept running into was: "those diseases don't exist there." Among the medical community, scientific community, and the policy community, almost everyone believed that it was impossible for these diseases of poverty to exist within the United States because we are a wealthy country; we do not have that kind of poverty here. Thus, this project was born. We wanted to examine what poverty, water and sanitation infrastructure, and healthcare looked like in the United States to demonstrate that it was, in fact, possible for NTDs to exist here. The result is the book you are now reading.

When the project began, I had no idea what to expect. But I can definitively say that it has changed the way I view the world. This project, and the people that participated in it, taught me about struggle, sacrifice, hope, and love. They taught me about understanding and forgiveness; compassion and determination. At a national level, poverty, healthcare, and infrastructure are heated political issues, but this book was not written to be political. During my time working on this project, I spoke with atheists and deeply religious people who devoted their time to the social issues discussed; I watched Baptists and Catholics work hand-in-hand to improve their communities; and I sat in conference rooms in Washington, DC with staffers from Democratic and Republican offices who were equally concerned about the data I brought them. The reality that I encountered is that most people find it unacceptable to allow fellow Americans to live on less than $2/day or in houses with the roof caving it. Most people find it unacceptable to have children who cannot read or do not know where their next meal is coming from.

What I also learned is that most people, even those who argue vehemently for the elimination of injustices and oppression in the American system, have no idea of the reality faced by individuals living in poverty. I did not when I started this project. And, even now, I have only scratched the surface of understanding. This is not to say that these communities need saviors to swoop in, because they do not. The savior complex we employ in most of our do-gooding, strips those we are "saving" of their autonomy and underestimates their skills, knowledge, and abilities. Rather, poor communities throughout the United States have many smart, innovative, and motivated people that need resources and individuals to work *with* them to improve their communities.

This book was written to expose the reality of poverty, the lack of healthcare access, and failing infrastructure in this country. It was not written to point fingers. We are *all* responsible, each and every one of us, for the suffering that exists. And lastly, it is not meant for shock factor. The people living in the communities that participated in this study are strong, creative, and kind. The communities might have challenges, but they are people's homes and the residents of each and every community we worked with love their home and are proud of their town. It was our hope with this book that we could shed light on the issues, while also conveying the beauty of each community. My biggest take away from this project is that, at a basic level, we are more united on these issues than national debate would have us believe and that we must work together on these real and serious challenges that must be addressed.

Christine Crudo Blackburn

Acknowledgments

Christy would like to thank the Bush School of Government and Public Service at Texas A&M University for providing the funding and flexibility to carry out the research necessary to produce this book. Thank you to Rojelio Mejia for both inspiring and teaching me about the challenges of NTDs in the United States. Thank you to Bill Sischo, you played a central role in helping me understand the importance of showing up in-person and building relationships with people who participate in research projects. Thank you to Michael Johnson Jr. for walking me through literature from the social sciences and humanities that I was unfamiliar with and helping me to craft the best possible study design. Thank you also for reviewing and providing feedback on earlier editions of this book. Thank you to Amanda Taffy for all the hard work you did over a summer to help us gather data. Thank you to Paul Lenze for your feedback and support throughout the writing process and for continuing to be a sounding board throughout my career. Thank you to Leslie Ruyle and Lauren Zajicek for keeping me sane. Thank you to all the residents of the communities we worked with on this project. Without your openness this project would not have been possible. Thank you to Anne Hanisch for her consistent friendship and willingness to let me think out loud about the difficult elements of American society that I experienced first-hand while researching this book. Thank you to my family, specifically Eric and Blake, for continuously supporting me and spending countless hours traveling with me to conduct the work necessary for this book. Finally, I would like to thank Macey for her dedication to this project, her compassion for the residents of the communities in this project, and for the many hours of conversation. Your perspective and friendship have truly made me a better person. I could not have asked for a better partner on this project.

Macey would like to thank the Scowcroft Institute of International Affairs. While a student at the Bush School of Government and Public Service, you made it possible to participate in research and take classes that inspired me to explore a new career field. For all of the community members that welcomed us, thank you for sharing the beauty, resilience, strength, and complexity of the places you call home. My parents, Bobbie Jill and Calder Lively, for always encouraging me to follow my dreams, and for the countless sacrifices you made to help them come true. Your love of faith, learning, and serving others with your whole heart has impacted the lives of many, and I am so proud to be your daughter. Edward Bock, for always making time for me and for sharing many of life's greatest lessons. Caryn Belikoff, for teaching me not to be afraid to take the road less traveled. Sandee Bloom, for your confidence and for showing me how wonderful life can be when you pay attention to details and take time to smell the tulips. Judy Meeks, for being someone I can confide in. You always know how to make me smile. Bill Meeks, for taking me on adventures that I will treasure forever and for showing me that each life, no matter how great or small, is unique and beautiful. Alice and Rich Feldman for being part of my family, and for providing a wealth of wisdom. Rachel Paige-Casey, for your steadfast friendship. Your strength in the face of adversity is a constant source of admiration. Leslie Ruyle, for showing me that a small-town girl can become a strong woman with unlimited potential if she has the courage and determination to venture outside. Alexandra Ding, for inspiring me with your intelligence and love of reading and writing. Cory Raney, for being someone I could count on during the times of uncertainty or celebration, and for endless laughter. All of my family and friends for your love and unconditional support. Finally, thank you Christy Blackburn for being my greatest mentor and friend when I needed it the most. My life would look very different without your guidance and support. Our road trips are among my favorite memories, and I learned so much about tackling life's obstacles, finding purpose, and pursuing my passions by watching you. Thank you for your dedication to this book and to bringing out the best in your students!

Introduction

In April of 1964 President Lyndon B. Johnson began the first in a series of "Poverty Tours" that would last approximately four months.[1] Some of the photos from these tours are iconic: Johnson squatting on the front porch of an Appalachian home with no running water, surrounded by young children. A few years later, Bobby Kennedy took a poverty tour of his own, visiting Eastern Kentucky and the Mississippi Delta. Again, photographs abound of hungry children and makeshift front porches. While the efforts of both President Johnson and Senator Kennedy were heart-felt, these poverty tours did little to change the economic outcomes of the residents they visited. Almost seventy years later, the Appalachia and Mississippi Delta remain the poorest areas of this country. Their residents face shrinking job prospects, underfunded schools, and widespread food insecurity. Just like in the 1960s, many homes still do not have clean water or proper sanitation. While social safety nets have improved, providing some level of security that was previously not possible, poverty is still pervasive and relentless in many rural communities throughout the United States.

The extent and depth of poverty in the modern-day United States is a central topic of this book because we are interested in diseases which thrive in areas of extreme poverty; areas that have been all but forgotten by higher income members of society. These diseases, called Neglected Tropical Diseases (NTDs), lead to negative health and economic outcomes. Many of them push people deeper into the cycle of poverty. Despite their significant and well-known impacts, relatively little work has been conducted on these diseases in the United States. The reason for this neglect is complicated and simplistic at the same time. It is both a refusal to acknowledge that the poor are suffering among the wealthy and a blame-oriented narrative, crafted over more than a century. It is a fear of dividing already scarce resources in states that do not collect enough tax money to support basic services and the American mantra that we should all pull ourselves up by our bootstraps. Whatever the reason for our denial, and no matter how hard we try not to look, the facts remain the same. There are people in America that live on less than $2/day. There are children who do not have a safe place to sleep at night or food on their table. There are people who do not have running water, have houses full of mold, and who run human waste out into their backyard because of a lack of sanitation infrastructure.

We know these things are true not because we read a New York Times article about them or heard about them from a pundit on TV. We know these things are true because we witnessed them with our own eyes and we heard the stories of people who live these realities on a daily basis. These stories are highlighted in chapter 4 of this book. This level of poverty and the diseases that it cultivates are not an abstraction. Millions of American adults and children are cold and hungry in the same country where other Americans are purchasing $700 cell phones every few months because only the newest version will do and reality TV stars spend $50,000 on their three year old's birthday party. Pope Francis stated, "These days there is a lot of poverty in the world, and that's a scandal when we have so many riches and resources to give everyone."[2] This statement applies globally, but could be specifically directed at the United States as well. There is extreme poverty in the United States and it coexists with excessive wealth. It is this very dichotomy that allows NTDs to exist and for many American physicians to dismissively state, "We don't have those diseases here."

In this book, we set out to catalog the realities of poverty in the poorest places in the United States and to highlight the risk factors that all but guarantee that these diseases *do* exist here. Until we can accept, as a nation, that the level of poverty necessary to sustain NTDs does not just exist in Africa, but exists right in our backyard, we cannot effectively address the millions of infected Americans.

WHAT IS A NEGLECTED TROPICAL DISEASE?

The NTDs are a grouping of various communicable diseases prevalent in regions with tropical and subtropical climates. Therefore, climate change influences the geographic spread of NTDs, as increasingly warmer temperatures create more environments hospitable to certain parasites. NTDs share several common attributes, but their most prominent trait is how closely these diseases are enmeshed with the cycle of poverty. Oftentimes, individuals are coinfected with multiple NTDs at once. Several of the diseases are caused by infection with various viruses, parasites, or bacteria, and although an estimated one-sixth of the world's population is infected with at least one NTD, the diseases remain largely outside of the public eye.[3] The names of these NTD's are often long and difficult to pronounce, adding yet another layer of mystery to these already obscure infections.[4]

The following diseases are categorized as NTDs by the World Health Organization: Buruli ulcer, Chagas disease, Dengue, Chikungunya, Dracunculiasis, Echinococcosis, Foodborne trematodiases, Human African trypanosomiasis, Leishmaniasis, Leprosy, Lymphatic filariasis, Mycetoma/chromoblastomycosis/other deep mycoses, Onchocerciasis, Rabies, Scabies and other ectoparasites, Schistosomiasis, Snakebite envenoming, Taeniasis/Cysticercosis, Trachoma, Yaws, and Soil-transmitted helminthiases (ascariasis, toxocariasis, and hookworm). They are a global problem, with 149 countries around the world serving as endemic regions for at least one type of infection.[5] NTDs are attributed as the cause of death for approximately half a million people each year, but the mortality rate of these diseases is vastly overshadowed by their prevalence.[6]

CHARACTERISTICS OF NTDS

A unique characteristic of NTDs, in comparison with other more "newsworthy" threats, are that these diseases are often chronic and can sometimes take years or even decades before an infected individual begins to suffer from symptoms caused by the diseases. Because of this, NTDs do not garner the flurry of media coverage prompted by more grotesque, quickly transmissible, and deadly infectious diseases such as Ebola.[7] In contrast with emerging infectious diseases, most NTDs have infected humans for centuries. Similar symptoms of some NTDs are described in ancient texts such as the Bible, Talmud, Vedas, Egyptian medical papyri, and works by Hippocrates.[8] Another compounding factor contributing to the lack of media coverage regarding NTDs is the tendency of these diseases to infect the poorest and most isolated members of society.[9] It follows, then, that those most impacted by these diseases are often those who are least able to access resources for prevention and treatment, but also to mitigate the risk factors that cause them.

While there is a strong association between NTD prevalence and poverty in general, this is especially true for rural poverty. Because NTDs are particularly prevalent in low-income, rural communities, those infected typically remain invisible to those with wealth and influence. This factor is compounded by preexisting social determinants of health care, such as the marginalization of residents who lack political clout and physical access to healthcare facilities. Another characteristic of many NTDs that contributes to the isolation of those infected are symptoms that cause visible disfigurements. Angry rashes, bulging sores, swollen lymph nodes, disfigured limbs, blindness, and even worms dangling from the skin are all possible physical manifestations of various NTD infections. These disfigurements can result in alienation from the individual's community and family. They can cause negative outcomes for employment opportunities and even marriage prospects and relationships. Some cultures even consider these symptoms as signs that the individual may be cursed.[10] Those who are infected may experience humiliation, discouraging them from getting treatment for fear of further embarrassment or worries that news of their condition may spread to others. All of these factors contribute to increased stigmatization of infected individuals, and exemplify how NTDs can have negative consequences far surpassing health outcomes alone. They create a barrier to economic security, health access, and community acceptance, which serves to further exacerbate the cycle of poverty. Other NTD symptoms have similar poverty-promoting effects that limit development, productivity, and contribute to an increase in the loss of disability-adjusted life years (DALYs), which are used to measure an estimated number of years that are lived with a disability or lost due to a disease.[11] The 2010 Global Burden of Disease study found that over 26 million DALYs were attributed to NTDs.[12] Because NTDs are often chronic, the symptoms continue to weaken the body over time, and can have a permanent impact on the development of young children in particular.

The physical impact can be partly explained by a phenomenon called the life-history theory, in which organisms prioritize the designation of the nutrients they intake to perform tasks that maximize their survival and fitness.[13] Several NTDs create a competitive environment within the body of an infected individual. Parasites and bacteria readily absorb nutrients consumed by the human host, whose body begins to expend more energy for immune responses intended to fight off the infection. An individual carrying a heavy disease burden will often become malnourished. As the body is further weakened by this reduction in energy, the individual becomes increasingly vulnerable to illness.[14] In low-income areas already lacking access to nutritious food, NTDs intensify the struggle individuals face to adequately fuel their bodies to perform basic functions at school and work each day. Malnutrition can result in impaired immune responses, prolonged illness recovery, anemia, infertility, osteoporosis, and can have psychosocial consequences such as depression.[15] If anemia endures for a prolonged period of time, the individual could also suffer from physical growth retardation, impaired memory, and delays in cognitive development. This is especially true for young children who would otherwise be growing and developing at a rapid pace. Additionally, anemia poses a unique risk to pregnant women, as it can lead to low birth weight and increased maternal morbidity and mortality.[16] For these reasons, NTDs disproportionately impact mothers and children, who are oftentimes the most vulnerable populations in areas of poverty and conflict.

The most severe consequences of NTDs include organ impairment or failure, as well as death. Patients with severe symptoms are incapacitated or have limited mobility, potentially causing infected individuals to be unable to attend work or school. Even if they were able to carry out their everyday activities, their productivity and performance are likely limited.

NTD INTERVENTIONS UNDERTAKEN BY THE UNITED STATES ABROAD

In 2000, the United Nations General Assembly issued the UN Millennium Declaration, establishing goals for development and poverty eradication. Of these resolutions, one was to have "halted and begun to reverse, the spread of HIV/AIDS, the scourge of malaria and other major diseases that afflict humanity."[17] The ambiguity of this Millennium Development Goal is reflective of the way these "other diseases" would receive few intervention efforts and little funding in comparison with diseases such as malaria.

The U.S. Congress first designated funds for combating NTDs in November 2005. In response, the U.S. Agency for International Development (USAID) created an integrated approach known as the NTD Control Program to leverage the resources donated by private companies by effectively distributing treatments to 40 million people in 15 countries.[18] Since then, the United States has contributed to NTD control abroad by providing funding and support through USAID to targeted programs such as ENVISION, which resulted in the delivery of 1.4 billion treatments from 2012 to 2018.[19]

On October 27, 2009, the first National Summit on Neglected Infections of Poverty, another commonly used term for NTDs, was held in Washington, DC. Four key areas for follow-up were identified by summit participants. These areas included the advancement and improved understanding of outreach and mobilization, data and surveillance needs, economic impact of NTDs, and research and development needs.[20] Another $350 million was allocated through the U.S. Presidential Initiative for NTDs in 2008. This initiative gave an additional five years of support for NTD control internationally.[21]

In 2012, the World Health Organization published an NTD Roadmap to develop a strategy for the control, elimination, and eradication of seventeen NTDs by the year 2020, which has now been expanded to 2030.[22] These intentions were echoed by target 3.3 of the Sustainable Development Goals established by the United Nations in 2015.[23] Although the WHO's NTD Roadmap strategy proposes elimination for most NTDs, this will remain impossible until safe water, waste disposal and treatment, basic sanitation, and improved living conditions are made accessible to all populations currently at risk. The Roadmap also outlines other areas of progress that would lead to reductions in NTD prevalence. The ability to define successful NTD elimination varies enormously depending on each country's assessment of the significance of the public health problem posed by the NTD.[24] While some NTDs near eradication entirely, such as dracunculiasis, others continue to increase in prevalence, such as Dengue and cutaneous leishmaniasis.[25]

Internationally, NTDs are often treated through the use of mass drug administration (MDA) campaigns, where at-risk populations have medications delivered to them on an annual or semi-annual basis.[26] Over 700 million people receive these treatments annually.[27] These MDA campaigns are capable of providing either prevention or treatment for up to seven NTDs at once. Diseases targeted by current MDA campaigns include trachoma, onchocerciasis, lymphatic filariasis, schistosomiasis, ascariasis, trichuriasis, and hookworm infection.[28] However, medications available through MDA campaigns are only accessible during the time frame of the campaign. If individuals are diagnosed with an NTD at a time when these medications are not available, there is a good chance their regular healthcare provider will be unable to provide them with treatment in a timely manner.[29] Additionally, lack of consistent access to these medications could result in individuals becoming reinfected. As long as the risk factors for NTDs exist, these diseases will continue to be a problem despite interventions focused on treatment.

At an estimated cost of 50 cents per person annually, MDA campaigns provide an affordable option for treatment in low-income countries. Residents of wealthy countries, however, may not be so lucky when seeking treatment for an NTD infection.[30] A common treatment for hookworm infection often included in MDA campaigns, Albendazole, carries an average cost of $400.43 for those looking to purchase the drug in the United States.[31] This sharp contrast in affordability and accessibility highlights a major problem. Although a great deal of research, funding, and interventions have been directed toward communities infected with NTDs in low-income countries, much less is available concerning the impact of NTDs in wealthy countries.

In his book *Blue Marble Health*, Peter Hotez discusses his realization that, "in addition to Nigeria, most of the world's neglected diseases are actually also found in the wealthiest economies, including the Group of 20 (G20) nations."[32] This idea of the poorest of the poor living among the wealthy is what makes the existence and proliferation of NTDs in even the wealthiest of countries possible. As globalization increases and the world grows increasingly interconnected, it is naïve to believe wealthy countries are immune to NTDs as long as conditions cultivated by prolonged poverty persist and the climate remains favorable to these diseases. The United States is no exception, and a long history of endemicity for some NTDs still found in certain states today should be a sufficient indicator that although these diseases may be forgotten, they are not yet gone from American soil.

NEGLECTED INFECTIONS OF POVERTY: AN AMERICAN AFFLICTION

NTDs are prevalent throughout North America. They exist in the United States, Mexico, and even in the Arctic regions of Canada.[33] Historically, the American slave trade caused tropical diseases such as hookworms, whipworms, amebae, malaria, yellow fever, and schistosomiasis to flourish to a degree previously unknown in the New World. Even when slavery was no longer permitted in the United States, NTDs compounded this past tragedy by continuing a legacy of affliction among the country's most vulnerable populations as they struggled to gain equal access to education, housing, and employment opportunities. The areas most impacted include communities in the Mississippi Delta, Appalachia, southern border region, and inner cities.[34] Residents of these areas experience many of the risk factors that make individuals vulnerable to NTDs given the appropriate climate. Issues such as healthcare and housing inaccessibility, inadequate sanitation, food insecurity, education and employment inequity, increased exposure to natural disasters, and the presence of stray animals not only perpetuate the cycle of poverty, but they leave millions at risk of negative health outcomes due to infection with NTDs.

As we will discuss at length in chapter 1, several NTDs are prevalent in the United States. For example, a review of studies conducted from the 1960s to the 1980s, found that the soil-transmitted helminth causing strongyloidiasis was prevalent in central Appalachia.[35] Additionally, Hotez estimated that 68,000–110,000 Appalachian residents may be infected today.[36] In low-income urban areas, leptospirosis, an infection spread by rat urine, has caused incidents of Weil's disease among low-income residents in the communities of Baltimore and Detroit.[37] Homeless populations in urban areas have been infected with bartonellosis, a bacterial disease.[38] Refugee populations from African countries have carried with them infections such as schistosomiasis, that continue to negatively affect their health if left untreated once they have crossed borders.[39] Cysticercosis, a disease prevalent along the U.S.-Mexico border caused by the consumption of pork tapeworms, is responsible for an estimated 10 percent of seizures in Los Angeles emergency rooms.[40] Native Americans living in low-income conditions on tribal lands also experience NTD infections such as cystic echinococcosis and trachoma.[41] Even Native Alaskans, living in isolated Alaskan and Arctic regions, are at risk of NTDs such as toxoplasmosis and trichinellosis from consuming infected food.[42]

Across race, ethnicity, culture, and region, NTDs thrive as long as poverty exists. Despite this diversity, for the purposes of this book, we focus primarily on NTDs with links to rural and systemic poverty in the Southern United States. The communities chosen for this study, therefore, were selected according to this criteria.

PUBLIC HEALTH IN THE UNITED STATES

A number of times throughout history mankind has seemed to turn the tide in the battle against infectious disease. Advancements in medicine and technology have both reduced the impact of many diseases and provided society with a false sense of security. This dichotomy was never better demonstrated than in 1969 when U.S. Surgeon General William Stewart testified to Congress that "the time [had] come to close the book on infectious disease."[43] With this declaration, public health research seemed to shift accordingly, away from infectious disease and toward chronic diseases with an invigorated emphasis on cancer, heart disease, and stroke.[44] Despite the pivot away from infectious diseases, this time period was marked with several victories in public health, such as the last reported cases of wild polio virus in the United States and the eventual success of the World Health Organization's smallpox eradication campaign. It was not until the 1980s and the emergence of HIV/AIDS, however, that the American public health system was forced to reevaluate its false sense of superiority over nature.

The history of public health in America is a series of ups and downs. During the early-1900s, with the development of Germ Theory, an individualistic approach to health protection gave way to a focus on the greater social good.[45] The federal government began to fund large-scale sanitation projects and address outbreak control through an organized effort. Unfortunately, the "Great Depression killed more than lives and economies: it rang the death knell for the public health revolution."[46] Today, the public health system again tends to view health protection as the responsibility of the individual, but much of the degradation of the system is occurring in silence. As described in Christoffel and Gallagher (2006), "Overt resistance to public health is rare. On the contrary, public health has been subject to the death of a thousand cuts, some of them noticed, others not."[47]

Today, it is clear that America's most vulnerable populations are suffering disproportionately from the decline of public health. Arguably, this disparity is nowhere greater than in the South. In the American South, like many other areas of the country, the poor live among the wealthy. "Although American medical skill is among the best in the world, we have an abominable system in this country for the delivery of healthcare, with gross inequalities towards the poor—particularly the working poor."[48] In other words, the individualistic nature of health in the United States means some people get top quality health care while others might suffer with none at all.

It is tempting to think that the health of low-income Americans is not our problem, but health, and infectious disease specifically, is not the problem of any one person. As the Nobel Prize winning molecular biologist Joshua Lederberg famously stated, "The world is really just one village. And our tolerance of disease in any place in the world is at our peril."[49] In this statement, Lederberg was speaking about global health broadly, but the reality is that tolerance of disease among the poorest Americans is to the peril of our entire country. And nowhere is this health inequality seen more clearly than in the prevalence of NTDs.

BOOK OVERVIEW

The purpose of this project was to answer the questions: How common are the risk factors and how underestimated are NTDs in the United States? While these question might seem broad, they are truly important to the conversation of domestic prevalence of NTDs. As we have mentioned, and will mention throughout this book, the most common argument against developing surveillance, prevention, and treatment measures for NTDs domestically is that they are not a problem here in the United States. Thus, to counter such an argument and move the conversation surrounding NTD transmission in the United States forward, it is necessary to show that this is a significant issue in this country.

We sought to answer the question by first examining the history of NTDs in the Southern United States, where they were most prevalent. To do this, in chapter 1, we conducted an extensive review of the peer-reviewed literature, government reports, and newspaper reports to demonstrate the prevalence of NTDs in the United States over the past hundred years. In chapter 2, we examine poverty in the United States and the link between poverty and health in order to demonstrate that the extent of poverty that is commonly associated with NTD infection exists in the United States.

In chapter 3, we examined the modern-day risk factors for NTD infection with the United States including improper waste disposal and the challenges of maintaining proper infrastructure. Chapter 4 tells the stories of some of America's most at-risk communities with the goal of helping readers understand the social and economic risk factors for NTD infection. The conclusion chapter discusses what steps should be taken moving forward to reduce the risk of infection from NTDs and, hopefully, eliminate the suffering of millions of Americans.

NOTES

1. "The Poverty Tours (1964)," Texas Archive of the Moving Image, accessed August 1, 2018, https://texasarchive.org/2010_00054.

2. Babulal Sethia and Parveen Kumar (eds), *Essentials of Global Health*, 97 (Amsterdam: Elsevier Health Sciences, 2019).

3. "Neglected Tropical Diseases," World Health Organization, accessed March 15, 2019, http://www.who.int/neglected_diseases/diseases/en/.

4. "Neglected Tropical Diseases," NIH: National Institute of Allergy and Infectious Diseases, last modified on July 11, 2016, https://www.niaid.nih.gov/research/neglected-tropical-diseases.

5. Centers for Disease Control and Prevention, "Neglected Tropical Diseases (NTDs)," last modified September 14, 2018, https://www.cdc.gov/globalhealth/newsroom/topics/ntds/index.html.

6. World Health Organization Department of Control of Neglected Tropical Diseases, *Sustaining the Drive to Overcome the Global Impact of Neglected Tropical Diseases: Second WHO Report on Neglected Diseases* (World Health Organization, 2013), https://www.who.int/neglected_diseases/9789241564540/en/; P. J. Hotez et al., "Incorporating a Rapid-Impact Package for Neglected Tropical Diseases with Programs for HIV/AIDS, Tuberculosis, and Malaria," *PLoS Medicine* 3, no. 5 (2006): e102.

7. George Dvorsky, "Why 'Neglected Diseases' Are Becoming A Global Danger," *Gizmodo*, published November 20, 2014, https://io9.gizmodo.com/why-neglected-diseases-are-becoming-a-global-danger-1660705505.

8. Peter Hotez, *Forgotten People, Forgotten Diseases: The Neglected Tropical Diseases and their Impact on Global Health and Development* (Sterling, Virginia: ASM Books, 2008), 6.

9. Aline Guio Cavaca et al., "Diseases Neglected by the Media in Espírito Santo, Brazil in 2011–2012," *PLOS Neglected Tropical Diseases* 10, no. 4 (2016): e0004662.

10. Hotez, *Forgotten People, Forgotten Diseases*, 9.

11. John P. Harris, Miren Iturriza-Gomara, and Sarah J. O'Brien, "Estimating Disability-Adjusted Life Years (DALYs) in Community Cases of Norovirus in England," *Viruses* 11, no. 2 (2019): 184, https://doi.org/10.3390/v11020184.

12. Peter J. Hotez et al., "The Global Burden of Disease Study 2010: Interpretation and Implications for the Neglected Tropical Diseases," *PLOS Neglected Tropical Diseases* 8, no. 7 (2014): e2865.

13. Samuel S. Urlacher, Peter T. Ellison, Lawrence S. Sugiyama, Herman Pontzer, Geeta Eick, Melissa A. Liebert, Tara J. Cepon-Robins, Theresa E. Gildner, and J. Josh Snodgrass, "Tradeoffs between Immune Function and Childhood Growth among Amazonian Forager-Horticulturalists," *Proceedings of the National Academy of Sciences* 115, no. 17 (2018): e3914–3921; Anthony J. Zera and Lawrence G. Harshman, "The Physiology of Life History Trade-Offs in Animals," *Annual Review of Ecology and Systematics* 32, no. 1 (2001): 95–126.

14. Diane Duong, "What Do Neglected Tropical Diseases Have to Do With Nutrition?" *Global Citizen*, published August 15, 2018, https://www.globalcitizen.org/en/content/neglected-tropical-diseases-ntds-nutrition/.

15. "Nutrition Support for Adults: Oral Nutrition Support, Enteral Tube Feeding and Parenteral Nutrition," National Collaborating Centre for Acute Care (UK), London: National Collaborating Centre for Acute Care, no. 32 (2006), https://www.ncbi.nlm.nih.gov/books/NBK49258/.

16. Hotez, *Forgotten People, Forgotten Diseases*, 7.

17. "United Nations Millennium Declaration General Assembly Resolution 55/2," The United Nations Human Rights Office of the High Commissioner, published September 8, 2000, https://www.ohchr.org/EN/ProfessionalInterest/Pages/Millennium.aspx.

18. "Neglected Tropical Disease Control Program Final Report," USAID and RTI International (2012), 9, http://www.ntdenvision.org/sites/default/files/docs/ntdcp_report_lo_update.pdf; "The U.S. Government and Global Neglected Tropical Disease Efforts," KFF, published January 28, 2020, https://www.kff.org/global-health-policy/fact-sheet/the-u-s-government-and-global-neglected-tropical-diseases/.

19. "The Envision Impact Final Report," USAID and RTI International, published December 31, 2019, https://www.ntdenvision.org/sites/default/files/docs/PA00WB3N.pdf.

20. Peter Hotez et al., "National Summit On Neglected Infections of Poverty in the United States," *Emerging Infectious Diseases* 16, no. 5 (2010): e1, https://wwwnc.cdc.gov/eid/article/16/5/09-1863_article.

21. World Health Organization, "Accelerating Work to Overcome the Global Impact of Neglected Tropical Diseases: A Roadmap for Implementation" (2012), https://unitingtocombatntds.org/wp-content/uploads/2017/11/who_ntd_roadmap.pdf.

22. World Health Organization, "Accelerating Work to Overcome the Global Impact of Neglected Tropical Diseases: A Roadmap for Implementation."

23. "Sixty-Ninth Session of the United National General Assembly. Draft Outcome Document of the United Nations Summit for the Adoption of the Post-2015 Development Agenda," United Nations General Assembly, published August 12, 2015, http://www.un.org/ga/search/view_doc.asp?symbol=A/69/L.85&Lang=E.

24. World Health Organization, "Accelerating Work to Overcome the Global Impact of Neglected Tropical Diseases."

25. Sharon L. Reed and James H. McKerrow, "Why Funding for Neglected Tropical Diseases should be a Global Priority," *Clinical Infectious Diseases* 67, no. 3 (2018): 323–326.

26. "Mass Drug Administration," USAID Neglected Tropical Disease Program, last modified 2019, https://www.neglecteddiseases.gov/about/what-we-do/mass-drug-administration.

27. Joanne P. Webster, David H. Molyneux, Peter J. Hotez, and Alan Fenwick, "The Contribution of Mass Drug Administration to Global Health: Past, Present and Future," *Philosophical Transactions of the Royal Society B: Biological Sciences* 369, no. 1645 (2014): 20130434.

28. Moses J. Bockarie, Louise A. Kelly-Hope, Maria Rebollo, and David H. Molyneux, "Preventive Chemotherapy as a Strategy for Elimination of Neglected Tropical Parasitic Diseases: Endgame Challenges," *Philosophical Transactions of the Royal Society B: Biological Sciences* 368, no. 1623 (2013): 20120144.

29. Jackie Marchildon, "Neglected Tropical Diseases: The Most Dangerous Diseases You've Never Heard Of," *Global Citizen*, published January 18, 2018, https://www.globalcitizen.org/en/content/neglected-tropical-diseases/.

30. "Annual Report 2012," The END Fund, published 2013, https://end.org/cms/assets/uploads/2018/01/2012-Annual-Report.pdf.

31. Phineas Rueckert, "Millions of Poor Americans Are Contracting These 'Diseases of Poverty' – But Can't Afford Pills to Cure Them," *Global Citizen*, published December 11, 2017, https://www.globalcitizen.org/en/content/hookworm-drug-prices-poverty-alabama/; "Albendazole Prices and Albendazole Coupons," GoodRx, accessed August 19, 2019, https://www.goodrx.com/albendazole.

32. Peter Hotez, *Blue Marble Health: An Innovative Plan to Fight Diseases of the Poor Amid Wealth* (John Hopkins University Press, 2016).

33. Peter Hotez, "Neglected Diseases Amid Wealth in the United States and Europe," *Health Affairs* 28, no. 6 (2009): 1720–1725.

34. Peter Hotez, "Neglected Infections of Poverty in the United States of America," *PLOS Neglected Tropical Diseases* 2, no. 6 (2008): e256.

35. Charles D. Ericsson, Robert Steffen, Afzal A. Siddiqui, and Steven L. Berk, "Diagnosis of Strongyloides Stercoralis Infection," *Clinical Infectious Diseases* 33, no. 7 (2001): 1040–1047.

36. Hotez, "Neglected Infections of Poverty in the United States of America"; Hotez, *Forgotten People, Forgotten Diseases*, 117.

37. Vinetz et al., "Sporadic Urban Leptospirosis," *Annals of Internal Medicine* 125, no. 10 (1996): 794–798; A. B. Thiermann, and R. R. Frank, "Human Leptospirosis in Detroit and the Role of Rats as Chronic Carriers," *International Journal of Zoonoses* 7, no. 1 (1980): 62–72; Raymond Y. Demers, Robert Frank, Paul Demers, and Melvin Clay, "Leptospiral Exposure in Detroit Rodent Control Workers," *American Journal of Public Health* 75, no. 9 (1985): 1090–1091.

38. David H. Spach et al., "Bartonella (Rochalimaea) quintana Bacteremia in Inner-City Patients with Chronic Alcoholism," *New England Journal of Medicine* 332, no. 7 (1995): 424–428; Lisa A. Jackson et al., "Seroprevalence to Bartonella quintana among Patients at a Community Clinic in Downtown Seattle," *Journal of Infectious Diseases* 173, no. 4 (1996): 1023–1026; Philippe Brouqui and Didier Raoult, "Arthropod-borne Diseases in Homeless," *Annals of the New York Academy of Sciences* 1078, no. 1 (2006): 223–235.

39. Carlos Franco-Paredes et al., "Persistent and Untreated Tropical Infectious Diseases among Sudanese Refugees in the United States," *The American Journal of Tropical Medicine and Hygiene* 77, no. 4 (2007): 633–635; Drew L. Posey et al., "High Prevalence and Presumptive Treatment of Schistosomiasis and Strongyloidiasis among African Refugees," *Clinical Infectious Diseases* 45, no. 10 (2007): 1310–1315.

40. Samuel Ong et al., "Neurocysticercosis in Radiographically Imaged Seizure Patients in US Emergency Departments," *Emerging Infectious Diseases* 8, no. 6 (2002): 608.

41. David T. Rearwin, J. H. Tang, and James W. Hughes, "Causes of Blindness among Navajo Indians: An Update," *Journal of the American Optometric Association* 68, no. 8 (1997): 511–517; Joel A. Ludlam, "Prevalence of Trachoma among Navajo Indian Children," *American Journal of Optometry and Physiological Optics* 55, no. 2 (1978): 116–118; P. M. Schantz et al., "Epidemiologic Investigation of Echinococcosis in American Indians Living in Arizona and New Mexico," *The American Journal of Tropical Medicine and Hygiene* 26, no. 1 (1977): 121–126.

42. Hotez, *Forgotten People and Forgotten Diseases*, 122.

43. Ross Upshur, "Ethics and Infectious Disease," *Bulletin of the World Health Organization* 86 (2008): 577–656.

44. Tony Pugh, "Shift from Infectious Diseases has Left the U.S. More Vulnerable," *McClatchy DC Bureau*, published May 25, 2007, https://www.mcclatchydc.com/latest-news/article24452836.html.

45. Laurie Garrett, *Betrayal of Trust: The Collapse of Global Public Health* (New York: Hyperion, 2000).

46. Garrett, *Betrayal of Trust*, 308.

47. Tom Christoffel and Susan Scavo Gallagher, *Injury Prevention and Public Health: Practical Knowledge, Skills, and Strategies* (Jones & Bartlett Learning, 2006), 23.

48. Garrett, *Betrayal of Trust*, 372.

49. Garrett, *Betrayal of Trust*, 279.

Chapter 1

Yesterday and Today

Neglected Tropical Disease in the Southern United States

Although mostly forgotten, tropical diseases have played a central role in social and economic aspects of the American South's history. Prior to the Civil War and for the decades that followed it, communities throughout the Southern United States battled against microscopic foes. The warm, humid weather and abundant rainfall combined with mostly rural, agrarian economies in states like Louisiana, Mississippi, Alabama, Georgia, North Carolina, South Carolina, Tennessee, Kentucky, and Arkansas to create a perfect storm for disease prevalence and spread. Almost every Southern state was plagued by hookworm, malaria, Dengue fever, Yellow fever, and more. Many of these diseases arrived on the American continent as a result of the Trans-Atlantic slave trade and once here, spread throughout port cities and up the Mississippi River—hitching rides on trade ships. Deadly infectious diseases, as well as chronic, debilitating diseases were an ongoing threat to Southerners well into the twentieth century.

The impact of tropical diseases on the Southern economy cannot be underestimated as many parts of the South continue to lag behind their Northern counterparts. Changes in the twentieth century—such as air conditioning, indoor plumbing, and the mechanization of agriculture—reduced Americans' environmental exposure to NTDs, but did not eliminate them. As the country advanced, many of America's poorest areas still struggled with the same problems. Unfortunately, "as tropical diseases faded from medical consciousness in the rich countries of the world, they also vanished from public awareness."[1] Today, in the contemporary South, many of the risk factors still exist that allowed infectious diseases to wreak havoc on the Southern population. Most importantly, "poverty is a critical factor. But the American South's hot and humid climate, the influx of insects that carry diseases, and the ever-increasing movement of humans have combined with the region's high poverty levels to create a perfect storm of disease."[2]

Although there is a perfect storm of circumstances that exist in the South, there is a lack of attention to NTDs. "Despite tremendous advances in other types of illness in recent decades," Arnold (2015) argues, "tropical medicine remains stubbornly stuck in the 1950s, leaving the USA as unprepared as low-income nations to treat any significant number of cases."[3] Additionally, and as we will state repeatedly throughout this book, not looking for something is not the same as it not existing, which is to say that we cannot maintain the refrain that NTDs are not a problem in the United States if we do not have any surveillance, reporting, or tracking of infections.

In this chapter, we will examine the history of NTDs and other infectious diseases in the Southern United States to demonstrate the forgotten historical prevalence of these diseases. This chapter examines the historical and modern-day impacts of hookworm, toxocariasis, ascariasis, Dengue fever, yellow fever, Chagas, and trichomoniasis. We detail the destructive history of these diseases and the impact they had on the development of the Southern states. Additionally, we will show that many of these diseases were never eliminated, just reduced, and relegated inclusively to communities of poverty.

DISEASE HISTORY OF THE SOUTHERN UNITED STATES

Hookworm

Hookworm is a soil-transmitted helminth, or parasitic worm, that was once widespread in the United States. Larvae and adult worms live in the small intestines of those infected and severe infections can cause abdominal pain, diarrhea, fatigue, and anemia.[4] There are two kinds of hookworm: *Ancylostoma duodenale* and *Necator americanus*. The type found most commonly in the American South is *Necator americanus*. It is estimated that there are 576–740 million people infected with hookworm globally.[5] An individual becomes infected when they come into contact with contaminated soil, which most commonly occurs when the individual is walking barefoot.[6] In optimal conditions, hookworm is able to live in the soil for months. Once it finds a host and enters their intestines, it is able to live for about five years and the severity of infection depends on the number of worms an individual is infected with.[7] There is evidence that hookworm has been infecting humans for centuries.[8] The ancient Egyptians painted hieroglyphs that described the anemic symptoms of severe hookworm infection and some ancient Greeks were said to eat rocks and dirt because of a disease.[9] The first modern-day mass hookworm infection was not discovered until 1880, however, when it was found that many Italian miners were suffering from severe infection.[10] While the earliest evidence of infection stems from North African and Southern Europe, hookworm eventually made its way to the United States. The disease is said to have arrived in the North American due to the Trans-Atlantic slave trade.[11] The climate of the Southern United States was perfect for hookworm and the disease quickly found a new home in the sandy Southern soil. Early in American history it was known as "ground itch" and was common enough that Harper Lee referred to it in her Pulitzer Prize winning book *To Kill a Mockingbird.*[12] In the late 1800s and up through the mid-1900s, hookworm infection was perpetuated by a lack of sanitation, the use of night-soil, and the fact that many children did not wear shoes.[13]

Today, hookworm is often referred to as a "disease of poverty" because it most commonly affects individuals living in extreme poverty, both in the United States and globally. Risk of hookworm infection increases in warm climates where there is poor sanitation and hygiene because infection requires direct contact with contaminated soil and hookworm thrives in warm temperatures.[14] Patterns of hookworm infection in the United States are similar to patterns of infection throughout the rest of the world in that, historically, the highest rates of infection have gone hand-in-hand with high rates of poverty.[15] Beginning in the 1980s, politicians, public health professionals, physicians, and the lay public began to believe that hookworm had been eliminated from the United States, although it had never been shown to be eradicated—only reduced—anywhere in the United States.[16] We disagree with this assumption. We concur with the growing voice of infectious disease researchers who believe that pockets of hookworm infection still exist in communities of extreme poverty in the United States. Indeed, some evidence for this exists.[17] We will detail our argument for this later in the book, but in the next several sections of this chapter, we will examine the history of hookworm in the Southern United States.

Hookworm Infection in the South 1800s—Early 1900s

The Trans-Atlantic slave trade in the 1800s first brought hookworm to the United States from Africa.[18] Once it arrived, it persisted quietly throughout the Southern United States, remaining completely undetected until the early 1900s. A central reason for the lack of detection was that "[I]t rarely killed its victims outright but rather left them feeling weak, listless, out-of-sorts: hence its later identification in the popular press as the 'germ of laziness'."[19] Hookworm was so pervasive that "millions of those bloodsucking parasites lived, fed, multiplied, and died within the guts of up to 40 percent of populations stretching from southeastern Texas to West Virginia . . . It was nearly impossible for the rural poor—the majority back then—to avoid hookworms."[20] In the early 1900s it was estimated that 7.5 million people, or roughly 30 percent of the Southern population were infected.[21]

Hookworm was able to thrive in the Southern United States for a number of reasons. One reason, as mentioned earlier, was that the climate was perfect for the worms. Ideal environmental conditions for the parasite are warm, humid climates, exactly like what is found throughout the South.[22] Due to these favorable environmental conditions, once hookworm arrived with the Trans-Atlantic slave trade, it found the climate and soil of the Southern United States a hospitable new home. Other reasons that hookworm thrived once it arrived in the United States was due to the lack of outhouses, the use of night-soil, and the lack of shoe-wearing among children in the Southern United States.[23] In 1902, Charles Wardell Stiles, a zoologist who first took up the cause of hookworm in the United States, proclaimed, "There is . . . not the slightest room for doubt that uncinariasis is one of the most important . . . diseases of . . . the South, especially on farms and plantations in sandy districts, and . . . that much of the trouble popularly attributed to 'dirt-eating' . . . and even some of the proverbial laziness of the poorer classes of the white population are . . . manifestations of uncinariasis."[24]

Most people mocked Stiles for his comments. Both Northerners and Southerners alike found it ridiculous that a worm could be responsible for tiredness or laziness. To most, particularly the elites of the time period the "laziness" of low-income Southerners was the result of moral failings. The idea of widespread hookworm infection was not as crazy as it was made out to be, however. At the turn of the century, approximately 80 percent of the churches and schools in the rural South did not have outhouses and an even greater number of farmhouses had no outhouse.[25] Unfortunately, discussion of this lack of sanitation only further angered Southerners. Many during the time period felt that it was undignified to discuss outhouses, night-soil, or other issues of sanitation. In fact, some residents of small towns throughout the South were so angered by these topics that they chased Stiles out of town.[26]

While Stiles' investigation of hookworm in the Southern United States brought public attention and Rockefeller funds to the issue, the parasite had already had a measurable impact on American history. Specifically, it is believed to have played an important role in the Civil War. As Rebecca Kreston (2011) explains, "The popular image during the American Civil War of the lazy Southern redneck with 'sallow skin, bare feet, scrawny neck, protuberant abdomen, retarded intelligence, and shiftless habits' undoubtedly derived from endemic hookworm infection and its debilitating symptoms."[27] Confederate soldiers were often barefoot and, at the time of the Civil War, the number of hookworm parasites in the Southern soil was so immense that anyone walking barefoot was sure to become infected.[28] Union soldiers wore boots, and, therefore, did not have the same risk of infection. "Hookworms had their heyday during the Civil War, when levels of infection exploded due to substandard living conditions, poor health and lack of sanitary infrastructure."[29]

Hookworm likely played a significant and decisive role in the Civil War, but once the war ended infections did not decrease. In fact, they only got worse in the years following the war. "Garland Brinkley . . . argues that hookworm disease worsened in the years following the Civil War, thanks to deteriorating conditions and economic setbacks, and that the rise of these parasites only served to slow recovery even further."[30] Put differently, the economic destruction, combined with physical destruction that accompanied the Civil War created an even more fertile environment for hookworm throughout the South. As Ettling (1981) states, "Between 1865 and 1910, more and more Southerners in each succeeding generation fell victim to the hookworm, until as much as 40 percent of the region's population harbored the parasite.[31] So prevalent was hookworm infection and for so long had it been a feature on the Southern landscape that people mistook the physical appearance of its sufferers for the peculiar badge of an unfortunate economic and social class."[32]

The physical destruction that hookworm wrecked on many Southerners perpetuated the stereotypes and further confirmed, in the mind of Northerners, that the South was a backward place. In turn, when Stiles turned his attention to hookworm infection in the South and the Rockefeller Foundation funded an eradication campaign, many Southerners viewed it as Yankee condemnation and responded with anger and hostility. The early years of the eradication campaign faced intense opposition throughout Southern communities as many remained in denial.[33] In the decades that hookworm silently infected the rural poor in the American South, it also hindered both economic and educational progress of the population. In the next section, we discuss the economic impacts that hookworm infection had on the Southern United States prior to the eradication campaign by the Rockefeller Sanitary Commission.

Economic Impacts

Although the magnitude of the impact is not always recognized, hookworm had a substantial, long-term impact on the economic development of the Southern United States. Over the decades, numerous scholars have sought to quantify the economic impact of hookworm, not only on the South as a whole, but on the places with the worst level of infection compared to lower infection levels. As Bleakley (2007) observes, "hookworm played a major role in the South's lagging behind the rest of the country."[34]

There are a number of ways that hookworm disease impacted the economic development of Southern states, but the most noticeable impacts came in agricultural productivity (and productivity more broadly) and educational attainment. As we have discussed previously, hookworm disease, particularly if it is severe, causes anemia, fatigue, and other symptoms that make it difficult for an individual to work quickly or for extended hours. These symptoms are specifically what led to the stereotype of the "lazy" Southerner. High rates of hookworm infection among the Southern workforce meant that production in the Southern states depressed compared to what it might have been with a healthy workforce. Additionally, hookworm reduced the number of individuals that were healthy enough to participate in the workforce at all, meaning that there were fewer available workers than there might otherwise have been. In his 2007 article on the economic impacts of hookworm, Bleakley observed that the largest impact comes from infection in children.[35] Hookworm infection in a child can impact the overall total number of years a person is able to work, which if significantly reduced, can affect both the individual's lifetime earnings and their contribution to the state's economy.

In order to accurately demonstrate the economic impact of hookworm, Bleakley (2007) analyzed the level of responsibility the disease holds for the economic disparities between the Northern and Southern United States. Through this analysis he finds "the hookworm infection rate could account for around half of the literacy gap and about 20 percent of income differences."[36] In a subsequent study, he also found that "persistent childhood hookworm infection depressed adult income by 43 percent."[37] When the economic impacts of hookworm and malaria are combined, they account for one-third of the economic disparity between the North and South.[38]

While it has been demonstrated the hookworm infection played a role in slowing economic development in the Southern states and increasing the economic disparity between the North and South following the Civil War, the burden of hookworm in different locations can also explain why some Southern states were more prosperous than others. "If you compare places in the South with the worst versus the least hookworm problem, you're talking differences in income of maybe 25%."[39] What this means is that, while the overall economic development of the South was depressed due to hookworm infection, areas with higher rates of infection were more significantly depressed. These areas fell behind economically even in relation to the other Southern states. "There are lots of reasons why the South had a different development path than the rest of the country, and while disease is not the whole story, it was certainly part of it."[40]

An individual's inability to enter the workforce and be productive was a significant reason for slow economic growth, but hookworm disease also impacted an individual's ability to attend school and be successful in their studies—which impacts their overall future earning potential. In the next section, we will discuss the educational and cognitive impacts of hookworm infection in the South.

Educational and Cognitive Impacts of Hookworm Infection

In conjunction with the economic impacts of, and indeed a contributing factor to decreased economic prosperity, hookworm infection in the Southern United States throughout the 1800s and into the early to mid-1900s had a notable impact on educational attainment. In fact, "modern researchers have correlated cognitive delay with hookworm disease, and the zoologist Stiles noted that children with hookworm were likely to be behind their appropriate grade in school or tracked into the lowest-performing strata of their grades."[41]

The relationship between hookworm infection and cognitive delays has been understood and was regularly discussed throughout the hookworm eradication campaigns of the early and mid-1900s. Nuwer (2016) notes, "A 1926 study of Alabama school children found that the greater the number of worms that students harbored, the lower their IQ."[42] Multiple studies over the course of many decades have demonstrated the cognitive impacts of hookworm infection and shown a linkage between the level of infection (i.e., number of worms) and the level of cognitive impairment.

As the burden of hookworm infection decreased throughout the Southern United States, there was a measurable improvement in school attendance and literacy. Numerous studies have shown that the Rockefeller Sanitary Commission campaign, which took place in the early 1900s and will be discussed in the next section, led to increased school enrollment and attendance. This, in turn, led to an increase in literacy rates.[43] What these findings demonstrate is that the educational lags of the Southern poor were not were due largely to the disease and not personal or moral failings, as was a common narrative then (and still is now). The anemia and fatigue, along with other symptoms that accompany hookworm infection make it difficult for children to attend school in the first place. Poor school attendance, or a complete lack of enrollment, put students further behind and compounded the challenges created by the impact of hookworm infection on cognitive development.

It is important to note that educational attainment and economic development are intrinsically linked within the story of hookworm infection in the South. Children with cognitive delays and learning disabilities, combined with low school enrollment and attendance, and low literacy rates made it difficult for Southerners to keep up in the changing economy. Additionally, the level of hookworm infection was much greater among Southerners living in poverty, exacerbating their educational and economic disadvantages. Lastly, there was likely a significant impact on populations of color, though most of the work on hookworm in the early to mid-1900s focused exclusively on the white population. The lack of attention to the issue among communities of color could be part of the reason that NTD infection rates are higher among such communities today.

Rockefeller Sanitary Commission

In the late 1800s and early 1900s, no one in the South, or throughout the United States for that matter, had heard of hookworm. It was not until Stiles began drawing attention to the disease in the Southern United States that anyone considered it an issue. Even for years after he started spreading the word about hookworm, many people, including doctors and politicians, did not believe it existed. When Stiles first began advocating for public and government attention for hookworm in the 1890s, many found the idea ridiculous.[44] Northern newspapers printed accounts that ridiculed Stiles and Southerners. This ridicule made it even more difficult for Stiles to gain traction in the South.[45] As Ettling (1981) explains, "Echoes of derisive Yankee laughter must have dogged Stiles's footsteps through dusty little Southern towns and drowned out his warnings in the ears of touchy farmers whose pride was greater even than their degree of hookworm infection."[46]

Through persistence and determination, Stiles was able to convince the Rockefeller Institute to donate $1 million to fight hookworm in the United States.[47] The effort was termed the Rockefeller Sanitary Commission and as the Commission began its work, it sought to partner with states and their existing agencies. Unfortunately, "the Sanitary Commission found most of the state public health agencies inadequate to meet the demands of a rigorous state-wide campaign of the type necessary to do battle with the hookworm."[48] Additionally, most individuals serving on public health boards in the Southern United States were political appointees without any medical background or knowledge of health. Ultimately, the Commission decided to focus on improving state and county public health boards in addition to raising awareness of hookworm among the public.

Getting the public to pay attention to the campaign was another difficult obstacle that the Commission fought to overcome.[49] Public health services in the Southern states were inconsistent, meaning not every state had one, and underfunded. "Southerners had come to regard their public health services as relief-bringing agencies, arriving on the scene of an epidemic or natural disaster to repair the damage and ameliorate the suffering."[50] This public perception meant that the Commission had to increase public health infrastructure throughout the South and change perceptions of the role of public health in society.[51]

The Commission's presence in the South was an unwelcome development in the minds of Southerners. Resentments still lingered following the Civil

War and the idea that Northerners were going to come save them from, what they believed was, an imaginary disease, only made tensions worse. The *Macon Telegraph* wrote, "Where was this hookworm or lazy disease when it took five Yankee soldiers to whip one Southerner?"[52] Other newspapers painted the issue as propaganda designed to disparage the South or claimed that Rockefeller was going into the shoe business and was using the campaign to sell more shoes. Still others viewed the campaign as "a Trojan Horse designed to take over Southern education."[53]

Even among those who were less skeptical of the existence of hookworm, resentment for Rockefeller and the Northerners behind the campaign was obvious. The *Raleigh News and Observer* commented that "many of us in the South are getting tired of being exploited by advertisements that exaggerate conditions. They are most harmful. As to hookworm, this paper has accepted the statement of the widespread prevalence of that disease with many grains of allowance. Let us not canonize Standard Oil Rockefeller by putting laurels on his head because he seeks to buy the appreciation of the people whom he has been robbing for a quarter of a century."[54] Put differently, even Southerners not resistant to the idea that there was hookworm infection did not want to praise Rockefeller for his donation. They felt that if there was a problem, then they could deal with it themselves. Many were vocal that they did not need the scorn, pity, or mockery of Northerners.

Due in large part to the strong resistance the Commission experienced at the beginning of the campaign, progress was slow. Once they adopted the structure and feeling of a Southern tent revival to distribute treatment and raise awareness, however, the campaign took off.[55] Over the next five years, nearly 500,000 people were treated at dispensaries throughout the South.[56] While this was a large number of individuals, it was only a fourth of the two million people the Commission had identified as suffering from hookworm and an even smaller proportion of the 7.5 million the Commission believed to be infected. Unfortunately, the program was terminated suddenly and by unilateral decision, with no explanation other than it was time for the South to begin taking care of their own health.[57]

The success of the Hookworm Eradication campaign was mixed. In the success category, awareness of hookworm had been substantially increased among government officials and the public and half a million people had been treated.[58] The increased awareness hookworm led to its official incorporation into the medical school curriculum. Lastly, the Commission was successful in creating an entire network of state and local public health agencies that were proactive and focused on conducting continuous public health work.[59]

Despite these important successes, however, there were a number of states that had high incidences of hookworm infection in which the Commission had not even begun work. Some of these places had high concentrations of sandy soil, which has been proven to have a profound impact on the prevalence of hookworm.[60] Additionally, the campaign had not "eradicated" hookworm as it had promised. "In fact, the Sanitary Commission had failed to eradicate hookworm anywhere in the South."[61]

Hookworm Today

Hookworm remained a problem in the Southern United States following the dissolution of the Rockefeller Sanitary Commission, though significant progress had been made in raising awareness of the disease and strengthening public health infrastructure. As late as the 1940s and 1950s, however, some areas of the South were still referred to as the "Hookworm Belt."[62] Throughout the 1950s "it was nearly impossible for the rural poor—the majority back then—to avoid hookworms, and although there is an absence of data, most people believed that hookworm was eradicated in the United States sometime between the 1950s and the 1980s."[63]

The perceived eradication of hookworm did not occur because of any policy directed at addressing the disease. It "disappeared" because of technological advancement, urbanization, and improved sanitation infrastructure.[64] With the widespread use of indoor plumbing alone, the risk of hookworm infection decreased drastically. The mechanization of farming also reduced the need for people to come into frequent contact with the soil. What all these changes have in common, however, is reduction of environmental exposure rather than reduction of the parasite itself and as one recent study found, reduced risk of environmental exposure does not mean that hookworm is eradicated from the United States.[65]

The study, conducted by McKenna et al. (2017), found evidence of hookworm in residents of Lowndes County, Alabama—a finding that shocked many.[66] "'I was very surprised by this,' says Dr. David Diemert, a hookworm expert at George Washington University. 'There has not been any documentation of people being infected in the US for the past couple of decades; we thought there was no more local transmission of hookworm in the US'."[67] But as we will discuss at length in this book, not looking for or reporting something does not mean that it is not there. There are still many places throughout Texas, the Gulf Coast, and other parts of the South that exhibit all the risk factors for hookworm and other NTDs. The hookworm problem of today was expressed best by Smith (2018) when he stated, "The disease may never have left . . . It likely persisted in this region, alongside dire poverty, as the country grew wealthier and wealthier and eventually turned its back."[68] Given the social and environmental risk factors that exist throughout the South, "it is likely that hookworm persists to some degree in the contemporary South."[69]

Seemingly overnight, residents of Lowndes County found themselves in the national spotlight. A spotlight based on a discovery brought about by the McKenna et al. study and one woman's fight against the impoverished conditions in her community. Catherine Flowers, the founder of the Alabama Center for Rural Enterprise, noticed one day that a mysterious rash had appeared on her body. Her doctor tried a variety of treatments to get rid of the rash, but none of the treatments had any effect. She asked her doctor, "Could it possibly be something here that American doctors don't test for?"[70] When the doctor expanded the diseases they were testing for, it was discovered that she was infected with hookworm. Upon the diagnosis, Flowers reached out to researchers at the Baylor College of Medicine to further investigate the prevalence of hookworm in Lowndes County.[71]

If "neglected diseases mainly afflict neglected communities," then Lowndes County certainly fits the criteria.[72] The county is known as much for its poverty as it is for its violent Civil Rights history. Today, approximately 73 percent of the population of Lowndes County is African American. The county struggles to attract new businesses to solve the crippling 6.6 percent unemployment rate, but attracting businesses is difficult when the county lacks the infrastructure necessary to make business prosperity feasible.[73]

Philip Alston, the UN's Special Rapporteur on extreme poverty and human rights, toured Lowndes County. When shown the raw sewage flowing through backyards and children's play areas, Alston condemned the "unwillingness of state and local governments to help people with no access to basic services like sewage management."[74] With nearly a third of its residents living in poverty, Lowndes County has scarce funding to provide such services.[75] The state of Alabama is not in a much better position to begin funding private infrastructure. As the sixth most impoverished state in the nation, Alabama already lacks critical resources to deal with many of the problems the state faces.[76]

In 2011, a UN report cited Alabama Department of Public Health estimates that between 40 and 90 percent of households in Lowndes County have either inadequate or no septic systems.[77] Installing a proper septic system can cost between $10,000 and 30,000, which, when compared to the median household income for Lowndes County residents of $27,000, is an insurmountable cost.[78] The cost to install a septic tank in Lowndes County is high compared to other regions of the country due to the impermeable soil associated with the Southern Black Belt. Even when new septic systems are installed, they often fail anyways due to the soil conditions. Due to the costs and likely failure of septic systems, many residents resort to straight piping, which refers to using PVC pipes to redirect waste into holes or other areas of their land.[79] Straight piping, along with sewage backup, and septic tank overflow, leaks into homes and yards. When combined with heavy rainfall and flooding, residents are exposed to the raw sewage puddled around and inside their homes on a regular basis.[80] In these households, the odor of the sewage is the least of their concerns. The sewage serves as a medium by which parasites, viruses, and bacteria proliferate before coming into contact with unsuspecting men, women, and children going about their daily life.

The taboo and humiliating nature of this problem is a source of embarrassment and stigmatization for residents who use straight piping. The threat of legal prosecution and jail time creates an additional layer of fear and complexity. In the state of Alabama, it is a criminal misdemeanor to build, maintain, or use an unsanitary system such as the straight piping techniques used by many residents. Failing to obtain a permit for a septic tank is another violation. Both of these violations can lead to fines and jail time.[81] Those whose septic tanks fail can also be fined and prosecuted. The criminalization of this problem breeds increasing levels of mistrust between residents and the local and state government, and furthers the cycle of poverty by punishing residents for being poor with fines they cannot afford and potentially even incarceration, which robs them of their ability to maintain employment.

The sanitation issues plaguing Lowndes County may be the worst kept secret in Alabama, but the issue reached a climax when the McKenna et al. (2017) study mentioned earlier was published. Out of the twenty-four households that took part, 42.4 percent said they had been exposed to sewage within their home.[82] Additionally, nineteen of the fifty-five stool samples collected from residents tested positive for hookworm. This means over a third of the residents participating in the study were infected.[83] The hookworm infections likely resulted from residents coming into contact with hookworm while walking outside with bare feet or ankles, or walking barefoot in their homes on flooring that had been exposed to contaminated soil from outside. The study brought Lowndes County's sanitation issues to the forefront as a public health crisis, and proved to many that developed countries are not excluded from NTD infections when many of their residents still live in the same impoverished conditions as those in low-income nations.

A notice by the Alabama Department of Public Health denounced the study, stating that there "is currently no evidence of an increased incidence of gastrointestinal (GI) outbreaks in [the ADPH District (which include, among others, the counties of Lowndes, Dallas, Hale, Perry, Wilcox, Marengo, Choctaw, and Sumter) than in other parts of Alabama."[84] The notice criticized the study for using experimental PCR technology that is not FDA approved to test the samples. Furthermore, ADPH claims that nine individuals who had received positive results of the study submitted samples to the CDC for examination. Using microscopy-based techniques, the CDC found no specimens tested positive for hookworm.[85]

Dr. Rojelio Meija, one of the scientists leading the study, responded to ADPH's notice by emphasizing the fact that there is currently no FDA-approved test for hookworm infection. This means the microscopy-based technique utilized by the CDC, a much less sensitive and accurate test in comparison to the DNA testing used by the Baylor College of Medicine research team in the Lowndes County study, has also not been approved by the FDA. In fact, one infectious disease researcher at the University of Washington stated that persisting to use microscopes in lieu of more advanced existing technology could "perpetuate the neglect" of underserved communities already lacking adequate access to healthcare.[86]

In terms of treating those infected with hookworm, a single dose of Albendazole, which consists of two 200 milligrams pills that cost approximately $400, can eradicate an infection.[87] However, this does little to solve the problem of potential reinfection. Until sanitation improves, it is unlikely that hookworm will cease to be a problem. Additionally, hookworm is not just a problem in Alabama. The perfect storm of unsanitary conditions, lack of healthcare access, and tropical climate exists in communities across the United States, meaning dozens, if not hundreds, of communities are possibly harboring hookworms.

Though hookworms are perhaps the most controversial NTD in the United States, they are not the only ones lurking in the soil of the Southern United States. *Toxocara cati/canis* and *Ascaris lumbricoides* are two helminths with equally troubling health effects. Helminths consists of three different groups of parasitic worms, which include flukes, tapeworms, and roundworms.[88] Despite contributing to approximately 45 percent of the global burden of NTDs, helminths garner little attention in the United States. Unlike hookworm, toxocariasis, the disease caused by infection with *Toxocara* species, and ascariasis, the disease caused by infection with *Ascaris lumbricoides*, have received little media coverage to call attention to their troubling presence.

TOXOCARIASIS

The Disease and Symptoms

Although *Toxocara* is often associated with developing countries, it may also be the most common parasitic worm infection found in humans in the United States.[89] Toxocariasis is a disease that results from infection with the *Toxocara* parasite, and it affects both humans and animals. The *Toxocara* parasite thrives in tropical, subtropical, and temperate climates across the world, making the Southern United States a perfect environment.[90] Humans contract the infection primarily from exposure to dog and cat roundworms, or the parasites *Toxocara cani* and *T. cati*. Infection typically occurs when humans come into contact with soil contaminated with *Toxocara* eggs from infected cat or dog feces and ingest these eggs. These microscopic eggs are undetectable to the human eye, so individuals would be unaware that they are consuming them. Children are particularly at risk of infection, as they have a great deal of contact between their hands and mouth while playing in contaminated soil from yards, playgrounds, and sandboxes.[91] Thus, children living in poverty, particularly in areas of environmental degradation, are particularly susceptible to contracting the disease.

Once ingested, the *Toxocara* eggs hatch larvae, which then travel throughout the individual's organs. The larvae make their way to the lungs, liver, brain, and eyes. There are four main types of *Toxocara* infection. These infections are classified as either ocular toxocariasis, visceral toxocariasis, neurotoxocariasis, or covert/common toxocariasis. Ocular toxocariasis occurs when the larvae cause inflammation in the eye of the patient, which can lead to permanent injury to the eye. Symptoms of ocular toxocariasis can include retinal detachment, formation of subretinal granulomatous masses or scars, and often leads to blindness. Visceral toxocariasis occurs mainly in children and is a result of the larvae damaging the body's organs. Typically, this manifests in liver or pulmonary damage. It can cause enlargement and necrosis of the liver and enlargement of the spleen.[92] Visceral toxocariasis can also occasionally lead to seizures, psychiatric symptoms, and encephalopathy, which can cause outcomes ranging from memory loss and subtle personality changes to coma and death.[93] Eosinophilic meningitis, pericardial effusion, and myocarditis also occasionally result from *Toxocara* infection.

Covert toxocariasis is the most common form of toxocariasis, and often features similar manifestations to the visceral form of toxocariasis. It is considered a primarily benign infection, with many individuals being asymptomatic or experiencing limited symptoms.[94] These symptoms could include wheezing, pulmonary infiltrates, and eosinophilia. As these symptoms are often associated with childhood asthma or allergies, more research is needed to determine to what extent some cases may be linked to toxocariasis.[95] It is currently not well understood why some infected with *Toxocara* remain asymptomatic, while others develop symptoms that have a wide range of severity and location of impact within the human body.[96]

There are a vast range of clinical outcomes attributed to *Toxocara* infections, including respiratory, gastrointestinal, and neurologic illnesses, and occasionally death. *Toxocara* is also associated with diminished lung function, cognitive changes, and adverse neuropsychological effects.[97] Additionally, some symptoms shown in the central nervous system as a result of toxocariasis have been linked with occult seizures, mental retardation, and developmental delays.[98] One study found that young children who tested seropositive for *Toxocara* had lower scores on the Wechsler Intelligence for Children-Revised and the Wide Range Achievement Test-Revised than children that tested seronegative. This correlation existed independent of socioeconomic status, ethnicity, gender, or rural residence.[99]

Toxocariasis Infection in the United States

The CDC has conducted two major national surveys useful for studying the prevalence of toxocariasis in the United States. The first study, which used samples collected during the first Health and Nutrition Examination Survey from 1971 to 1973, found that the overall prevalence of toxocariasis was between 4.6 and 7.3 percent nationally.[100] However, some areas in the South had prevalence for toxocariasis as high as 10 percent and African American children were found to be disproportionately impacted by toxocariasis with over 30 percent seroprevalence.[101] The study also found that higher seroprevalence was associated with low socioeconomic status, poverty, crowding, and the head of the household attaining a lower educational level.[102]

Because toxocariasis can impact cognitive development, these risk factors are particularly disturbing. The same risk factors that cause individuals to be more exposed to the disease continue to amass and negatively impact their lives in alongside the symptoms of the disease itself. Put differently, not only will a child living in poverty be more at risk for becoming infected with toxocariasis, but once infected the disease could continue to impair the child's mental function and physical capabilities for the remainder of their life, further plunging the individual into poverty. This highlights another major shortfall in our current body of knowledge regarding toxocariasis. Little is known about the economic cost of toxocariasis, particularly in terms of DALYs, and the economic burden the disease presents on a national scale.[103] In order to develop a proper understanding of the economic burden, however, there must be more accurate figures depicting the number of Americans currently infected with toxocariasis.

Data collected from 1988 to 1994 as part of the 3rd National Health and Nutrition Examination Survey was again used to analyze seroprevalence for toxocariasis. In 2008, the CDC reported that results from the survey indicated an overall seroprevalence of 13.9 percent for toxocariasis.[104] Again, the seroprevalence was distinctly higher among African Americans and individuals living in poverty. Based on this information, one study came to the conclusion that an estimated 2.8 million Africans Americans living in poverty may be infected with toxocariasis.[105] With evidence suggesting a high number of Americans are infected with toxocariasis, it is staggering to consider that the majority of toxocariasis cases remain completely undiagnosed.

In 2009–2010, the number of patients diagnosed with ocular toxocariasis was highest in the Southern United States, with Georgia, Florida, California, Texas, and Alabama ranking in the top five states.[106] Currently, toxocariasis is not a disease that is nationally reportable, and there is no surveillance system utilized to document cases. More population-based studies are necessary in order to establish a baseline and a better understanding of the epidemiologic characteristics of *Toxocara* infections, as well as the prevalence and incidence of these infections within various demographics and regional groups. Without this data, it is more difficult to determine precise risk factors that result in higher rates of *Toxocara* infections.[107]

Toxocariasis Diagnosis and Treatment

Toxocariasis is typically diagnosed through the use of a serologic test known as ELISA, or enzyme-linked immunosorbent assay. However, this method of testing is not widely available in the United States due to limited demand for parasitic disease diagnosis and the scarcity of an antigen produced from the larvae. Additionally, low test sensitivity has proven to be a problem for assays currently in use. The low sensitivity means that many people who are infected receive a false negative, meaning that cases are going undiagnosed. This further contributes to a vast underestimate of the prevalence of toxocariasis.[108] Providing further complication, the ELISA method is not capable of distinguishing between an active or past infection.[109] Moving forward, it will be critical to develop a diagnostic test that is able to make this distinction.

Treatment for toxocariasis typically requires the infected individual to take either Albendazole or Mebendazole. However, as of 2014 there had yet to be a randomized controlled treatment study to determine the best drug dose and treatment duration for those diagnosed with toxocariasis.[110] Additionally, even a tried and true treatment for toxocariasis needs to begin with proper diagnosis of the disease in clinics and hospitals. Doctors and healthcare providers often have a weak knowledgebase regarding toxocariasis. This means that oftentimes asthma-like symptoms, cognitive deficits, and pulmonary dysfunction are diagnosed without recognition of the infection as the underlying cause.[111] A study assessing pediatrician knowledge of toxocariasis in the United States found that 85 percent of participants were not confident that their knowledge of toxocariasis was current.[112] Besides medical professionals, practicing veterinarians also play a key role in identifying the risks of contracting toxocariasis.

Toxocariasis and Animal Populations

Veterinarians are a vital factor in raising awareness of toxocariasis. They are in an ideal position to promote educational awareness among their clients and community by encouraging deworming and the proper disposal of pet waste. Preventing the spread of toxocariasis must also involve preventative veterinary care of owned dogs and cats, as well as outreach efforts to deworm stray populations. A meta-analysis of studies done on toxocariasis seemed to indicate that animal ownership itself did not present a greater risk for toxocariasis.[113] Instead, the study suggested that pet care is a key determinant of whether the owner is more or less at risk for contracting the disease. For instance, dogs that are owned and well-cared for have a greater chance of being dewormed compared to feral dogs, which eat a more unconventional diet and live primarily outdoors.[114] Owned animals that receive inadequate veterinary care, however, can put their owners at risk of toxocariasis.

In *Blue Marble Health,* Hotez recalls, "driving through poor areas of Houston and elsewhere in Texas and the American South, [he is] struck by the frequent sight of stray dogs, often traveling in packs," and that the numerous *Toxocara* eggs are "practically ubiquitous in areas of environmental degradation, including play areas across poor urban and rural landscapes."[115] Each year, the American Society for the Prevention of Cruelty to Animals (ASPCA) estimates that animal shelters in the United States receive approximately 3.3 million dogs and 3.2 million cats.[116] Such a large stray population roaming the streets, playgrounds, and yards of American households certainly poses a risk for the spread of toxocariasis infection. A key factor in mitigating the role of stray dogs and cats in spreading the disease is reducing the stray pet populations in communities.

One such way is through the promotion of spay and neuter surgeries to reduce the number of unwanted pets born in these communities. In contrast to Northeast and Northwestern United States, rural states and the South typically have less strict spay-neuter laws for dogs and cats.[117] While some city and local governments have enacted mandatory spay-neuter ordinances, many cities operating on limited resources place the issue at the bottom of their list of priorities.[118] The risk of dogs and cats spreading toxocariasis by means of environmental contamination is worsened by the fact that there is no effective way of eliminating the *Toxocara* eggs systematically in contrast with vector elimination campaigns directed at killing off the disease before it reaches the host.[119] Because of this, accurate diagnosis and treatment of toxocariasis is vitally important. This is also true for ascariasis, another disease caused by soil-transmitted helminths.

ASCARIASIS

The history of ascariasis in the United States dates back to prehistoric times. Van Buren County, Tennessee, is home to an incredible archaeological discovery where human feces found in Big Bone Cave contained the parasite *Ascaris lumbricoides*, with radiocarbon-dating indicating the material was over 2,000 years old.[120] *Ascaris* species and other soil-transmitted helminths were present in high levels in the Southern United States and Appalachia in the 1980s, where sanitation and poverty were considered to be the root problem of the infections.[121]

Today, it is estimated that over 1.4 billion people worldwide suffer from infection with the parasite *Ascaris lumbricoides*. Ascariasis, the disease that occurs from infection with the parasite, can also result from exposure to *Ascaris suum*, a species which typically dwell in pig hosts, but are capable of infecting humans.[122] Ascariasis is the third most common type of helminthic infection present in the United States.[123] If you look up "Ascariasis" on the CDC's webpage, a bold statement stands out at the end of the last paragraph, which reads, "Ascariasis is now uncommon in the United States."[124] This statement echoes the same story told about many NTDs—that ascariasis was left behind in American history and is now only a disease which predominantly impacts developing countries with inadequate hygiene and sanitation. This perception contributes to misinformation regarding the current epidemiology of the disease in America. One estimate pointed to the potential existence of 4 million cases of ascariasis in the United States.[125] Currently, ascariasis infection is not a reportable condition by state or national standards.[126] However, the warm climate and impoverished status of many communities in the American South makes it difficult to assert that this endemic disease has disappeared as a public health concern.

The Disease and Symptoms

Ascaris lumbricoides is a roundworm known for its characteristically large size, with females capable of reaching up to 40 centimeters.[127] Infection with the parasite occurs when eggs are ingested through contact with contaminated soil, food, or water. These eggs remain viable for only eighteen days before they become infertile. Once consumed, the larvae hatch in the small intestine, where they eventually break through the intestinal wall before traveling to the right side of the heart and finally reach the lungs.[128] Afterward, the larvae breach the network of capillaries referred to as the capillary bed and continue on to the tiny air sacs of the lungs known as the alveolar space.[129] The larvae go through a molting process twice before resuming their journey up the throat, where the larvae are swallowed. Once returned to the small intestine, the larvae stay there into adulthood. Here, they continue to produce eggs for approximately six months. These eggs are then excreted along with the human's feces.[130] Within two to four weeks, the embryos develop into infective larvae.[131]

Many *Ascaris lumbricoides* infections are asymptomatic. However, those with a high worm load experience more severe health complications. Pulmonary ascariasis manifests in a form of pneumonia resulting in cough, labored breathing (dyspnea), fever, and occasionally hemoptysis, or coughing up blood. Intestinal ascariasis is typically found in individuals appearing asymptomatic. Symptoms of intestinal ascariasis can include abdominal pain and/or distention, nausea, and diarrhea. Heavier worms loads can create masses resulting in intestinal obstruction, which can lead to further intestinal complications Hepatobiliary and pancreatic ascariasis is rare in children, but can result in biliary colic, inflammation of the gallbladder without gallstones (acalculous cholecystitis), acute inflammation of the bile duct (cholangitis), acute pancreatitis, and liver abscess. Peritoneal Ascariasis creates a complication causing acute inflammation of an abdominal membrane (peritonitis) or chronic intra-abdominal lesions known as peritoneal granulomas.[132]

While the majority of the symptoms caused by ascariasis infection tend to remain chronic unless treated, life-threatening complications resulting from ascariasis can occur.[133] Ascariasis can have a particularly heavy burden on children, as the infection can cause poor food digestion. This results in malnutrition, and ultimately, has the potential to cause growth retardation.[134] Additionally, iron-deficiency caused by ascariasis infection can lead to anemia. This results in reduced energetic efficiency, decreased endurance, and fatigue, which limits productivity and participation at work, school, and within families and social circles.

Disease Diagnosis and Treatment

There are multiple methods capable of diagnosing individuals with ascariasis. Currently, Kato-Katz thick smears are the most common means of diagnosing the infection. Other methods such as FLOTAC ®, Mini-Flotac, the McMaster egg counting technique, and molecular diagnostics are all possible alternatives, all with varying sensitivities, intensities, costs, timing, and energy source complications. A study analyzing all of these methods concluded that there is a "paucity of data on novel, convenient diagnostics for ascariasis, even compared to other NTDs."[135] The study encouraged more investment for developing a simple and cost-effective diagnostic tool for detecting ascariasis infections. Ultrasounds, CT MRI, endoscopy, and molecular diagnostics also serve as methods to detect ascariasis infection.[136]

Because ascariasis is rarely considered by physicians and pediatricians in developed countries, it is imperative that medical professionals become more familiar with ascariasis. One example of this is the story of a six-year-old boy, who lived in Yokohama, an urban Japanese city. He was taken to the pediatric emergency room due to repeated episodes of bilious vomiting, abdominal colic, and a fever.[137] Several diagnostic tests failed to produce evidence of ileus, a lack of intestinal movement, which they had been suspected to be the culprit. The boy's symptoms vanished the next day, but a capsule endoscopy performed three days after his admission revealed a live roundworm measuring at least 10 centimeters long.[138] The following day the boy received treatment and his feces contained another roundworm.[139] While this is a single, isolated case of ascariasis, it provides a shocking example of the havoc a small number of roundworms can wreak on the body of a young child. Additionally, this instance provides a stellar example of how difficult it can be to identify ascariasis infection in a high-income country, where NTDs rarely receive consideration.

While higher worm burdens can cause health complications requiring extensive care, most infections can be treated using antihelminth medical therapy aimed at ridding the body of adult worms. Because of this, treatment must be repeated one to three months later to ensure that larvae in the body at the time of the original treatment have time to mature into adulthood to be vulnerable to the medication. Typically, the medications Albendazole or Mebendazole are used to complete this treatment. However, in cases where pregnancy is involved, the patients are often administered the medication Pyrantel Pamoate.[140] Chemotherapy has been introduced as a quick and efficient way to reduce heavy worm burdens at a "relatively low cost."[141]

Risk Factors

Ascaris lumbricoides has been known to infect humans by spreading through contact with soil intermingled with contaminated pig feces, as recorded in an instance of pig farmers living in Maine.[142] However, it is more likely that humans will come into contact with the parasite through exposure to raw sewage containing eggs. Because of this, poverty is a major risk factor for ascariasis. Poor socioeconomic conditions are one of the leading risk factors for increased prevalence of ascariasis.[143]

As seen with hookworm, crumbling sanitation infrastructure and lack of access to affordable options for waste disposal creates the perfect breeding ground for soil-transmitted parasites like *Ascaris lumbricoides*. A study conducted in Assam, India found that ascariasis was more prevalent in crowded households.[144] This provides yet another example of how poverty creates living conditions that cause individuals to be more at risk for disease infection. Many low-income households throughout the United States experience overcrowding, as individuals and families join incomes and pool resources together in an effort to make housing more affordable.

Additionally, a study examining ascariasis infections in college students in Kabul, Afghanistan, determined that using well water, eating street food, and consuming unwashed vegetables resulted in higher ascariasis prevalence.[145]

Risk factors such as these highlight the importance of accessibility to clean water, which many low-income communities in the United States lack. Additionally, education and health promotion are necessary to inform community members about practicing safe food preparation and consumption.

In Summary of Soil-Transmitted Helminths

Diseases caused by soil-transmitted helminths like hookworm, *Toxocara* species, and *Ascaris lumbricoides* present several public health challenges for low-income communities across the Southern United States. With nearly one in every two people in the developing world estimated to be infected with at least one intestinal nematode worm, the impact of these diseases cannot be underestimated or viewed as an isolated problem of low-income countries.[146] Globally, soil-transmitted helminth infections have claimed 5.18 million DALYs, a figure higher than any other NTD.[147] These diseases are quite literally sucking the productivity and potential out of children and adults already struggling to survive in low-income communities against all odds.

Another attribute that hookworm, toxocariasis, and ascariasis all have in common is that the parasites cannot reproduce and multiply within the host's body. Because of this, high levels of parasitic infection are caused by continuous exposure and reinfection amassing in the host's body over time. The risk of high rates of post-treatment reinfection makes the prospect of a vaccine to prevent soil-transmitted helminth infections an appealing solution to work toward. In addition to working on the Human Hookworm Vaccine, the Sabin Vaccine Institute Product Development Partnership is currently developing a Pan-anthelmintic vaccine with goal of someday preventing infection due to exposure to ascariasis, trichuriasis, and hookworm.[148] Such a vaccine would be an innovative milestone in NTD treatment, as current vaccines are only effective against bacteria and viruses. However, developments such as these are still years in the making. In the meantime, improved diagnostics, increased health promotion and educational awareness, and addressing the lack of resources and infrastructure in low-income communities will continue to be vital in the struggle to prevent the proliferation of soil-transmitted helminths and other NTDs in the Southern United States.

DENGUE

While hookworm has the most well-documented history in the United States, another prominent disease foe of many Southerners was Dengue. Dengue is a viral disease caused by one of four strains—characterized as DEN 1, DEN 2, DEN 3, and DEN 4.[149] It is antigenically related to a number of other serious viruses including, St. Louis Encephalitis, Yellow Fever, West Nile

Virus, and Japanese B Encephalitis. Dengue is a vector-borne disease, transmitted to humans via mosquitoes and can manifest in several ways. These manifestations include classical Dengue Fever, Dengue Hemorrhagic Fever, and Dengue Shock Syndrome.[150] It is estimated that there are 50 million new Dengue infections globally every year.[151]

Classical dengue fever looks very similar to flu and includes symptoms such as joint pain, nausea, vomiting, and rash.[152] Dengue Hemorrhagic Fever (DHF) is a more severe form of classical Dengue infection. In this form, however, the disease can cause severe bleeding and a sudden drop in blood pressure. This sudden drop in blood pressure can lead to the most severe form of Dengue—Dengue Shock Syndrome (DSS). Both DHF and DSS can be fatal.[153] Though there is still limited understanding as to why most cases of Dengue are asymptomatic while others progress to DSS, it appears that the majority of severe cases are caused by the DEN 2 serotype.[154]

Overall, Dengue is an ancient disease. The earliest recorded history of Dengue symptoms were published during the Chin Dynasty (265 AD–420 AD) (Gubler 1998). The Chinese referred to the disease as "water poison" and believed that it was caused by insects closely associated with water, which was an impressive early understanding of the mosquito-borne disease.[155] The first recorded incidents of likely Dengue epidemics occurred in Indonesia and Egypt in 1779 and the United States in 1780.[156] Thus, by the time Dengue arrived in the United States it was already a global threat.

Endemic Dengue in the United States

The earliest recorded case of Dengue in the United States was observed in Philadelphia, Pennsylvania in 1780.[157] Following its first emergence, Dengue became a regular threat to American public health with outbreaks occurring throughout the 1800s and into the 1900s.[158] Part of the reason that Dengue took hold so easily in the United States is because the United States—particularly the Southern US—"has the conditions for autochthonous (i.e., locally acquired) transmission of dengue virus."[159] Most importantly, Dengue infection is possible anywhere that the *Aedes aegypti* mosquito exists.

Roughly forty years after the initial cases of Dengue in Philadelphia, the disease had established itself as an endemic infection in many parts of the United States. In 1827 there was an outbreak in New Orleans, Savannah, Pensacola, and Charleston that is often attributed to Dengue, though more recently it has been suggested that the outbreak may have been chikungunya instead.[160] Throughout the mid-1800s "sporadic outbreaks were mentioned in the Gulf and Atlantic seaports in the United States, being the largest in 1873 in New Orleans, with 40,000 people affected, and followed by another large epidemic in several Southern United States port cities between 1878 and 1880."[161] Specifically, Dengue moved into Texas in 1885 and "was responsible for 16,000 clinical cases in Austin, which was nearly three-quarters of the city's population at the time."[162] By 1887 the disease had spread throughout the entire state of Texas.[163]

The problem only continued to grow in the early 1900s with outbreaks throughout the Southern United States. As Beaumier et al. (2014) describe, "Outbreaks also occurred in the Texas gulf coast cities of Houston, Galveston and Brownsville in 1907 and again in 1918 with the compounding factor being once again military units travelling from endemic regions, this time returning from the West Indies."[164] As with many other diseases throughout history, Dengue was perpetuated, in part, by military movements throughout the world and the heavy concentration of military personnel in certain areas of the United States. In a 1971 article by Ehrenkranz et al., they state that the, "Propagation of dengue appears to be directly dependent on human populations with a sufficient number of susceptible members to support infection."[165]

Following the end of World War I, the disease showed no signs of disappearing in the United States. The opposite was true, in fact. In the years following the war, the number of people infected in outbreaks grew. In 1922 there were approximately 500,000 cases of Dengue in Texas alone.[166] Twelve years later, in 1934, an outbreak in Florida infected approximately 10 percent of the population of Miami.[167] Large-scale Dengue outbreaks continued for another two decades until mosquito eradication campaigns began in the late 1940s. "The last historical outbreak within the continental USA occurred in the gulf cities of Texas in 1941 and Louisiana in 1945."[168] The last historical outbreak in Hawaii occurred in 1944.[169]

DDT and Mosquito Eradication Campaigns

Beginning in 1901, William Gorgas of Havana, began the first effort to eliminate the *Aedes aegypti* mosquito.[170] And although the focus of this work was to control or eliminate Yellow Fever, reducing the incidence of Dengue infection was a positive additional consequence. In the 1940s, the Pan-American Health Organization (PAHO) began mosquito eradication efforts throughout the Americas.[171] The United State officially began their mosquito eradication program in 1947, though the initial elements of the program actually began in 1942 when the Office of Malaria Control in War Areas, a predecessor of the CDC, began working to prevent the spread of malaria and murine typhus around military bases in the South.[172]

They located the Office of Malaria Control in War Areas in Atlanta because the South had the highest rates of malaria transmission.[173] In 1947, this limited focused mosquito control was expanded and the National Malaria Eradication Program officially commenced.[174] The primary method of eradication was to spread DDT inside and around houses that were in areas of high malaria transmission. By 1949, malaria was declared to no longer be a major public health problem in the United States and in 1951 the CDC shifted from active eradication to surveillance.[175]

The National Malaria Eradication Program was considered a success. The number of malaria cases in the United States dropped to zero. A byproduct of this program was that it also eliminated Dengue, since the elimination of mosquitoes that transmit malaria also resulted in the elimination of mosquitoes that transmit Dengue. Efforts in the United States combined with efforts across Mexico, Latin America, and South America resulted in no more reported cases of Dengue. "For more than thirty years, it was believed that dengue had been eliminated from the Americas, until 1977–1979 when dengue reappeared in the Caribbean and Mexico."[176]

The Reemergence of Dengue in the United States

Like many infectious disease stories, however, with the elimination of transmission came complacency. "The deterioration of the eradication program over time was due mainly to the loss of political importance in most of the countries that had achieved eradication."[177] Put simply, as the number of reported cases dropped toward zero, politicians and public health officials did not see the need to continue investing in mosquito control and surveillance. Additionally, the realization that DDT was extremely toxic led the United States government to ban it from use. Banning DDT, while beneficial for the environment, made it more difficult to control the mosquito population. Some communities were more proactive than others. Galveston County, Texas began a mosquito surveillance program in 1977 specifically because of the high risk of Dengue reemergence.[178] Other communities, however, did not address the risk of reemergence. By 1980, health officials began to see locally acquired cases of Dengue along the Texas-Mexico border.[179] About half of the cases in the 1980 outbreak were acquired on the U.S. side of the border in the counties of Cameron, Hidalgo, Starr, and Willacy, demonstrating that the disease had re-established itself in that area of the United States.

After the initial reemergence in 1980, Dengue outbreaks have continued to occur in the United States. In 2005, there was a DEN 2 outbreak in Brownsville, Texas though some researchers have hypothesized that there have been additional outbreaks of Dengue throughout Texas prior to 2005; they have just gone unrecognized.[180] As Beaumier et al. (2014) explained, "Investigators in Houston, Texas were also concerned about underdiagnosis of dengue in the region, and as a consequence, they conducted a retrospective study to retest all specimens of DENV that were submitted between 2003-2005 for West Nile virus testing."[181] When conducting tests on 3,768 specimens they found forty-seven samples positive for Dengue[182] suggesting that Dengue was circulating at higher rates than was recognized. Between 2003 and 2012, the Texas Department of Health and Human Services reports

154 cases of Dengue in the state.[183] Cameron County has had the most cases, followed by Harris County and Travis County.[184]

Texas is not the only place Dengue has reappeared. In 2009, Florida experienced its first Dengue outbreak in several decades. The outbreak occurred in Key West, Florida and had three confirmed cases, though researchers later found thirteen other residents that were seropositive for the disease.[185] This study estimated that approximately 3–5 percent of residents in Old Town Key West were infected with Dengue in the fall of 2009.[186] Key West is a popular tourist destination, which increased the concerns of public health officials across the country who feared tourists may become infected and cases of Dengue could turn up elsewhere in the United States. In 2019, Florida has experienced twelve cases (as of this writing) of locally acquired Dengue, mostly in Miami-Dade County.[187]

In 2010, Dengue was placed on the list of Nationally Notifiable Infectious Conditions, but the most concerning outbreak was still ahead.[188] In 2015–2016 there was an outbreak of Dengue in the Hawaiian Islands. This was the first outbreak in Hawaii in fifty-seven years and it was the first recognized outbreak where the disease was spread by the *Aedes albopictus* mosquito.[189] The new vector is particularly concerning because *Aedes albopictus* has a much wider range in the United States than *Aedes aegypti*. The ability of the *Aedes albopictus* to transmit the virus means that many more Americans are at risk of infection. In all, the Hawaii outbreak had 1,644 suspected cases and 122 confirmed cases.

Dengue Prevalence into the Future

Over the last few decades Dengue has reemerged in the United States and has shown no signs of abating. The discovery that *Aedes albopictus* can transmit the disease only serves to complicate the picture, though a changing climate means that the natural range of the *Aedes aegypti* is also expanding into new regions. There is a strong need for the political will and resources to establish adequate Dengue surveillance and to develop effective mosquito control programs in the most at-risk areas. With the recent emergence of Zika in the United States and growing cases of West Nile Virus throughout both the Northern and Southern United States, it is possible that Dengue-control will again benefit from the fear of other mosquito-borne diseases.

YELLOW FEVER

Yellow Fever has played a central role in many pivotal points of American history. Arguably, the disease has had a greater impact on the path the country has taken than any other infectious disease from contributing to the acquisition of the Panama Canal and the Louisiana Purchase to changing the destiny of Memphis from a major American port city. Yellow Fever is entangled with the political and economic outcome of the United States and the Yellow Fever Commission was the first major effort in modern science to prevent and control an endemic disease in the United States.

Yellow Fever is an acute, vector-borne viral hemorrhagic disease that is endemic in forty-seven countries.[190] Although there are endemic countries throughout Africa, Central America, and South America, approximately 90 percent of all reported cases occur in sub-Saharan Africa.[191] Yellow Fever got its name from the jaundice that many infected individuals' experience in which they quite literally turn a yellowish color. Other symptoms include headache, muscle pain, fever, nausea, vomiting, and fatigue.[192] One of the most devastating elements of Yellow Fever's progression is that after the first few days of illness, infected individuals start to feel better and are believed to be on the mend. Then, for many, the disease comes back more severely than before. Only a small proportion of infected individuals develop severe symptoms but half of those that do die within seven to ten days.[193]

Yellow Fever is spread by the *Aedes* and *Haemogogus* genera of mosquitoes, with the *Aedes aegypti* responsible for the majority of cases. As we have discussed in previous sections of this chapter, the *Aedes aegypti* is widespread throughout the Southern United States and is also a host for several other severe vector-borne diseases. The *Haemogous* species of mosquito is found almost exclusively in the jungle and is not a possible disease vector in the United States.[194] There are a number of ways to prevent infection, including vaccination, mosquito control, and epidemic preparedness. Once an individual becomes infected, however, there is no antiviral treatment for Yellow Fever. Despite the lack of cure, early supportive treatment can improve survival rates for infected individuals.[195]

Most Americans likely do not know that Yellow Fever used to be a highly feared disease throughout the Southern United States. It caused multiple epidemics, thousands of deaths, and shaped the political and economic future of the country. In the next section, we will examine the history of Yellow Fever in the United States. We will discuss some of the largest epidemics, as well as the role the disease played in shaping the country.

The History of Yellow Fever in the United States

In the 1700 and 1800s, cities throughout the United States regularly experienced Yellow Fever epidemics. It was a normal, and terrifying, part of life. In spite of their regularity, the severity of Yellow Fever enabled a few large epidemics to alter the course of American history. The first such epidemic occurred in Philadelphia in 1793. At the time of the outbreak, Philadelphia served as the Nation's Capital, the seat of the new American government. When the first signs of Yellow Fever emerged in the summer of 1793, people began to flee in fear that if they stayed, they would become infected "Half the population left the city as an epidemic of Yellow Fever spread that muggy summer, claiming dozens of victims each day," Skwarecki explains.[196] Many of the young nation's leaders were among the fleeing individuals. George Washington, expecting the epidemic to be over shortly, "sparked a constitutional crisis when he left town."[197]

Many of the fleeing politicians may have believed that the epidemic would pass quickly, though historical experience with Yellow Fever would have told them otherwise. Evacuation of the country's officials meant that all governing came to a standstill. When constructing the new government, it had been decided that Congress would never be allowed to meet outside of Philadelphia. The purpose of this rule was to prevent what many colonists experienced with the British Parliament, which often moved meeting locations in order to rig a vote. Following the 1793 Yellow Fever epidemic, however, a law was passed that allowed Congress to relocate in case of emergency.[198] The change meant that the United States government would not come to a standstill if there was another disease outbreak in the Capital city.

Despite the importance of the 1793 Yellow Fever outbreak to the laws surrounding governing, epidemics in the late 1800s actually had a significantly larger impact on American history. The first was the 1878 epidemic in Memphis and the second was the continued epidemics in Panama throughout the 1880s. As of 1870, Memphis had a population of roughly 40,000 people, making it second only to New Orleans in the South.[199] The city was thriving and served as a major port along the Mississippi River. This all changed in 1878, however. "In the summer of 1878, the Mississippi River, the great artery of North America, would carry death in its bloodstream, spreading the worst yellow fever epidemic in American history."[200] Yellow Fever arrived in Memphis that summer aboard the *Emily B. Souder*, which had sailed from Cuba to New Orleans and then on to Memphis. The epidemic started slowly, but quickly spiraled out of control. Half the city fled to the countryside in hopes of avoiding infection. "The city collapsed, hemorrhaging its population, its income, its viability . . . A morbid calmness fell over Memphis, so still and quiet as to be serene if one didn't know it was simply a pallor of death."[201]

The city's population of 47,000 dropped by more than half and approximately 90 percent of those who remained where infected.[202] The city had gone from a vibrant, thriving port city to "only six months after the lavish Mardi Gras celebration, Memphis was a city of corpses."[203] More than 20,000 people lost their lives to Yellow Fever that summer and the federal government was blamed for not coming to the aid of the people.[204] President Hayes had stated during the epidemic that he felt accounts of the outbreak were greatly exaggerated, when in reality, "the toll on human life in Memphis alone surpassed the Chicago fire, San Francisco earthquake, and Johnstown flood combined. It was being called by some the worst urban disaster in American history."[205] Anger at the lack of federal support persisted and the large-scale death meant that the city was forever changed. What had once been a center of culture now provided a breeding ground for Protestant fundamentalism and white supremacy.[206] Memphis was also never able to regain its economic prominence. Memphis historian Gerald M. Capers would later write, "It can be suggested with some justification that Atlanta owes its present position as the 'New York of the South' more to the work of the *Aedes aegypti* in Memphis a half century ago than to any other cause'."[207] This is to say that following the 1878 Yellow Fever epidemic Memphis never recovered. Business and elite moved on from the city that had once promised to be one of the most influential cities in the United States. Its power forgotten to history.

The Panama Canal and the Yellow Fever Commission

The United States' relationship with Yellow Fever extends beyond its physical borders. In 1803, Yellow Fever played a central role in the rebellion of slaves and the independence of Haiti.[208] The lost rebellion was the beginning of the end for the French in the Caribbean, Panama, and the Southern United States. As Skwarecki (2016) describes, "France, unable to win a war in *Aedes aegypti* territory, withdrew from the area. A year later, it sold the Louisiana territory to the United States, changing the course of that nation's history"[209] Put simply, yellow fever, in combination with malaria, had completely driven the French from the region and when one looks at the losses suffered while attempting to build the Panama Canal, it is easy to see why.

After several years of exploration and debate, the French began construction of the Panama Canal in 1878. Unfortunately, with each year of construction, the number of workers dying of disease increased. In 1882, there were 400 workers who died from Yellow Fever or malaria. By 1884 there were 7,000 workers sick.[210] This totaled approximately one-third of the workforce. In fact, "during the time the French managed the Panama Canal construction project, more than 22,000 workers died."[211]

Around the same time that the French were losing interest in the project and the region, the United States was becoming increasingly interested. Due to the California Gold Rush and the United States increasing interest in Latin America and the Caribbean as a whole, Congress authorized a commission to negotiate a land deal with the French to gain control of the Canal.[212] Colombia was strongly opposed to U.S. control of the Canal, however, what ensued was U.S. support and encouragement of the Panamanian revolution against Colombia and recognition of the new Republic of Panama.[213] Two weeks after Panama gained independence, they granted the United States "permanent and exclusive" use of the Canal.[214]

The inability of the French to control Yellow Fever and malaria played a central role in the Louisiana Purchase and the United States gaining control of the Panama Canal; two pivotal moments in American history that allowed the country to expand coast to coast and become a world economic power. Americans were no less susceptible to Yellow Fever than the French, however, and the country's interest in endemic areas, including much of the Southern United States, pushed policy-makers and scientists to tackle the disease head on.

The Yellow Fever Commission

In the late 1800s and early 1900s, Cuba had become America's new frontier. Its location and central importance during the Spanish-American War were significant reasons for America's interest in Cuba, but also of great significance was Cuba's role as the place of origin for many of the major epidemics in the United States.[215] Cuba had numerous disease challenges including malaria and dysentery, but the United States was most interested in Yellow Fever. Thus, following the devastating epidemic of 1878, the National Board of Health organized the Havana Yellow Fever Commission and sent them to Cuba in 1879.[216] The Commission included experts Dr. Stanley E. Chaillé, Dr. George M. Sternberg, and Dr. Juan Guitéras.[217] Dr. Chaillé was from New Orleans and had experienced the most recent Yellow Fever outbreak there. Dr. Sternberg was from the U.S. Army Medical Corps and a pioneering bacteriologist. Dr. Guitéras was from the Marine Hospital Service and was born in Cuba. The members of the Commission partnered with Dr. Carlos Finlay, a Cuban-born doctor who believed that Yellow Fever was spread by *Aedes* mosquitoes, a radical idea for its time. He had presented this theory to the Royal Academy in 1881 and the world's leading scientists ridiculed him, calling him a "crazy old man" for this theory, which would later turn out to be correct.[218]

Beginning in 1900, the U.S. military took an interest in Cuba and decided to re-energize their efforts to fight Yellow Fever. One important reason for this interest was that deployed soldiers were not able to return home if there was an outbreak of Yellow Fever in their camps, which occurred frequently.[219] For this renewed effort, the United States sent Walter Reed to Havana and allowed him to choose his own team of scientists to work on the problem. He chose James Carroll, Aristides Agramonte, and Jesse Lazear. The scientists worked to determine how Yellow Fever was transmitted. Many years later and following the loss of Jesse Lazear to the disease (he is believed to have experimented on himself by letting a mosquito captured from the yellow fever hospital bite him), the Commission was successful. "The tests conducted in the Infected Mosquito Building demonstrated that exposure to *Aedes aegypti* mosquitoes carrying yellow fever—and only exposure to those mosquitoes—spread the virus."[220] The work Reed's commission proved definitively that Yellow Fever was spread by mosquitoes and made Walter Reed one of the most famous names in medicine.

The work conducted by Reed and his colleagues laid the groundwork for American and international campaigns to eliminate Yellow Fever. Major William C. Gorgas developed a campaign to eradicate the *Aedes aegypti* from Havana and later from Panama and the United States used the findings to work on eliminating the mosquito from the South.[221] Eventually, a vaccine was developed and the epidemics that were a normal part of Southern life, became forgotten history.

Yellow Fever Today

Today, many Americans have likely never heard of Yellow Fever. The disease has been eliminated from the United States, but the favorable environmental conditions and the *Aedes aegypti* still exist throughout the South. Cases do still occur in the United States, but are typically a result of foreign travel. In particular, most cases that occur in the United States are a result of travel to South America.

Internationally the disease was well-controlled until decreased use of the vaccine led to its reemergence, particularly in Africa, in the 1970s and 1980s. Recently the World Health Organization has partnered with UNICEF and Gavi, the Vaccine Alliance to ensure that vaccines get to people in the most high-risk areas. This project is termed, "Eliminate Yellow Fever Epidemics Strategy." The need for vaccines is especially great due to the resurgence of epidemics in Africa and South America.

It might be easy for Americans to look at Yellow Fever as a disease of the past; something that we have defeated and no longer must concern ourselves with. This is a false mindset. The climate, conditions, and vectors that allowed Yellow Fever to be so deadly throughout the 1800s still exist in the modern South. And, "viruses have taught us one thing throughout history, and it is this: That their will and ability to survive may be stronger than ours."[222]

CHAGAS DISEASE

Chagas is a disease resulting from infection with the parasite *Trypanosoma cruzi* by one of several species of triatomines. Although the disease is found in a number of places throughout the world, WHO estimates that the highest burden on the *T. cruzi* parasite is found in Latin America.[223] Specifically, individuals living in rural areas of Latin America are the most likely to be infected with *T. cruzi*. Although it is difficult to determine the exact number of infected individuals, it is estimated that there are 7.5–10 million people infected globally.[224] Of these infected individuals, approximately 11,000 die every year from Chagas-related heart complications.[225] In North America, it is estimated that 40,000 pregnant women are infected, putting their babies at risk of congenital transmission.[226] It is important to note that all these numbers are estimates. The burden could be higher due to the asymptomatic nature of the disease when it has not yet progressed to heart or liver failure.

Chagas disease is spread by triatomines, commonly known as kissing bugs, which infect an individual or animal when they bite them and defecate near the wound. The parasite *T. cruzi* then enters the bloodstream when an individual scratches the fecal matter into the wound. While vector-borne transmission accounts for the majority of human cases, 1–10 percent of infants born to infected mothers will contract the parasite through congenital transmission, approximately 3 percent of transmission comes as a result of organ transplant, and 10–25 percent of cases result from transfusion.[227] Most recently, cases in Brazil and Venezuela have shown that individuals can become infected with *T. cruzi* through oral transmission. In these cases, individuals, mostly children, became infected through contaminated sugar cane and fruit juices.[228] There are over 130 triatomine species in the Americans and the majority of them are infected *T. cruzi*.[229] This means that almost anywhere that has triatomines likely has the *T. cruzi* parasite.

Once an individual becomes infected, the parasite incubates for one to two weeks before progressing to the acute phase.[230] The acute phase lasts eight to twelve weeks but most individuals in this phase are asymptomatic. If infected individuals do show symptoms, they are usually mild and non-descript, most commonly edema or flu-like symptoms.[231] The chronic phase is also typically asymptomatic, with 30 percent of cases leading to fatal cardiac disease, however, the disease can also be fatal in the acute phase.[232] In addition to a lack of symptoms, there are other barriers to diagnosis, particularly in the United States. "Much bigger barriers to diagnosis are social and cultural. Many patients lack health insurance. Others are undocumented immigrants fearing deportation. Health literacy and language barriers are huge."[233] Put differently, social, economic, and legal barriers often stand in the way of diagnosis. Lastly, even outside the United States, Chagas Disease is associated with poverty.[234] The stigma associated with the disease prevents many people from getting tested.

The asymptomatic nature of Chagas Disease combined with its disproportionate impact on immigrants and individuals living in poverty, means that many cases of Chagas go undiagnosed. In the next section, we will discuss the history of Chagas in the United States and the challenges the country faces today in controlling the disease.

History of Chagas Disease in the United States

While Americans, including doctors and public health officials, often consider Chagas Disease to be an emerging disease in the United States, it actually has a long history here. Archaeologists have found evidence of Chagas-infected individuals in the Rio Grande Valley of Texas dating back 1150 years.[235] There are eleven species of triatomines present in the United States and the triatomine species found in the United States, which include *Triatoma gerstaeckeri, T. incrassata, T. indictiva, T. lecticularia, T. neotomae, T. protracta, T. recurva, T. rubida, T. rubrofasciata, T. sanguisuga, and Paratriatoma hirsuta*, with *T. gerstaeckeri,* are commonly the cause of infections in Texas.[236] Studies conducted over a seventy year period found triatomines present in twenty-eight states.[237] The highest triatomine burden exists in Texas, Arizona, and New Mexico.[238] Out of the 28 states, *T. cruzi* infected triatomines have been found in 10.[239] As Bern et al. (2011) describe, "*T. gerstaeckeri* is one of the most frequently collected and tested species in the United States; 57.7 percent (1,038/1,800) of tested specimens were found to harbor T. cruzi."[240] The majority of infected *T. gerstaeckeri* are found in Texas and New Mexico.

Despite this presence of the disease for centuries, the first documented case in the United States did not occur until the mid-1930s.[241] A study done by Packchanian (1939) documented household triatomine infestations in Texas and found that 92 percent of the triatomine they collected were infected with *T. cruzi.*[242] Following these findings, the Texas Department of Health conducted a study on *T. cruzi* prevalence in the 1940s and found an infection rate of 0.05 percent.[132] Though the infection rate was low, studies were published throughout the 1940s to raise awareness among Texas doctors.[243]

Studies of the prevalence of triatomines and triatomine bites in Texas continued throughout the 1950s and 1960s. The first case of autochthonous transmission occurred in Corpus Christi, Texas in 1955.[244] This first case occurred in a ten-month-old girl and a few months later a second case appeared in a six-month-old child in Houston.[245] Throughout the early 1960s, a number of larger-scale studies of Chagas took place. One of the most prominent of these examined seven children and two adults in the Corpus Christi, Texas area who were positive for *T. cruzi.* They determined that 57 percent of the triatomines collected from the homes were infected.[246]

The focus on Chagas in Texas did not last, however. There were only a handful of studies conducted in the 1970s, though one such study determined a 2.4 percent prevalence of *T. cruzi* in long-time residents of the Rio Grande

Valley in Texas.[247] Throughout the 1980s, 1990s, and early 2000s there were limited studies on Chagas, but there was growing concern within the medical community about *T. cruzi* in the blood supply.[248] It was not until many years later, however, that screening for *T. cruzi* became a normal part of the blood donation process. Prior to these screenings, donors were screened with questions such as whether they had visited one of the countries where Chagas' is endemic, or if they had ever slept in a thatched hut.[249] Additionally few hospitals had the capability of ordering or processing diagnostic tests. Many infected individuals discover they are infected from participating in blood donation after blood supply screening began.[250] The United States did not begin screening the U.S. blood supply for Chagas' disease until 2007.[251] This screening has increased awareness of Chagas among the population of Texas, as many seemingly healthy people have been positive for the parasite. Garcia et al. (2015) state that "Over the first 5 years of routine blood donor screening in Texas, confirmed positive donors have come from 109 different ZIP codes."[252]

A troubling trend in these blood screen results is a statistic provided by the American Red Cross indicating only 26.5 percent of blood donors identified as positive followed up with a physician.[253] Even when patients do follow up, their concerns can sometimes be dismissed by physicians. A study of patients who had positive serological test results for Chagas Disease found that some of the patients' physicians had assumed the test was a false positive.[254]

The Challenge of Chagas Today

Since the implementation of blood donation screening for Chagas, Texas has also declared Chagas a notifiable disease. There is evidence that the disease may affect as many as 1 of every 6,500 residents throughout the state.[255] Additionally, a 2015 study found that 41 percent of Chagas-infected donors who were presumed healthy, actually showed signs of cardiac disease.[256] Lastly, there is an increasing amount of evidence that shows autochthonous transmission in Texas. This means that the disease is likely endemic with large percentages of local triatomines infected. There are an estimated 300,000 cases of Chagas among the immigrant population alone in the United States and there have been thirty documented cases of local transmission.[257] These numbers indicate that Chagas is not a small problem in the United States.

While individuals living in poverty, particularly those with substandard housing, are most likely to become infected, there is a new risk group emerging: hunters. Hunters are particularly at risk in Texas, as they are likely to spend a greater amount of time outdoors compared to the rest of the population. Time outdoors means greater exposure to triatomines that could be carrying *T. cruzi*. It is important for this high-risk population to be aware of their exposure to triatomines and take the proper precautions, such as wearing insect repellent.

Although Texas has the highest number of cases and the majority of autochthonous transmission, it is not the only state at risk. In fact, "Multiple publications have highlighted the Southern United States as an area where autochthonous infection occurs, especially due to the high proportion of low-income residents living in substandard housing infested by triatomines."[258] Thus, anywhere in the United States that has the presence of *T. cruzi* infected triatomines and a higher proportion of low-income residents is at risk for Chagas.

For those that do become infected, there is treatment, though the effectiveness is not as high as one might like. Individuals diagnosed with Chagas receive Benznidazole, an antiparasitic, directly from the CDC under investigational protocols because the drug is not FDA approved.[259] Unfortunately, even after the drug is acquired, it only helps 15–35 percent of patients who take it.[260] Additionally, a study by Morillo et al. (2015) found that while Benznidazole reduces or eliminates the parasite from the person, it does not have any significant impact on the development of cardiac disease.[261] Put differently, you can be treated for the parasite but there is no way to prevent an individual who has been infected from developing Chagas cardiomyopathy or other Chagas-related cardiac complications. Lastly, the genotype of the *T. cruzi* infection, which is related to geographic location, impacts the effectiveness of treatment. For example, Benznidazole has the lowest level of effectiveness against *T. cruzi* infections originating from Columbia and El Salvador.[262]

Despite the lack of completely effective treatment, there are some positives. The CDC covers the cost of confirmatory diagnostic testing or provides low-cost diagnostic testing for uninsured patients. It also covers the cost of procuring and distributing Benznidazole/Nifurtimox to physicians. However, patients must pay for all costs associated with treatment-related visits or hospitalization for secondary events.[263] Additionally, the toxicity of Benznidazole and Nifurtimox, and the harsh side effects associated with them, raises concern among physicians that their patients may require hospitalization, potentially incurring additional costs.[264]

However, physicians and healthcare practitioners are oftentimes unaware of the threat of Chagas. A study conducted by Medscape in 2008 surveyed primary care, infectious disease, cardiology, obstetrics/gynecology, and transplantation medicine physicians to determine their basic knowledge and consideration of Chagas disease. Of those surveyed, 29–60 percent "never consider the risk for Chagas disease in their patients," and even fewer are confident in their knowledge of Chagas.[265] An area of particular concern is the low levels of knowledge of Chagas among those in the obstetrics/gynecology physicians, who deal first-hand with congenital Chagas transmission from mother to child.[266]

Pharmacists also represent an area of missed intervention opportunity. As pharmacists play a critical role in the prevention of congestive heart failure, it opens the door for possible interventions to promote awareness of Chagas Disease among patients who may benefit from diagnosis and subsequent treatment. A 2014 publication in the American Journal of Health-System Pharmacy called for increased pharmacist awareness of Chagas disease, noting that Chagas had yet to be described in the official journals of the American Pharmacists Association, American College of Clinical Pharmacy, or American Society of Health-Systems Pharmacists.[267] With such limited prospects for diagnostics and awareness among physicians, pharmacists, and patients, working toward preventing Chagas is just as important as raising awareness and improving prospects for treatment. The Texas Chagas Taskforce has made great strides to increase awareness among physicians over the past five years, but there is still a great deal of progress to be made. Currently, the Sabin Vaccine Institute Product Development Partnership and the Texas Children's Hospital Center for Vaccine Development are working toward developing a vaccine for Chagas disease in collaboration with CINVESTAV and Birmex.[268] The development of a vaccine would allow infections to be altogether prevented.

Despite these efforts, it is likely an impossible task to eliminate Chagas from the United States given that infected triatomines have been discovered in over a dozen states, but actions can be taken to reduce an individual's risk of infection, to raise awareness, and to educate high-risk populations. Immigrant communities and other vulnerable populations remain at the highest risk for infection within the United States, and many of these individuals lack health insurance or access to health care. To help these individuals and reduce the burden of Chagas in the United States, we must continue screening and surveillance.

Relative to the disease burden of Chagas in the United States, our comprehensive epidemiological understanding of the disease remains sparse. Increased surveillance and developing knowledge of the epidemiology of Chagas is vital to creating effective disease prevention methods. One of the leading projects in improving this conundrum is Data Tri, a database ranging across twenty-four countries from the United States to southern Chile. It provides the first integrated public geographical and ecological compilation data for 135 different species of American triatomines.[269] The data are sourced from public repositories, data provided by colleagues, and personal fieldwork ranging from the years 1904 to 2017.[270] Other projects seek to promote involvement from ordinary people throughout the course of their day-to-day life.

In 2012, a research team led by Dr. Sarah Hamer from Texas A&M University began a program which encourages people throughout the United States to become citizen scientists by submitting triatomines they find around their communities to Dr. Hamer's laboratory. The program provides information about the submitted bugs and the incidence of Chagas Disease among them. Additionally, it maps the geographic locations of the submissions, providing a visual guide of Chagas prevalence in the Southern United States.[271] In an interview, Dr. Hamer stated that the citizen science approach has allowed her lab to receive and analyze an unprecedented sample size of triatomines in the United States.[272] Most importantly, the bugs submitted are those posing the highest risk because they are the ones who have come into contact with humans during their everyday activities.[273] Despite increased awareness of triatomines and Chagas Disease, several kinds of bugs, such as leaf-footed bugs, wheel bugs, stink bugs, or other types of assassin bugs, are oftentimes mistaken for triatomines, which can cause undue panic for the individuals that encounter them.[274]

Another important project, the Virtual Vector Project at the University of Kansas, utilizes artificial intelligence to analyze photographs of bugs. The program has demonstrated an accuracy rate of 95.8–98.9 percent in recognizing various species of triatomines.[275] This recognition ability helps overcome obstacles in species identification and allows scientists to better understand the ecology of the triatomine. The project aims to develop an application or web platform that would be able to provide users with instant identification feedback.[276] Increased funding and grants for research and projects such as these will prove significant in improving our understanding of Chagas.

This is important because *T. cruzi* does not just infect humans. To date, there are over 100 different types of mammals that have been shown to serve as a natural host for the parasite. In the United States, the most common reservoirs are wood rats, opossums, and armadillos.[277] Additionally, forty-eight breeds of domestic dogs in the United States have been documented with the parasitic infection.[278] The plethora of mammalian reservoirs means that the parasite has greater opportunities to persist in communities and eventually infect humans. Indoor infestations of triatomines are likely to coincide with areas of rodent infestation, pet resting areas, and in bedrooms near mattresses.[279] Because of this, dog owners should be aware of triatomines that may be found in pet bedding and areas outdoors where the pet spends time.

A study of the prevalence of Chagas Disease in dogs residing in animal shelters across the state of Texas determined a conservative statewide average of 8.8 percent of dogs testing positive for Chagas Disease.[280] Having a pet with Chagas Disease could potentially increase a person's risk of becoming infected, as an insect that bites an infected dog could then spread the parasite to a human.[281] More often, however, it is simply an indicator that the parasite is present in vectors in the area and that humans are more likely to become infected with the disease. Although there is currently no preventative vaccine or treatment for Chagas infection among pets, veterinarians have a critical role.[282] In some cases, veterinarians are seeing cases of Chagas disease in dogs more frequently and are more familiar with Chagas disease than physicians.[283] Because of this, veterinarians are in a unique position to raise awareness about Chagas disease in their communities.

In general, Chagas has received intermittent attention as a public health concern since the early 2000s. Recently, a statement released by the American Heart Association in conjunction with the Inter-American Society of Cardiology called for providers to increase their knowledge of the origins, epidemiology, pathogenesis, diagnostic characteristics, and treatment options for Chagas cardiomyopathy.[284] Soon after, news sources and social media flooded with a rush of articles about the spread of kissing bugs and the disease they carry. Delaware. California. Pennsylvania. Each bug spotting drew more and more attention to Chagas. This led many to believe Chagas was a "recently emerging disease" despite the disease's long history in the United States.[285] This misconception likely has a great deal to do with the misconception that Chagas only exists in developing countries.

Another major factor that contributes to the lack of reporting, diagnosis, and care-seeking for Chagas in the United States is the harsh stigmatization that surrounds the disease. In Latin American countries, intense social stratification causes Chagas to be a divisive topic. Because inadequate housing is a leading cause of kissing bug infestations that infect humans, Chagas disproportionately impacts those living in poverty. This is compounded by other factors associated with poverty, such as lack of healthcare, health education, and environmental management.[286] Chagas Disease does not manifest itself through physical attributes that are visible to others. Additionally, the potential for performance to be limited as a result of Chagas Disease contributes to the misconception that those with Chagas Disease may be lazy or unproductive workers.[287]

Furthermore, increased political tensions over border control and immigration law cause additional problems. Because immigrants constitute many Chagas Disease cases in the United States, due to environmental factors, immigrants from Latin American countries experience further stigmatization. Some media sources and blogs focus solely on the rates of Chagas infection among individuals who have immigrated to the United States, oftentimes using inflammatory language and inaccurate facts. They falsely claim Chagas only comes to the United States through migration, and that keeping out migrants would, in turn, keep out the disease. This is simply not true. Chagas is, and has been, endemic in areas of South and Central Texas for decades.

Immigrant populations in the United States are already a vulnerable population, with limited screening and treatment options due to lack of health insurance and the constant threat of deportation. Posing Chagas Disease as an immigrant problem will not only cause further stigmatization against those already disadvantaged, but it perpetuates the myth that others are not vulnerable to the disease. The perpetuation of this myth can have devastating consequences for all those infected with Chagas, regardless of race or ethnic background. As one woman was told by a nurse when she arrived at the Center of Excellence for Chagas Disease for treatment, "You don't have Chagas — you're white."[288] Public awareness regarding the threat of Chagas will never improve if it is characterized as a disease that only impacts a marginalized population. With the economic burden of Chagas disease costing an estimated $27,684 per person—a result of healthcare costs and the cost of DALYs—there is a strong economic incentive to minimize the impact of Chagas throughout the entire population of the United States, regardless of citizenship or income level.[289]

TRICHOMONIASIS

Another parasitic disease that is highly prevalent in the United States and represents a large economic burden is the sexually transmitted infection trichomoniasis. Trichomoniasis is a result of infection with a protozoan parasite called *Trichomonas vaginalis*. Both men and women can be infected with trichomoniasis, but the symptoms of the disease have a greater impact on women. *T. vaginalis* flourishes in an environment where the pH of the vagina is greater than 5, or less acidic.[290] However, the protozoa is remarkably adept at evading the body's immune response, as well as withstanding enormous changes in the micro-environment of the vagina throughout the menstrual cycle.[291] Unlike other non-viral STIs, the rate of infection of trichomoniasis increases with age.[292] Because many cases of trichomoniasis are asymptomatic, the high prevalence of trichomoniasis among older individuals likely indicates that the disease persisted over time because the individual was not diagnosed or treated at the time of infection. A study conducted in a metropolitan area found that women ages fifty-one to sixty represented the population with greatest prevalence of trichomoniasis.[293] Because men with trichomoniasis are frequently asymptomatic, it is likely that they are unaware they have the disease or the risk the infection poses to those they come into sexual contact with. The most frequent symptom associated with trichomoniasis in males is inflammation of the prostate gland (prostatitis) and inflammation of the urethra (urethritis), which can result in painful urination, itchiness of the prostate and urethra, and discharge containing pus or mucus.[294]

Among women, infection with *T. vaginalis* can also be asymptomatic, sometimes taking years to become visible to those infected.[295] In total, an estimated 85 percent of trichomoniasis cases are asymptomatic.[296] For women who are symptomatic, trichomoniasis results in inflammation of the cervix and vagina, as well as itchiness or pain during urination or sexual activity.[297] An infected woman may notice their vaginal discharge appears to have an abnormal color, texture, or odor. A rarer condition, which occurs in approximately 2–5 percent of cases, is "strawberry cervix."[298] This name is derived from the strawberry-like appearance of the cervix, as several hemorrhagic lesions cover the ectocervix.

Trichomoniasis is associated with a variety of other negative health outcomes. For example, infection with *T. vaginalis* makes an individual more susceptible to the transmission of HIV.[299] The potential for trichomoniasis to promote HIV infection could have massive implications for those already vulnerable to the risk of contracting HIV. As such, it is important that those testing positive for HIV also be screened for trichomoniasis to prevent further disease spread.[300] Additionally, individuals that are coinfected with HIV and trichomoniasis experience a decrease in HIV genital shedding as a result of treatment.[301] Because of these benefits, the CDC recommends that women who are HIV positive receive screening for trichomoniasis.[302]

Trichomoniasis can also result in adverse pregnancy outcomes. Most notable is the tendency for infected individuals to give birth prematurely.[303] Additionally, trichomoniasis is associated with low birth weights.[304] Treatment with metronidazole, the medication typically used to treat the disease, failed to reduce preterm labor in two different studies, and may have even contributed to increasing the risk.[305] More importantly, however, a study found that women with trichomoniasis were significantly more likely to give birth to a child with an intellectual disability, and that, "second-trimester trichomoniasis was associated with more than a three-fold increase in the odds a child was identified as trainable mentally handicapped or profoundly mentally handicapped in the public school system, or was receiving ID services from DDSN."[306]

Trichomoniasis in History

Trichomoniasis was discovered nearly 200 years ago by Alfred François Donné, who sketched the protozoan's features and size. While he failed to determine the pathological significance of the parasite, he did record that it was found "in purulent fluids and secretions of genital organs from Men and Women."[307] Nearly half a century later in 1883, the parasite's behavior inside the female urinary tract was documented by a researcher named Kunstle.[308] In 1894, records claim that a man was found to have trichomoniasis due to the infection of his urinary tract.[309] However, it was not until 1939 that such an event was documented in a medical journal in Great Britain. Despite the early discovery of trichomoniasis, knowledge of effective treatment for the parasite remained scarce for decades.

Initially, vaginal discharges caused by a variety of ailments were treated by local application of various concoctions. One such treatment involved the application of arsenic in the form of vaginal insert tablets or powder. High doses of such treatments had the potential to cause overdose, and often resulted in frequent relapses in the presence of the disease. Later, Metronidazole was developed as a treatment, with oral administration in lieu of the local application of other products. This method of treatment proved effective in 1960. For women, the opportunity to receive treatment for trichomoniasis through oral medication was a significant improvement in their quality of life over previous methods that were repetitive, invasive, uncomfortable, and expensive over the course of time.

Although the affliction of trichomoniasis has spanned across almost two centuries, the neglected nature of this disease makes for a short history lesson. Even today, minimal attention has been shifted toward trichomoniasis and progress toward research and development of other treatment and prevention methods have been relatively stagnant. Healthy People 2020, which establishes the national objectives for improving the health of Americans within the span of a decade, failed to mention trichomoniasis altogether in its list of Sexually Transmitted Disease objectives.[310] This is a shocking exclusion given that trichomoniasis is more prevalent than both chlamydia and gonorrhea.[311]

Trichomoniasis Today

Of all the human parasitic infections in the United States, trichomoniasis is among the most prevalent, with an estimated 3.7 million Americans impacted by the disease.[312] Of these infections, approximately 2.3 million are present in women and 1.4 million in men.[313] When compared to other sexually transmitted infections, or STIs, trichomoniasis is the most prevalent non-viral infection impacting Americans today. A study of the prevalence of trichomoniasis used PCR to analyze the presence of the parasite in vaginal fluids collected from swabs as part of the National Health and Examination Survey cycles 2001–2004.[314] The results found an overall prevalence of 3.1 percent among non-Hispanic white women and Mexican Americans had prevalence rates of 1.3 percent and 1.8 percent respectively.[315] Prevalence of trichomoniasis was highest among non-Hispanic black women, with an astonishing rate of 13.3 percent.[316] Another study also examined the prevalence rates of trichomoniasis in young adult men, finding an overall prevalence rate of 1.7 percent.[317]

Native American men had the highest rates of prevalence at 4.1 percent.[318] Black men are also disproportionately impacted by trichomoniasis, with a prevalence rate of 3.3 percent in comparison of 1.3 percent of white men.[319]

There are no known biological or physiological reasons why various races or ethnicities are more at risk for trichomoniasis infection. Socioeconomic status, however, is a key determinant in all aspects of sexual health, with STI rates particularly affected by unemployment, low mean income, and low levels of education.[320] So, the increased prevalence of trichomoniasis and other STIs among some ethnic and racial minorities overlaps with the same populations who are at increased vulnerability to income inequality, poverty, and limited economic opportunity.

In comparison with the rest of the United States, the Southern United States has the highest prevalence of trichomoniasis.[321] Although urban areas have been historically regarded as centers for STI transmission, rural areas have recently seen a shift toward increasing STI case numbers. Oftentimes, rural health departments are struggling with federal and state budget cuts, diminishing already limited resources to provide services to cover the needs of a vast expanse of counties. Access to health clinics and hospitals is already problematic in rural areas, especially for those without access to transportation. Lower patient-to-doctor ratios in rural areas also limit the accessibility of receiving care.[322] Additionally, these rural areas often grapple with stigmatization rooted in socially conservative perceptions of sex and sexual orientation based on religious and political beliefs.[323] All of these factors reduce the likelihood that an individual would be willing or able to seek and successfully access affordable care and treatment for trichomoniasis. While this holds true for all STIs, the lack of awareness and education regarding trichomoniasis compared to other STIs such as chlamydia, gonorrhea, and syphilis makes the proliferation of this disease even more frightening.

Similar to some other STIs, condom usage prevents the transmission of trichomoniasis between sexual partners.[324] However, the affordability, accessibility, and education to promote the use of condoms may be lacking in low-income, rural communities. A CDC study of Youth Risk Behavior found that compared to Hispanic and white teenagers, condom usage was most prevalent among black males and females.[325] Other circumstances may also play a role in whether a female uses condoms. One study found a 50 percent reduction in condom usage among women at six to twelve months if their boyfriend was the primary provider for their source of spending money.[326] In rural areas with limited job prospects, financial dependency in instances such as this may be a factor leading to increased risk of contracting an STI such as trichomoniasis.

The economic impact of trichomoniasis infections in the United States, although likely underestimated due to asymptomatic or undiagnosed infections, is estimated at approximately $24 million annually.[327] This estimate is based solely on the direct medical costs related to the infection itself, and not any indirect costs that might result from infection such as costs associated with pregnancy complications resulting from the infection. Another overlooked cost is the greater likelihood of HIV infection in individuals with preexisting trichomoniasis infection. This alone carries a burden of an annual lifetime cost estimated at nearly $167 million.[328]

Screening and Diagnosis

Despite the prevalence of trichomoniasis, it is not a reportable condition in the United States. While individual states have the authority to decide whether or not a disease is required to be reported, the Council of State and Territorial Epidemiologists is responsible for recommending which conditions states should report to the CDC.[329] However, formal criteria to designate such conditions has yet to be published. Because many cases of trichomoniasis go undiagnosed, there is still a great deal that remains unknown about the disease, such as the overall costs associated with the infection, its severity, and more expansive prevention methods. Additionally, there is little awareness of trichomoniasis among the general public, and, therefore, little interest.

The CDC guidelines recommend that healthcare providers conduct screening for trichomoniasis for all women experiencing unusual vaginal discharge. Typically, healthcare providers have the final say in who gets tested. This usually means only symptomatic women will have access and can afford to use to this service. Wet mount preparation tests, which examine samples for the presence of *T. vaginalis* using microscopy, are the most common and cost-effective way to test for trichomoniasis. Low sensitivity is a drawback of this diagnostic method, as it varies from 38 to 82 percent depending on the size of the protozoa.[330] Because this is an in-office procedure and trichomoniasis is not a reportable condition, laboratories do not have estimates of the prevalence or other epidemiological information regarding the disease.[331] Another method of diagnosis is the broth culture technique.[332] Although it is more time-consuming, given the two to seven day time span necessary to complete, the method is highly sensitive. It is also more expensive, however, which may explain why the method has only been used in a small number of studies.

Another area for improvement in the diagnosis and treatment of trichomoniasis involves raising awareness of the disease among obstetricians and gynecologists. A 2016 survey of American College of Obstetricians and Gynecologists members revealed that less than half of participants screen HIV-positive patients for trichomoniasis either "always" or "most of the time."[333] Additionally, less than a tenth of participants retested their patients after the three months following their treatment for trichomoniasis to check for incidence of reinfection.[334] The response of participants to both survey questions indicate a serious lack of knowledge of trichomoniasis and the risks posed by the disease. Without a solid foundation of necessary diagnosis and screening procedures for at risk populations, many of these patients will fail to receive the medication necessary to treat the disease or prevent reinfection.

Treatment

Nitroimidazoles are antimicrobial medications used to treat trichomoniasis. Of the two nitroimidazoles, tinidazole is typically more expensive than metronidazole. It has a cure rate of approximately 92–100 percent in contrast with metronidazole's approximate cure rate of 84–92 percent.[335] The CDC recommends for doses of metronidazole to be taken orally three times a day for a week.[336] Throughout the duration of this treatment, the individual is also able to engage in intercourse with a sexual partner without risk of immediate reinfection. However, the partner must also receive treatment to prevent future reinfection. Studies have examined various methods to encourage those infected with trichomoniasis to notify their partner for the purpose of encouraging them to seek treatment. One such study found that repeat infections were lower when the partners were able to deliver therapy to each other in contrast to a public health disease intervention, which involves health officials contacting the partner and administering treatment.[337]

Aside from Metronidazole or Tinidazole, there are no alternative treatments for trichomoniasis that have been approved by the Food and Drug Administration. For this reason, antimicrobial resistance to Nitroimidazole represents a serious cause for alarm. An estimated 5 percent of all clinical cases of trichomoniasis are the result of infection with a strain of *T. vaginalis* that is resistant to Metronidazole.[338] Although many of these strains display low levels of resistance, this could present a major obstacle moving forward if resistance develops at an increasing rate. There have already been some cases trichomoniasis that have required treatment with higher doses of metronidazole than recommended, which results in an increased risk that the individual suffers from side effects of the drug.[339] Because both Metronidazole and Tinidazole are Nitroimidazoles, incidences of cases with cross-resistance to *T. vaginalis* are possible and would have serious implications. In contrast with some other NTDs, such as Chagas and hookworm, vaccine prospects for trichomoniasis are grim. Progress in vaccine development has been impeded by little knowledge of the host's immune response to trichomoniasis, as well as the lack of an appropriate animal model to utilize in studies.[340]

An Additional Risk Factor—Incarceration

Incarceration is yet another potential risk factor for NTDs, as it often traps inmates and their families in a cycle of poverty. Incarceration disproportionately impacts ethnic and racial minorities and those of low socioeconomic status. The United States has had the highest incarceration rate in the world since 2002.[341] Although mass incarceration strategies were scaled up with the intention of reducing crime among both first-time and repeat offenses, recidivism rates remain high.[342] Incarceration rates in the American South have historically been higher than other areas, with Louisiana's rates representing the highest in the nation.[343] Nationwide, African Americans are 5.1 times more likely to be incarcerated in a state prison compared to whites, and Latinos have a rate 1.4 times the incarceration rate of whites.[344] Low educational attainment, literacy, and skill levels are also associated with incarceration.[345] Those who are incarcerated face further disadvantages upon their release as a result of structural discrimination. Oftentimes, they face increased difficulty accessing housing, public benefits, employment opportunities, and education.[346] The accumulation of these factors leads to diminishing upward mobility, which may explain the motivation behind those who re-offend due to financial pressures.[347]

Several studies point to high-risk behaviors that connect incarceration with high rates of STIs, as well as lack of access to health-related services.[348] Additionally, some incarcerated women engage in prostitution in exchange for food, shelter, drugs, or were coerced into having sex prior to their arrest.[349] The CDC's Sexually Transmitted Disease Guidelines, published in 2010, states that "screening for T. vaginalis in women can be considered in those at high risk for infection (i.e., women who have new or multiple partners, have a history of STIs, exchange sex for payment, and use injection drugs)."[350] The National Commission on Correctional Health Care has previously recommended offering universal, routine screening to incarcerated populations.[351] Despite this, the majority of correctional facilities, especially jails, do not routinely conduct screening for STIs.[352]

This represents a significant missed opportunity to not only improve the health of inmates suffering from STIs, but also to protect the health of the general population who will interact with these inmates upon their eventual release. Additionally, early intervention and treatment could improve health outcomes for both the inmate, their current or future partners, and their children, as a result of improved pregnancy outcomes.

Several studies demonstrate the need for such services. The HIV Epidemiology Research Study enrolled female participants from April 1993 to January 1995 in 4 urban centers, of which 33 percent had been incarcerated at least once.[353] In contrast with chlamydia, gonorrhea, and syphilis, a strong independent association linked trichomoniasis with incarceration among the study's cohort of women with high-risk sexual behavior.[354] A study examining the prevalence of trichomoniasis among inmates incarcerated at the San Francisco County Jail found that 25 percent of women age 18–25 and 38 percent of women 26–35 percent were infected with trichomoniasis.[355] In a Rhode Island study, 26 percent of pregnant inmates tested positive for trichomoniasis infection.[356] Similarly, 47 percent of pregnant inmates in New York tested positive.[357] Another study comparing the association between incarceration and trichomoniasis infection found no evidence that the acquisition of trichomoniasis among the inmates occurred during their time at the facility.[358] Instead, the study suggests there may be multiple other confounding variables that contribute to the association between the two variables. These could include higher numbers of sexual partners, higher rates of drug and alcohol use, decreased condom use prior to incarceration, or factors after incarceration such as problems within their family or community and new partnerships.[359]

Although those who have been incarcerated are often part of the population most vulnerable to the risk factors of contracting trichomoniasis, many of these individuals lack access or resources to afford STI testing and treatment. Routine STI screening of this population is a potentially cost-saving or cost-effective program, as diagnosing and treating STIs early reduces the burden of disease, as well as costs incurred from the expensive treatment of more advanced symptoms and health problems caused by these diseases.[360] Some facilities, such as jails, experience the comings and goings of more transient inmates. As such, the testing, diagnosis, and treatment of these inmates would have to be conducted and administered more quickly. Because of the burden this may place on limited resources, collaborations would be necessary to achieve this goal. Community organizations and healthcare providers may need to be involved. Despite these challenges, conducting routine STI testing presents a unique opportunity for a health intervention targeting some of the populations most vulnerable to STIs like trichomoniasis—a population that is clearly in need of such interventions.

Lessons from Fighting Disease in the South

The examples we have discussed throughout this chapter show the American experience with NTDs. These are diseases that played a central role in our history, affecting everything from the Constitution to the Civil War to migration, trade, and blood bank screening. The invention of flush toilets, window screens, and air conditioning reduced the impact of these NTDs in the United States, lulling many Americans into a false sense of security. For the past several decades it has been believed, even by medical professionals, that these diseases no longer exist here. The narrative that NTDs are gone from the United States and only affects developing countries is a false one. NTDs are and always have been right here in the United States. Today, their impact is limited mostly to the country's poorest communities. Thus, the more appropriate title for these diseases are "diseases of poverty."

The diseases we discussed throughout this chapter, with the exception of Yellow Fever, are endemic in the United States today. They are allowed to persist because of a lack of adequate sanitation infrastructure, housing, and health access in low-income communities throughout the American South. Hot, humid temperatures, made worse by climate change, are helping vectors such as triatomines and the *Aedes aegypti* mosquito move into new regions of the United States. The movement of vectors ensures that these diseases will become more problematic in coming decades. To counter this expansion and provide relief to communities already suffering, policies must be created at the local, state, and national level to address issues of infrastructure, housing, and health access. Additionally, education and training of doctors and nurses, particularly in high-risk areas must be conducted to increase awareness of the disease among these groups. Increased awareness will help with timely and accurate diagnosis.

In this chapter, we have outlined the history of NTDs in the United States. Although these are not all the NTDs that have and continue to impact the American population, they are some of the most prominent and concerning ones. In the next chapter, we will examine poverty in the United States to further explore the social and economic factors suitable to NTDs.

NOTES

1. Carrie Arnold, "Can America Cope with a Resurgence of Tropical Disease?" *Wellcome Trust*, published August 10, 2015, https://mosaicscience.com/story/america-tropical-disease/.
2. Arnold, "Can America Cope with a Resurgence of Tropical Disease?"
3. Arnold, "Can America Cope with a Resurgence of Tropical Disease?"
4. Centers for Disease Control and Prevention, "Hookworm FAQs," published December 16, 2014, https://www.cdc.gov/parasites/hookworm/gen_info/faqs.html; Centers for Disease Control and Prevention, "Parasites—Hookworm," published January 10, 2013, https://www.cdc.gov/parasites/hookworm/index.html.
5. Centers for Disease Control and Prevention, "Parasites—Hookworm."
6. Centers for Disease Control and Prevention, "Hookworm FAQs."
7. John Ettling, *The Germ of Laziness: Rockefeller Philanthropy and Public Health in the New South* (Harvard University Press, 1981).
8. Allen Scott, "The Prevalence and Distribution of Hookworm Infection in Egypt," *American Journal of Epidemiology* 26, no. 3 (1937): 455–505; Wilhelm

Griesinger, "Klinische und anatomische Beobachtungen über die Krankheiten von Egypten," *Arch. Physiol. Heilkd* 13 (1854): 528–575.

9. Ettling, *The Germ of Laziness*.

10. Ettling, *The Germ of Laziness*; Angelo Dubini, "New Worm of the Human Intestine (Agchylostoma duodenale) Constituting a Sixth Genus of Nematodes Found in Man," *Tropical Medicine and Parasitology: Classic Investigations*, 2 vols., ed. B. H. Kean, Kenneth E. Mott, and Adair J. Russell (Ithaca, NY: Cornell University Press, 1978), 2: 287–291.

11. Philip RP Coelho and Robert A. McGuire, "Racial Differences in Disease Susceptibilities: Intestinal Worm Infections in the Early Twentieth-Century American South," *Social History of Medicine* 19, no. 3 (2006): 461–482; Rachel Nuwer, "How a Worm Gave the South a Bad Name," *PBS*, published April 27, 2016, https://www.pbs.org/wgbh/nova/article/how-a-worm-gave-the-south-a-bad-name/.

12. Nuwer, "How a Worm Gave the South a Bad Name"; Harper Lee, *To Kill a Mockingbird* (New York: Grand Central Publishing, 1960).

13. Rebecca Kreston, "Blood Money: Hookworm Economics in the Postbellum South," *Discover Magazine*, published April 25, 2011, https://www.discovermagazine.com/health/blood-money-hookworm-economics-in-the-postbellum-south.

14. Dipali Pathak, "Hookworms, Poverty, Poor Sanitation Linked in Rural Alabama," *Baylor College of Medicine*, published September 6, 2017, https://www.bcm.edu/news/school-of-tropical-medicine/hookworm-poverty-sanitation-alabama.

15. Hotez, "Neglected Infections of Poverty in the United States of America"; Peter J. Hotez and Sheila Jackson Lee, "US Gulf Coast States: The Rise of Neglected Tropical Diseases in 'Flyover Nation,'" *PLoS Neglected Tropical Diseases* 11, no. 11 (2017): e0005744.

16. Ettling, *The Germ of Laziness*.

17. Megan L. McKenna et al., "Human Intestinal Parasite Burden and Poor Sanitation in Rural Alabama," *American Journal of Tropical Medicine and Hygiene* 97, no. 5 (2017): 1623–1628.

18. Coelho and McGuire, "Racial Difference in Disease Susceptibilities"; Nuwer, "How a Worm Gave the South a Bad Name."

19. Ettling, *The Germ of Laziness*.

20. Nuwer, "How a Worm Gave the South a Bad Name," 24.

21. Kreston, "Blood Money: Hookworm Economics in the Postbellum South."

22. M. L. H. Mabaso et al., "The Effect of Soil Type and Climate on Hookworm (Necator americanus) Distribution in KwaZulu-Natal, South Africa," *Tropical Medicine & International Health* 8, no. 8 (2003): 722–727.

23. Ettling, *The Germ of Laziness*.

24. Ettling, *The Germ of Laziness*, 35.

25. Ettling, *The Germ of Laziness*.

26. Ettling, *The Germ of Laziness*.

27. Kreston, "Blood Money: Hookworm Economics in the Postbellum South."

28. Ettling, *The Germ of Laziness*.

29. Kreston, "Blood Money: Hookworm Economics in the Postbellum South."

30. Nuwer, "How a Worm Gave the South a Bad Name," 24.

31. Ettling, *The Germ of Laziness.*

32. Ettling, *The Germ of Laziness*, 2.

33. Ettling, *The Germ of Laziness.*

34. Hoyt Bleakley, "Disease and Development: Evidence from Hookworm Eradication in the American South," *The Quarterly Journal of Economics* 122, no. 1 (2007): 92.

35. Hoyt, "Disease and Development: Evidence From Hookworm Eradication in the American South," 92.

36. Hoyt, "Disease and Development: Evidence From Hookworm Eradication in the American South," 105.

37. Hoyt, "Disease and Development: Evidence From Hookworm Eradication in the American South," 220.

38. Hoyt, "Disease and Development: Evidence From Hookworm Eradication in the American South," 218–223.

39. Nuwer, "How a Worm Gave the South a Bad Name," 24.

40. Nuwer, "How a Worm Gave the South a Bad Name," 24.

41. Margaret Humphreys, "How Four Once Common Diseases were Eliminated from the American South," *Health Affairs* 28, no. 6 (2009): 1734–1744, https://www.ncbi.nlm.nih.gov/pubmed/19887414.

42. Nuwer, "How a Worm Gave the South a Bad Name," 6.

43. Kreston, "Blood Money: Hookworm Economics in the Postbellum South."

44. Ettling, *The Germ of Laziness.*

45. Cheryl Elman, Robert McGuire, and Barbara Wittman, "Extending Public Health: The Rockefeller Sanitary Commission and Hookworm in the American South," *American Journal of Public Health* 104, no. 1 (2014): 47–58.

46. Ettling, *The Germ of Laziness*, 38.

47. Mary Boccaccio, "Ground Itch and Dew Poison The Rockefeller Sanitary Commission 1909–14," *Journal of the History of Medicine and Allied Sciences* 27, no. 1 (1972): 30–53.

48. Ettling, *The Germ of Laziness*, 118.

49. Elman, McGuire, and Wittman, "Extending Public Health: The Rockefeller Sanitary Commission and Hookworm in the American South," 47–58.

50. Ettling, *The Germ of Laziness*, 120.

51. "Rockefeller Sanitary Commission (RSC)," Rockefeller Foundation, accessed January 26, 2019, https://rockfound.rockarch.org/rockefeller-sanitary-commission.

52. Ettling, *The Germ of Laziness*, 130.

53. Ettling, *The Germ of Laziness*, 131.

54. Ettling, *The Germ of Laziness*, 131.

55. Elman, McGuire, and Wittman, "Extending Public Health: The Rockefeller Sanitary Commission and Hookworm in the American South," 47–58.

56. Ettling, *The Germ of Laziness.*

57. Ettling, *The Germ of Laziness*; Rockefeller Foundation, "Rockefeller Sanitary Commission (RSC)."

58. Elman, McGuire, and Wittman, "Extending Public Health: The Rockefeller Sanitary Commission and Hookworm in the American South," 47–58.

59. Ettling, *The Germ of Laziness.*

60. Alice L. Anderson and Thomas Allen, "Mapping Historic Hookworm Disease Prevalence in the Southern Us, Comparing Percent Prevalence with Percent Soil Drainage Type Using Gis," *Infectious Diseases: Research and Treatment* 4 (2011): IDRT-S6762.

61. Ettling, *The Germ of Laziness*, 211.

62. Nuwer, "How a Worm Gave the South a Bad Name."

63. Nuwer, "How a Worm Gave the South a Bad Name."

64. Nuwer, "How a Worm Gave the South a Bad Name."

65. McKenna et al., "Human Intestinal Parasite Burden and Poor Sanitation in Rural Alabama."

66. McKenna et al., "Human Intestinal Parasite Burden and Poor Sanitation in Rural Alabama."

67. Nadia Whitehead, "The U.S. Thought it was Rid of Hookworm," Wrong. *NPR.org*, published September 12, 2017, https://www.npr.org/sections/goatsandsoda/2017/09/12/550387650/the-u-s-thought-it-was-rid-of-hookworm-wrong.

68. Dawn Smith, "The HIV Epidemiology Research Study, HIV Out-Patient Study, and the Spectrum of Disease Studies," *JAIDS Journal of Acquired Immune Deficiency Syndromes* 17 (1998): S17–S19.

69. Humphreys, "How Four Once Common Diseases were Eliminated from the American South."

70. Michael Harriot, "Lowndes County, Ala: The Place God Forgot," *The Root*, published April 27, 2018, https://www.theroot.com/lowndes-county-ala-the-place-god-forgot-1825483659.

71. Harriot, "Lowndes County, Ala: The Place God Forgot."

72. Paul Hunt, "The Human Right to the Highest Attainable Standard of Health: New Opportunities and Challenges," *Transactions of the Royal Society of Tropical Medicine and Hygiene* 100, no. 7 (2006): 603–607.

73. Jim Byard, "Workforce Information Lowndes County AL Unemployment Underemployment," *Lowndes County*, accessed October 3, 2018, https://lowndescountyedc.com/doing-business/workforce-information; Daniel Vock, "People Are Literally Being Poisoned: How Sewage Problems in Alabama Got So Bad–and Why Other States Should Worry," *Governing*, published July 17, 2018, https://www.governing.com/topics/transportation-infrastructure/gov-alabama-hookworm-sewage.html.

74. Philip Alston, "Report of the Special Rapporteur On Extreme Poverty and Human Rights on His Mission to the United States of America," *United Nations*, published May 4, 2018, http://digitallibrary.un.org/record/162953.

75. "Lowndes County, Al," Data USA, accessed November 27, 2018, https://datausa.io/profile/geo/lowndes-county-al/.

76. Vock, "People Are Literally Being Poisoned."

77. Catarina de Albuquerque, "Promotion and Protection of All Human Rights, Civil, Political, Economic, Social and Cultural Rights, Including the Right to Development" (United Nations General Assembly Human Rights Council, 2011), https://doi.org/10.1163/2210-7975_HRD-9970-2016149.

78. Catherine Flowers, "Opinion: A County Where the Sewer is Your Lawn," *The New York Times*, published May 22, 2018, https://www.nytimes.com/2018/05/22/opinion/alabama-poverty-sewers.htm; Nathalie Baptiste, "This Black Community Has Filed

a Civil Rights Complaint over Unsanitary Sewage Conditions," *Mother Jones*, published October 4, 2018, https://www.motherjones.com/environment/2018/10/this-black-community-has-filed-a-civil-rights-complaint-over-unsanitary-sewage-conditions/.

79. Mark Elliot, "Prevalence and Impacts of Failing Septic Systems and Straight Pipes in Rural Alabama," Presented at the UNC Water and Health Conference, Chapel Hill, NC, last modified May 10, 2018, https://cfpub.epa.gov/ncer_abstracts/index.cfm/fuseaction/display.abstractDetail/abstract/10779/report/F.

80. Flowers, "Opinion: A County Where the Sewer is Your Lawn."

81. Baptiste, "This Black Community Has Filed a Civil Rights Complaint over Unsanitary Sewage Conditions."

82. McKenna et al., "Human Intestinal Parasite Burden and Poor Sanitation in Rural Alabama."

83. McKenna et al., "Human Intestinal Parasite Burden and Poor Sanitation in Rural Alabama."

84. Mary McIntyre, "Notice: Environmental Study in Lowndes County, Alabama, Fails to Prove Hookworm Infection," *Alabama State Department of Health*, published April 9, 2018, http://www.alabamapublichealth.gov/infectiousdiseases/assets/hookworm-notice.pdf.

85. McIntyre, "Notice: Environmental Study in Lowndes County, Alabama, Fails to Prove Hookworm Infection."

86. Arielle Duhaime-Ross, "Scientists Think Alabama's Sewage Problem Has Caused a Tropical Parasite. The State Has Done Little About It," *Vice News*, published December 17, 2018, https://www.vice.com/en_us/article/pa5wdg/scientists-raised-the-alarm-about-hookworm-in-alabama-a-year-ago-the-state-has-done-little-about-it.

87. Whitehead, "The U.S. Thought it was Rid of Hookworm"; "Albendazole Prices and Albendazole Coupons," GoodRx, accessed 2019, https://www.goodrx.com/albendazole.

88. Gilbert A. Castro, "Helminths: Structure, Classification, Growth, and Development," in *Medical Microbiology*, 4th ed. (Galveston, TX: University of Texas Medical Branch at Galveston, 1996).

89. Peter J. Hotez and Patricia P. Wilkins, "Toxocariasis: America's Most Common Neglected Infection of Poverty and a Helminthiasis of Global Importance?" *PLoS Negl Trop Dis* 3, no. 3 (2009): e400.

90. Rajinder K. Chitkara and P. S. Sarinas, "Dirofilaria, Visceral Larva Migrans, and Tropical Pulmonary Eosinophilia," *Seminars in Respiratory Infections* 12, no. 2 (1997): 138–148.

91. Laura Beil, "The Parasite on the Playground," *The New York Times*, published January 16, 2018, https://www.nytimes.com/2018/01/16/health/toxocara-children-new-york-playgrounds.html.

92. Dickson Despommier, "Toxocariasis: Clinical Aspects, Epidemiology, Medical Ecology, and Molecular Aspects," *Clinical Microbiology Reviews* 16, no. 2 (2003): 265–272.

93. Despommier, "Toxocariasis: Clinical Aspects, Epidemiology, Medical Ecology, and Molecular Aspects."

94. J. Fillaux and J. F. Magnaval, "Laboratory Diagnosis of Human Toxocariasis," *Veterinary Parasitology* 193, no. 4 (2013): 327–336.

95. Hotez and Wilkins, "Toxocariasis: America's Most Common Neglected Infection of Poverty and a Helminthiasis of Global Importance?"

96. Dana M. Woodhall, Mark L. Eberhard, and Monica E. Parise, "Neglected Parasitic Infections in the United States: Toxocariasis," *The American Journal of Tropical Medicine and Hygiene* 90, no. 5 (2014): 810–813.

97. Despommier, "Toxocariasis: Clinical Aspects, Epidemiology, Medical Ecology, and Molecular Aspects."

98. Hotez and Wilkins, "Toxocariasis: America's Most Common Neglected Infection of Poverty and a Helminthiasis of Global Importance?"; Peter J. Hotez, "Visceral and Ocular Larva Migrans," *Seminars in Neurology* 13, no. 2 (1993): 175–179; Suchitra Nelson, Tom Greene, and Claire B. Ernhart, "Toxocara Canis Infection in Preschool Age Children: Risk Factors and the Cognitive Development of Preschool Children," *Neurotoxicology and Teratology* 18, no. 2 (1996): 167–174; C. Marx et al., "Toxocariasis of the CNS Simulating Acute Disseminated Encephalomyelitis," *Neurology* 69, no. 8 (2007): 806–807.

99. Michael G. Walsh and M. A. Haseeb, "Reduced Cognitive Function in Children with Toxocariasis in a Nationally Representative Sample of the United States," *International Journal for Parasitology* 42, nos. 13–14 (2012): 1159–1163.

100. Nira Herrmann et al., "Seroprevalence of Zoonotic Toxocariasis in the United States: 1971–1973," *American Journal of Epidemiology* 122, no. 5 (1985): 890–896.

101. Herrmann et al., "Seroprevalence of Zoonotic Toxocariasis in the United States: 1971–1973."

102. Herrmann et al., "Seroprevalence of Zoonotic Toxocariasis in the United States: 1971–1973."

103. Woodhall, Eberhard, and Parise, "Neglected Parasitic Infections in the United States: Toxocariasis."

104. Aaron Farmer, Thomas Beltran, and Young Sammy Choi, "Prevalence of Toxocara Species Infection in the US: Results from the National Health and Nutrition Examination Survey, 2011–2014," *PLoS Neglected Tropical Diseases* 11, no. 7 (2017): e0005818.

105. Hotez and Wilkins, "Toxocariasis: America's Most Common Neglected Infection of Poverty and a Helminthiasis of Global Importance?"

106. Centers for Disease Control and Prevention, "Ocular Toxocariasis–United States, 2009–2011," *MMWR: Morbidity and Mortality Weekly Report* 60, no. 22 (2011): 734.

107. Woodhall, Eberhard, and Parise, "Neglected Parasitic Infections in the United States: Toxocariasis."

108. Hotez and Wilkins, "Toxocariasis: America's Most Common Neglected Infection of Poverty and a Helminthiasis of Global Importance?"

109. Woodhall, Eberhard, and Parise, "Neglected Parasitic Infections in the United States: Toxocariasis."

110. Woodhall, Eberhard, and Parise, "Neglected Parasitic Infections in the United States: Toxocariasis."

111. Guangxu Ma et al., "Human Toxocariasis," *The Lancet Infectious Diseases* 18, no. 1 (2018): e14–e24.

112. Woodhall, Eberhard, and Parise, "Neglected Parasitic Infections in the United States: Toxocariasis."

113. Rachel M. Lee et al., "Toxocariasis in North America: A Systematic Review," *PLoS Neglected Tropical Diseases* 8, no. 8 (2014): e3116.

114. Lee et al., "Toxocariasis in North America: A Systematic Review."

115. Hotez, *Blue Marble Health: An Innovative Plan to Fight Diseases of the Poor Amid Wealth*, 130.

116. ASPCA, "Pet Statistics," accessed August 20, 2019, https://www.aspca.org/animal-homelessness/shelter-intake-and-surrender/pet-statistics.

117. AVMA, "Mandatory Spay/Neuter Laws," accessed August 20, 2019, https://www.avma.org/Advocacy/StateAndLocal/Pages/sr-spay-neuter-laws.aspx?mode=full.

118. Samantha Raphelson, "No 'Easy Answer' to Growing Number of Stray Dogs in the US, Advocate Says," *KPBS Public Media*, published December 29, 2017, https://www.kpbs.org/news/2017/dec/29/no-easy-answer-to-growing-number-of-stray-dogs-in/.

119. Jim C. Parsons, "Ascarid Infections of Cats and Dogs," *Veterinary Clinics of North America: Small Animal Practice* 17, no. 6 (1987): 1307–1339.

120. Charles T. Faulkner, Sharon Patton, and Sandra Strawbridge Johnson, "Prehistoric Parasitism in Tennessee: Evidence from the Analysis of Desiccated Fecal Material Collected from Big Bone Cave, Van Buren County, Tennessee," *The Journal of Parasitology* (1989): 461–463.

121. Leigh Ann Miller et al., "Ascariasis in Humans and Pigs On Small-Scale Farms, Maine, USA, 2010–2013," *Emerging Infectious Diseases* 21, no. 2 (2015): 332.

122. Peter Nejsum et al., "Ascariasis is a Zoonosis in Denmark," *Journal of Clinical Microbiology* 43, no. 3 (2005): 1142–1148.

123. Mohammed Sultan Khuroo, "Ascariasis," *Gastroenterology Clinics of North America* 25, no. 3 (1996): 553–577.

124. Centers for Disease Control and Prevention, "Parasites—Ascariasis," published February 15, 2018, https://www.cdc.gov/parasites/ascariasis/index.html.

125. Khuroo, "Ascariasis."

126. Miller et al., "Ascariasis in Humans and Pigs on Small-Scale Farms, Maine, USA, 2010–2013," 332.

127. Jessika Lora, "Ascariasis," last modified December 2004, https://web.stanford.edu/group/parasites/ParaSites2005/Ascaris/JLora_ParaSite.htm.

128. Lora, "Ascariasis."

129. Lora, "Ascariasis."

130. John H. Cross, "Enteric Nematodes of Humans," *Medical Microbiology* 4 (1996).

131. Lora, "Ascariasis."

132. Kalyan Kanneganti, Jasbir S. Makker, and Prospere Remy, "Ascaris Lumbricoides: To Expect the Unexpected During a Routine Colonoscopy," *Case Reports in Medicine* 2013 (2013).

133. Quan-yue Li et al., "Life-Threatening Complications of Ascariasis in Trauma Patients: A Review of the Literature," *World Journal of Emergency Medicine* 5, no. 3 (2014): 165–170.

134. Thein Hlaing, "Ascariasis and Childhood Malnutrition," *Parasitology* 107, no. S1 (1993): S125–S136.

135. Poppy H. Lamberton and Peter M. Jourdan, "Human Ascariasis: Diagnostics Update," *Current Tropical Medicine Reports* 2, no. 4 (2015): 196.

136. Li et al., "Life-Threatening Complications of Ascariasis in Trauma Patients: A Review of the Literature."

137. Shuichiro Umetsu et al., "Intestinal Ascariasis at Pediatric Emergency Room in a Developed Country," *World Journal of Gastroenterology: WJG* 20, no. 38 (2014): 14058.

138. Umetsu et al., "Intestinal Ascariasis at Pediatric Emergency Room in a Developed Country."

139. Umetsu et al., "Intestinal Ascariasis at Pediatric Emergency Room in a Developed Country."

140. Jamil Shah and Abul Shahidullah, "Ascaris Lumbricoides: A Startling Discovery During Screening Colonoscopy," *Case Reports in Gastroenterology* 12, no. 2 (2018): 224–229.

141. Cristiano Lara Massara and Martin Johannes Enk, "Treatment Options in the Management of Ascaris Lumbricoides," *Expert Opinion on Pharmacotherapy* 5, no. 3 (2004): 529–539.

142. Miller et al., "Ascariasis in Humans and Pigs on Small-Scale Farms, Maine, USA, 2010–2013."

143. P. O'lorcain and C. V. Holland, "The Public Health Importance of Ascaris Lumbricoides," *Parasitology* 121, no. S1 (2000): S51–S71.

144. Shuichiro Traub et al., "The Prevalence, Intensities and Risk Factors Associated with Geohelminth Infection in Tea-Growing Communities of Assam, India," *Tropical Medicine & International Health* 9, no. 6 (2004): 688–701.

145. Mohammad Yousuf Mubarak et al., "Hygienic Behaviors and Risks for Ascariasis Among College Students in Kabul, Afghanistan," *The American Journal of Tropical Medicine and Hygiene* 97, no. 2 (2017): 563–566.

146. Andrew Hall et al., "A Review and Meta-Analysis of the Impact of Intestinal Worms on Child Growth and Nutrition," *Maternal & Child Nutrition* 4 (2008): 118–236.

147. Christopher J. L. Murray, Theo Vos, Rafael Lozano, Mohsen Naghavi, Abraham D. Flaxman, Catherine Michaud, Majid Ezzati et al., "Disability-Adjusted Life Years (DALYs) for 291 Diseases and Injuries in 21 Regions, 1990–2010: A Systematic Analysis for the Global Burden of Disease Study 2010," *The Lancet* 380, no. 9859 (2012): 2197–2223.

148. Bin Zhan et al., "Advancing a Multivalent 'Pan-Anthelmintic' Vaccine Against Soil-Transmitted Nematode Infections," *Expert Review of Vaccines* 13, no. 3 (2014): 321–331.

149. Centers for Disease Control and Prevention, "Dengue," published February 14, 2002, https://www.cdc.gov/dengue/index.html?CDC_AA_refVal=https%3A%2F%2Fwww.cdc.gov%2Fdengue%2Ffaqfacts%2Findex.html.

150. Nidhi Bouri et al., "Return of Epidemic Dengue in the United States: Implications for the Public Health Practitioner," *Public Health Reports* 127, no. 3 (2012): 259–266.

151. Bouri et al., "Return of Epidemic Dengue in the United States: Implications for the Public Health Practitioner"; Felipe J. Colón-González et al., "The Effects of Weather and Climate Change on Dengue," *PLoS Negl Trop Dis* 7, no. 11 (2013): e2503.

152. Bouri et al., "Return of Epidemic Dengue in the United States: Implications for the Public Health Practitioner."

153. Duane J. Gubler, "Dengue and Dengue Hemorrhagic Fever," *Clinical Microbiology Reviews* 11, no. 3 (1998): 480–496.

154. Bouri et al., "Return of Epidemic Dengue in the United States: Implications for the Public Health Practitioner."

155. Gubler, "Dengue and Dengue Hemorrhagic Fever."

156. Gubler, "Dengue and Dengue Hemorrhagic Fever"; Dick et al., "The History of Dengue Outbreaks in the Americas," *The American Journal of Tropical Medicine and Hygiene* 87, no. 4 (2012): 584–593.

157. Gubler, "Dengue and Dengue Hemorrhagic Fever"; Dick et al., "The History of Dengue Outbreaks in the Americas"; Benjamin Rush, "An Account of the Bilious Remitting Fever: As It Appeared in Philadelphia, in the Summer and Autumn of the Year 1780," *The American Journal of Medicine* 11, no. 5 (1951): 546–550.

158. Dick et al., "The History of Dengue Outbreaks in the Americas."

159. Bouri et al., "Return of Epidemic Dengue in the United States: Implications for the Public Health Practitioner," 260.

160. Dick et al., "The History of Dengue Outbreaks in the Americas."

161. Dick et al., "The History of Dengue Outbreaks in the Americas."

162. Coreen Beaumier, Melissa N. Garcia, and Kristy O. Murray, "The History of Dengue in the United States and its Recent Emergence," *Current Tropical Medicine Reports* 1, no. 1 (2014): 33.

163. Beaumier, Garcia, and Murray, "The History of Dengue in the United States and its Recent Emergence," 32–35.

164. Beaumier, Garcia, and Murray, "The History of Dengue in the United States and its Recent Emergence," 33.

165. N. Joel Ehrenkranz et al., "Pandemic Dengue in Caribbean Countries and the Southern United States—Past, Present and Potential Problems," *New England Journal of Medicine* 285, no. 26 (1971): 1460.

166. Beaumier, Garcia, and Murray, "The History of Dengue in the United States and its Recent Emergence," 32–35.

167. Dick et al., "The History of Dengue Outbreaks in the Americas."

168. Beaumier, Garcia, and Murray, "The History of Dengue in the United States and its Recent Emergence," 33.

169. Bouri et al., "Return of Epidemic Dengue in the United States: Implications for the Public Health Practitioner."

170. Dick et al., "The History of Dengue Outbreaks in the Americas."

171. Dick et al., "The History of Dengue Outbreaks in the Americas."

172. Beaumier, Garcia, and Murray, "The History of Dengue in the United States and its Recent Emergence," 32–35; Centers for Disease Control and Prevention, "Elimination of Malaria in the United States (1947–1951)," published July 23, 2018, www.cdc.gov/malaria/about/history/elimination_us.html.

173. Centers for Disease Control and Prevention, "Elimination of Malaria in the United States (1947–1951)."

174. Centers for Disease Control and Prevention, "Elimination of Malaria in the United States (1947–1951)."

175. Centers for Disease Control and Prevention, "Elimination of Malaria in the United States (1947–1951)."

176. Beaumier, Garcia, and Murray, "The History of Dengue in the United States and its Recent Emergence," 33.

177. Dick et al., "The History of Dengue Outbreaks in the Americas," 585

178. Don W. Micks and William B. Moon, "Aedes Aegypti in a Texas Coastal County as an Index of Dengue Fever Receptivity and Control," *The American Journal of Tropical Medicine and Hygiene* 29, no. 6 (1980): 1382–1388.

179. Beaumier, Garcia, and Murray, "The History of Dengue in the United States and its Recent Emergence," 32–35.

180. Beaumier, Garcia, and Murray, "The History of Dengue in the United States and its Recent Emergence," 32–35.

181. Beaumier, Garcia, and Murray, "The History of Dengue in the United States and its Recent Emergence," 34.

182. Beaumier, Garcia, and Murray, "The History of Dengue in the United States and its Recent Emergence," 32–35.

183. Texas Department of Health and Human Services, "Data: Dengue Fever & Dengue Hemorrhagic Fever (DHF)," last modified April 3, 2019, https://www.dshs.texas.gov/IDCU/disease/dengue/Data.aspx.

184. Texas Department of Health and Human Services, "Data: Dengue Fever & Dengue Hemorrhagic Fever (DHF)."

185. Elizabeth G. Radke et al., "Dengue Outbreak in Key West, Florida, USA, 2009," *Emerging Infectious Diseases* 18, no. 1 (2012): 135–137.

186. Radke et al., "Dengue Outbreak in Key West, Florida, USA, 2009."

187. Centers for Disease Control and Prevention, "Statistics and Maps: Dengue Cases in the US," published March 13, 2020, https://www.cdc.gov/dengue/statistics-maps/index.html.

188. Bouri et al., "Return of Epidemic Dengue in the United States: Implications for the Public Health Practitioner."

189. Bouri et al., "Return of Epidemic Dengue in the United States: Implications for the Public Health Practitioner."

190. World Health Organization, "Yellow Fever," published May 7, 2019, https://www.who.int/en/news-room/fact-sheets/detail/yellow-fever.

191. World Health Organization, "Yellow Fever: Questions and Answers," published March 2, 2017, https://www.who.int/features/qa/yellow-fever/en/.

192. World Health Organization, "Yellow Fever."

193. World Health Organization, "Yellow Fever."

194. World Health Organization, "Yellow Fever."

195. World Health Organization, "Yellow Fever."

196. Beth Skwarecki, *Outbreak!: 50 Tales of Epidemics that Terrorized the World* (Avon, Massachusetts: Adams Media, 2016), 110.

197. Skwarecki, *Outbreak!*, 110.
198. Skwarecki, *Outbreak!*
199. Molly Crosby, *The American Plague: The Untold Story of Yellow Fever, The Epidemic That Shaped Our History* (New York, New York: Berkley Publishing Group, 2006).
200. Crosby, *The American Plague*, 41.
201. Crosby, *The American Plague*, 55.
202. Crosby, *The American Plague.*
203. Crosby, *The American Plague*, 57.
204. Crosby, *The American Plague.*
205. Crosby, *The American Plague*, 87–88.
206. Crosby, *The American Plague.*
207. Crosby, *The American Plague*, 103.
208. Skwarecki, *Outbreak!*
209. Skwarecki, *Outbreak!*, 126.
210. Irwin W. Sherman, *Twelve Diseases that Changed the World* (Washington, DC: ASM Press, 2007).
211. Sherman, *Twelve Diseases that Changed the World*, 153–154.
212. Sherman, *Twelve Diseases that Changed the World.*
213. Sherman, *Twelve Diseases that Changed the World.*
214. Sherman, *Twelve Diseases that Changed the World.*
215. Crosby, *The American Plague.*
216. Crosby, *The American Plague.*
217. Crosby, *The American Plague.*
218. Crosby, *The American Plague.*
219. Crosby, *The American Plague.*
220. Crosby, *The American Plague*, 229.
221. Crosby, *The American Plague.*
222. Crosby, *The American Plague*, 280.
223. Caryn Bern et al., "Trypanosoma cruzi and Chagas' Disease in the United States," *Clinical Microbiology Reviews* 24, no. 4 (2011): 655–681.
224. Melissa N. Garcia et al., "Historical Perspectives on the Epidemiology of Human Chagas Disease in Texas and Recommendations for Enhanced Understanding of Clinical Chagas Disease in the Southern United States," *PLoS Negl Trop Dis* 9, no. 11 (2015): e0003981.
225. Judy Stone, "Chagas: An Emerging Infectious Disease Threat in the U.S," *Forbes*, published October 1, 2015, https://www.forbes.com/sites/judystone/2015/10/01/chagas-an-emerging-infectious-disease-threat-in-u-s/#155348876530.
226. Stone, "Chagas: An Emerging Infectious Disease Threat in the U.S."
227. Bern et al., "Trypanosoma cruzi and Chagas' Disease in the United States."
228. Bern et al., "Trypanosoma cruzi and Chagas' Disease in the United States."
229. Bern et al., "Trypanosoma cruzi and Chagas' Disease in the United States."
230. Bern et al., "Trypanosoma cruzi and Chagas' Disease in the United States."
231. Bern et al., "Trypanosoma cruzi and Chagas' Disease in the United States."

232. Garcia et al., "Historical Perspectives on the Epidemiology of Human Chagas Disease in Texas"; Hanford et al., "Chagas Disease in Texas: Recognizing the Significance and Implications of Evidence in the Literature," *Social Science & Medicine* 65, no. 1 (2007): 60–79.

233. Stone, "Chagas: An Emerging Infectious Disease Threat in the U.S."

234. Stone, "Chagas: An Emerging Infectious Disease Threat in the U.S."

235. Hanford et al., "Chagas Disease in Texas: Recognizing the Significance and Implications of Evidence in the Literature."

236. Bern et al., "Trypanosoma cruzi and Chagas' Disease in the United States," 655–681.

237. Bern et al., "Trypanosoma cruzi and Chagas' Disease in the United States," 655–681.

238. Bern et al., "Trypanosoma cruzi and Chagas' Disease in the United States," 655–681.

239. Bern et al., "Trypanosoma cruzi and Chagas' Disease in the United States," 655–681.

240. Bern et al., "Trypanosoma cruzi and Chagas' Disease in the United States," 655–681.

241. Garcia et al., "Historical Perspectives on the Epidemiology of Human Chagas Disease in Texas," 659.

242. Ardzroony Packchanian, "Natural Infection of Triatoma gerstaker with Trypanosoma cruzi in Texas," *Public Health Reports (1896–1970)* (1939): 1547–1554.

243. Packchanian, "Natural Infection of Triatoma gerstakeri with Trypanosoma cruzi in Texas," 1547; Dorland J. Davis and T. D. Sullivan, "Complement-Fixation Tests for American Trypanosomiasis in Texas," *Public Health Rep* 61 (1946): 1083; Sherwin F. Wood, "New Localities for Trypannosoma cruzi Chagas in Southwestern United States," *American Journal of Epidemiology* 34, no. 1 (1941): 1–13; Ardzroony Packchanian, "Infectivity of the Texas Strain of Trypanosoma cruzi to Man," *The American Journal of Tropical Medicine and Hygiene* 1, no. 3 (1943): 309–314; Ardzroonv Packchanian, "The Problem of Chagas' Disease in Texas," *Texas State Journal of Medicine* 43, no. 3 (1947): 179–183; AF W., "Abstract of Discussion: Severe Reactions from Insect Stings," *Texas State Journal of Medicine* 46, no. 8 (1950): 640.

244. Norman C. Woody and Hannah B. Woody, "American Trypanosomiasis (Chagas' Disease); First Indigenous Case in the United States," *Journal of the American Medical Association* 159, no. 7 (1955): 676–677.

245. D. A. Greer, "Found: Two Cases of Chagas Disease," *Texas Health Bulletin* 9, no. 11 (1955).

246. Norman C. Woody, Noel DeDianous, and Hannah B. Woody, "American Trypano-somiasis. II. Current Serologie Studies in Chagas' Disease," *Journal of Pediatrics* 58, no. 5 (1961): 738–745.

247. J. E. Burkholder, T. C. Allison, and V. P. Kelly, "Trypanosoma cruzi (Chagas) (Protozoa: Kinetoplastida) in Invertebrate, Reservoir, and Human Hosts of the Lower Rio Grande Valley of Texas," *The Journal of Parasitology* (1980): 305–311.

248. Garcia et al., "Historical Perspectives on the Epidemiology of Human Chagas Disease in Texas."

249. Donald J. McNeil, "Rare Infection Threatens to Spread in Blood Supply," *The New York Times*, published November 18, 2003, https://www.nytimes.com/2003/11/18/science/rare-infection-threatens-to-spread-in-blood-supply.html.

250. Jennifer Manne-Goehler, Michael R. Reich, and Veronika J. Wirtz, "Access to Care for Chagas Disease in the United States: A Health Systems Analysis," *The American Journal of Tropical Medicine and Hygiene* 93, no. 1 (2015): 108–113.

251. Centers for Disease Control and Prevention, "Blood Donor Screening for Chagas Disease–United States, 2006–2007," *MMWR: Morbidity and Mortality Weekly Report* 56, no. 7 (2007): 141.

252. Garcia et al., "Historical Perspectives on the Epidemiology of Human Chagas Disease in Texas," 5.

253. Manne-Goehler, Reich, and Wirtz, "Access to Care for Chagas Disease in the United States: A Health Systems Analysis."

254. Garcia et al., "Historical Perspectives on the Epidemiology of Human Chagas Disease in Texas."

255. Garcia et al., "Historical Perspectives on the Epidemiology of Human Chagas Disease in Texas."

256. Garcia et al., "Historical Perspectives on the Epidemiology of Human Chagas Disease in Texas."

257. Susan P. Montgomery et al., "What Do We Know about Chagas Disease in the United States?" *The American Journal of Tropical Medicine and Hygiene* 95, no. 6 (2016): 1225–1227.

258. Garcia et al., "Historical Perspectives on the Epidemiology of Human Chagas Disease in Texas," 9.

259. Daisy Hernandez, "Northern Virginia: 'Ground Zero' for Kissing Bug Disease," *The Atlantic*, published July 24, 2014, https://www.theatlantic.com/health/archive/2014/07/northern-virginia-ground-zero-for-kissing-bug-disease/374383/.

260. Hernandez, "Northern Virginia: 'Ground Zero' for Kissing Bug Disease."

261. Carlos A. Morillo et al., "Randomized Trial of Benznidazole for Chronic Chagas' Cardiomyopathy," *New England Journal of Medicine* 373, no. 14 (2015): 1295–1306.

262. Morillo et al., "Randomized Trial of Benznidazole for Chronic Chagas' Cardiomyopathy."

263. Manne-Goehler, Reich, and Wirtz, "Access to Care for Chagas Disease in the United States: A Health Systems Analysis."

264. Manne-Goehler, Reich, and Wirtz, "Access to Care for Chagas Disease in the United States: A Health Systems Analysis"; I. Molina et al., "Toxic Profile of Benznidazole in Patients with Chronic Chagas Disease: Risk Factors and Comparison of the Product from Two Different Manufacturers," *Antimicrobial Agents and Chemotherapy* 59, no. 10 (2015): 6125–6131.

265. Kelly K. Stimpert and Susan P. Montgomery, "Physician Awareness of Chagas Disease, USA," *Emerging Infectious Diseases* 16, no. 5 (2010): 871.

266. Stimpert and Montgomery, "Physician Awareness of Chagas Disease, USA."

267. Matthew L. Romo, "Need for Pharmacist Awareness of Chagas Disease," *American Journal of Health-System Pharmacy* 71, no. 13 (2014): 1069–1070.

268. Eric Dumonteil et al., "Accelerating the Development of a Therapeutic Vaccine for Human Chagas Disease: Rationale and Prospects," *Expert Review of Vaccines* 11, no. 9 (2012): 1043–1055.

269. Soledad Ceccarelli et al., "DataTri, a Database of American Triatomine Species Occurrence," *Scientific Data* 5 (2018): 180071.

270. Ceccarelli et al., "DataTri, a Database of American Triatomine Species Occurrence."

271. Sarah A. Hamer, Rachel Curtis-Robles, and Gabriel L. Hamer, "Contributions of Citizen Scientists to Arthropod Vector Data in the Age of Digital Epidemiology," *Current Opinion in Insect Science* 28 (2018): 98–104.

272. Sarah Hamer, personal communication, December 5, 2018.

273. Hamer, personal communication, December 5, 2018.

274. Scott Friedman, "Identifying Kissing Bugs From Similar Bugs," *NBC 5 Dallas-Fort Worth*, last modified November 24, 2015, https://www.nbcdfw.com/investigations/Hidden-Threat-Identifying-Kissing-Bugs-From-Similar-Bugs-353226731.html.

275. Rodrigo Gurgel-Gonçalves et al., "Automated Identification of Insect Vectors of Chagas Disease in Brazil and Mexico: The Virtual Vector Lab," *PeerJ* 5 (2017): e3040.

276. Ali Khalighifar et al., "Deep Learning Algorithms Improve Automated Identification of Chagas Disease Vectors," *Journal of Medical Entomology* 56, no. 5 (2019): 1404–1410.

277. Caryn Bern et al., "Trypanosoma cruzi and Chagas' Disease in the United States," *Clinical Microbiology Reviews* 24, no. 4 (2011): 655–681.

278. S. A. Kjos et al., "Distribution and Characterization of Canine Chagas Disease in Texas," *Veterinary Parasitology* 152, nos. 3–4 (2008): 249–256.

279. Centers for Disease Control and Prevention, "CDC – Chagas Disease – General Information," published July 17, 2019, https://www.cdc.gov/parasites/chagas/gen_info/vectors/index.html.

280. Trevor D. Tenney et al., "Shelter Dogs as Sentinels for Trypanosoma cruzi Transmission across Texas," *Emerging Infectious Diseases* 20, no. 8 (2014): 1323–1326.

281. David Heflin, "Chagas Disease in Dogs," *TexVetPets*, published June 2014, https://www.texvetpets.org/article/chagas-disease-in-dogs/.

282. Heflin, "Chagas Disease in Dogs."

283. Texas State University, "Chagas Disease: A Silent Killer with a Cure," *Infection Control Today*, published April 18, 2019, https://www.infectioncontroltoday.com/infectious-diseases-conditions/chagas-disease-silent-killer-cure.

284. Maria Carmo Pereira Nunes et al., "Chagas Cardiomyopathy: An Update of Current Clinical Knowledge and Management: A Scientific Statement from the American Heart Association," *Circulation* 138, no. 12 (2018): e169–209.

285. Garcia et al., "Historical Perspectives on the Epidemiology of Human Chagas Disease in Texas."

286. Peter J. Hotez et al., "An Unfolding Tragedy of Chagas Disease in North America," *PLoS Neglected Tropical Diseases* 7, no. 10 (2013): e2300.

287. Karlijn Hofstraat and Wim H. van Brakel, "Social Stigma Towards Neglected Tropical Diseases: A Systematic Review," *International Health* 8, no. suppl_1 (2016): i53–i70.

288. Catharine Smith, "Why the U.S., One of the World's Richest Countries, Struggles with Diseases of Poverty," *Huffington Post*, last modified March 2, 2018, https://www.huffingtonpost.com/entry/america-diseases-of-poverty_us_5a69f610e4b0dc592a0fe66a.

289. Bruce Y. Lee et al., "Global Economic Burden of Chagas Disease: A Computational Simulation Model," *The Lancet Infectious Diseases* 13, no. 4 (2013): 342–348.

290. Dino Petrin et al., "Clinical and Microbiological Aspects of Trichomonas vaginalis," *Clinical Microbiology Reviews* 11, no. 2 (1998): 300–317.

291. Petrin et al., "Clinical and Microbiological Aspects of Trichomonas vaginalis."

292. Erik Munson et al., "Female Epidemiology of Transcription-Mediated Amplification-based Trichomonas vaginalis Detection in a Metropolitan Setting with a High Prevalence of Sexually Transmitted Infection," *Journal of Clinical Microbiology* 50, no. 12 (2012): 3927–3931.

293. Munson et al., "Female Epidemiology of Transcription-Mediated Amplification-based Trichomonas vaginalis Detection."

294. Centers for Disease Control and Prevention, "Diseases Characterized by Urethritis and Cervicitis – 2015 STD Treatment Guidelines," published June 4, 2015, https://www.cdc.gov/std/tg2015/urethritis-and-cervicitis.htm.

295. Catherine Lindsey Satterwhite et al., "Sexually Transmitted Infections among US Women and Men: Prevalence and Incidence Estimates, 2008," *Sexually Transmitted Diseases* 40, no. 3 (2013): 187–193.

296. Jenifer E. Allworth, Jane Alyce Ratner, and Jeffrey F. Peipert, "Trichomoniasis and Other Sexually Transmitted Infections: Results from the 2001–2004 NHANES Surveys," *Sexually Transmitted Diseases* 36, no. 12 (2009): 738.

297. H. Swygard et al., "Trichomoniasis: Clinical Manifestations, Diagnosis and Management," *Sexually Transmitted Infections* 80, no. 2 (2004): 91–95.

298. Pål Wølner-Hanssen et al., "Clinical Manifestations of Vaginal Trichomoniasis," *JAMA* 261, no. 4 (1989): 571–576.

299. Frank Sorvillo et al., "Trichomonas vaginalis, HIV, and African-Americans," *Emerging Infectious Diseases* 7, no. 6 (2001): 927.

300. Patricia Kissinger and Alys Adamski, "Trichomoniasis and HIV Interactions: A Review," *Sexually Transmitted Infections* 89, no. 6 (2013): 426–433.

301. Kissinger and Adamski, "Trichomoniasis and HIV Interactions: A Review."

302. Centers for Disease Control and Prevention, "Diseases Characterized by Urethritis and Cervicitis – 2015 STD Treatment Guidelines."

303. Mary Frances Cotch et al., "Trichomonas vaginalis Associated with Low Birth Weight and Preterm Delivery," *Sexually Transmitted Diseases* 24, no. 6 (1997): 353–360.

304. Cotch et al., "Trichomonas vaginalis Associated with Low Birth Weight and Preterm Delivery."

305. J. Christopher Carey et al., "Metronidazole to Prevent Preterm Delivery in Pregnant Women with Asymptomatic Bacterial Vaginosis," *New England Journal of Medicine* 342, no. 8 (2000): 534–540; Mark A. Klebanoff et al, "Failure of Metronidazole to Prevent Preterm Delivery among Pregnant Women with Asymptomatic Trichomonas vaginalis Infection," *New England Journal of Medicine* 345, no. 7 (2001): 487–493.

306. Joshua R. Mann et al., "Trichomoniasis in Pregnancy and Mental Retardation in Children," *Annals of Epidemiology* 19, no. 12 (2009): 891–899.

307. Alfred Donné, "Animacules observes dans les matieres purulentes et le produit des secretions des organes genitaux de l'homme et de la femme," *CR Acad Sci* 3 (1836): 385–386.

308. Stanford University, "History of Discovery," accessed August 2019, https://web.stanford.edu/group/parasites/ParaSites2002/trichomoniasis/History.html.

309. Robert Forgan, "History of the Treatment of Trichomoniasis," *British Journal of Venereal Diseases* 48, no. 6 (1972): 522.

310. HealthyPeople.gov, "Sexually Transmitted Diseases," last modified June 23, 2020, https://www.healthypeople.gov/2020/topics-objectives/topic/sexually-transmitted-diseases.

311. Madeline Sutton et al., "The Prevalence of Trichomonas vaginalis Infection among Reproductive-Age Women in the United States, 2001–2004," *Clinical Infectious Diseases* 45, no. 10 (2007): 1319–1326; Jenifer E. Allsworth, Jane Alyce Ratner, and Jeffrey F. Peipert, "Trichomoniasis and Other Sexually Transmitted Infections: Results from the 2001–2004 NHANES Surveys," *Sexually Transmitted Diseases* 36, no. 12 (2009): 738–744.

312. Satterwhite et al., "Sexually Transmitted Infections among US Women and Men."

313. Satterwhite et al., "Sexually Transmitted Infections among US Women and Men."

314. Sutton et al., "The Prevalence of Trichomonas vaginalis Infection among Reproductive-Age Women in the United States, 2001–2004."

315. Sutton et al., "The Prevalence of Trichomonas vaginalis Infection among Reproductive-Age Women in the United States, 2001–2004."

316. Sutton et al., "The Prevalence of Trichomonas vaginalis Infection among Reproductive-Age Women in the United States, 2001–2004."

317. William C. Miller et al., "The Prevalence of Trichomoniasis in Young Adults in the United States," *Sexually Transmitted Diseases* 32, no. 10 (2005): 593–598.

318. Miller et al., "The Prevalence of Trichomoniasis in Young Adults in the United States."

319. Miller et al., "The Prevalence of Trichomoniasis in Young Adults in the United States."

320. Miller et al., "The Prevalence of Trichomoniasis in Young Adults in the United States."

321. Miller et al., "The Prevalence of Trichomoniasis in Young Adults in the United States."

322. National Rural Health Association, "About Rural Health Care," accessed December 2019, https://www.ruralhealthweb.org/about-nrha/about-rural-health-care.

323. National Rural Health Association, "About Rural Health Care."

324. National Health Service, "Trichomoniasis – Prevention," last modified October 23, 2018, https://www.nhs.uk/conditions/trichomoniasis/prevention/.

325. Danice K. Eaton et al., "Youth Risk Behavior Surveillance–United States, 2011," *Morbidity and Mortality Weekly Report: Surveillance Summaries* 61, no. 4 (2012): 1–162.

326. Janet Rosenbaum et al., "Cash, Cars, and Condoms: Economic Factors in Disadvantaged Adolescent Women's Condom Use," *Journal of Adolescent Health* 51, no. 3 (2012): 233–241.

327. Kwame Owusu-Edusei et al., "The Estimated Direct Medical Cost of Selected Sexually Transmitted Infections in the United States, 2008," *Sexually Transmitted Diseases* 40, no. 3 (2013): 197–201.

328. Harrell W. Chesson, John M. Blandford, and Steven D. Pinkerton, "Estimates of the Annual Number and Cost of New HIV Infections among Women Attributable to Trichomoniasis in the United States," *Sexually Transmitted Diseases* 31, no. 9 (2004): 547–551.

329. Brooke E. Hoots et al., "A Trich-y Question: Should Trichomonas vaginalis Infection be Reportable?" *Sexually Transmitted Diseases* 40, no. 2 (2013): 113.

330. Gary E. Garber, "The Laboratory Diagnosis of Trichomonas vaginalis," *Canadian Journal of Infectious Diseases and Medical Microbiology* 16 (2005): 35–38.

331. Jill S. Huppert, "New Detection Methods for Trichomoniasis May Help Curb More Serious STIs," *Patient Care* 40, no. 5 (2006): 32–37.

332. Garber, "The Laboratory Diagnosis of Trichomonas vaginalis."

333. Eugene W. Liu et al., "Survey of Obstetrician-Gynecologists in the United States about Trichomoniasis, 2016," *Sexually Transmitted Diseases* 46, no. 1 (2019): 9.

334. Liu et al., "Survey of Obstetrician-Gynecologists in the United States about Trichomoniasis, 2016."

335. Fatu Forna and A. Metin Gülmezoglu, "Interventions for treating trichomoniasis in women," *Cochrane Database of Systematic Reviews* 2 (2003).

336. Centers for Disease Control and Prevention, "Diseases Characterized by Urethritis and Cervicitis – 2015 STD Treatment Guidelines."

337. Jane R. Schwebke and Renee A. Desmond, "A Randomized Controlled Trial of Partner Notification Methods for Prevention of Trichomoniasis in Women," *Sexually Transmitted Diseases* 37, no. 6 (2010): 392–396.

338. Sarah L. Cudmore et al., "Treatment of Infections Caused by Metronidazole-Resistant Trichomonas vaginalis," *Clinical Microbiology Reviews* 17, no. 4 (2004): 783–793.

339. Cudmore et al., "Treatment of Infections Caused by Metronidazole-Resistant Trichomonas vaginalis."

340. Petrin et al., "Clinical and Microbiological Aspects of Trichomonas vaginalis."

341. Tyjen Tsai and Paola Scommegna, "U.S. Has World's Highest Incarceration Rate," *Population Reference Bureau*, published August 10, 2012, https://www.prb.org/us-incarceration/.

342. Kelby Swanson, "WRITE TEAM: Rethinking Crime and Punishment," *The Times*, published September 25, 2019, https://www.mywebtimes.com/2019/09/24/write-team-rethinking-crime-and-punishment/ax0k4kt/.

343. Desiree Evans, "Doing Time in the South," *Facing South*, published March 5, 2009, https://www.facingsouth.org/2009/03/doing-time-in-the-south.html.

344. Ashley Nellis, "The Color of Justice: Racial and Ethnic Disparity in State Prisons," *The Sentencing Project*, published June 14, 2016, https://www.sentencingproject.org/publications/color-of-justice-racial-and-ethnic-disparity-in-state-prisons/.

345. Erwin James, "Most Offenders Have Low Skills and Prison Is the Place to Put That Right," *The Guardian*, published February 3, 2012, https://www.theguardian.com/society/joepublic/2010/feb/03/prison-education-training-low-skills.

346. Swanson, "WRITE TEAM: Rethinking Crime and Punishment."

347. Swanson, "WRITE TEAM: Rethinking Crime and Punishment."

348. Matthew Hogben and Janet S. St. Lawrence, "HIV/STD Risk Reduction Interventions in Prison Settings," *Journal of Women's Health & Gender-Based Medicine* 9, no. 6 (2000): 587–592; Robert P. Pack et al., "High Prevalence of Asymptomatic STDs in Incarcerated Minority Male Youth: A Case for Screening," *Sexually Transmitted Diseases* 27, no. 3 (2000): 175–177.

349. Catherine Ingram Fogel and Michael Belyea, "The Lives of Incarcerated Women: Violence, Substance Abuse, and at Risk for HIV," *Journal of the Association of Nurses in AIDS Care* 10, no. 6 (1999): 66–74.

350. Kimberly A. Workowski and Stuart M. Berman, "Sexually Transmitted Diseases Treatment Guidelines, 2015," *MMWR: Morbidity and Mortality Weekly Report: Recommendations and Reports* (2010), https://www.cdc.gov/mmwr/preview/mmwrhtml/rr5912a1.htm.

351. Julie R. Kraut-Becher et al., "Cost-Effectiveness of Universal Screening for Chlamydia and Gonorrhea in US Jails," *Journal of Urban Health* 81, no. 3 (2004): 453–471.

352. Centers for Disease Control and Prevention, "Assessment of Sexually Transmitted Diseases Services in City and County Jails–United States, 1997," *MMWR: Morbidity and Mortality Weekly Report* 47, no. 21 (1998): 429.

353. Karl Brown, "Managing Sexually Transmitted Diseases in Jails," *TheBodyPro*, published September 1, 2003, https://www.thebodypro.com/article/managing-sexually-transmitted-diseases-jails.

354. Brown, "Managing Sexually Transmitted Diseases in Jails."

355. Alexandra H. Freeman et al., "Prevalence and Correlates of Trichomonas vaginalis among Incarcerated Persons Assessed Using a Highly Sensitive Molecular Assay," *Sexually Transmitted Diseases* 37, no. 3 (2010): 165–168.

356. Denise M. Willers et al., "Prevalence and Predictors of Sexually Transmitted Infection among Newly Incarcerated Females," *Sexually Transmitted Diseases* 35, no. 1 (2008): 68–72.

357. Willers et al., "Prevalence and Predictors of Sexually Transmitted Infection among Newly Incarcerated Females."

358. Jeffrey D. Klausner et al., "Investigation of a Suspected Outbreak of Vaginal Trichomoniasis among Female Inmates," *Sexually Transmitted Diseases* 26, no. 6 (1999): 335–338.

359. Ank E. Nijhawan et al., "The Association between Trichomonas Infection and Incarceration in HIV-seropositive and At-risk HIV-seronegative Women," *Sexually Transmitted Diseases* 38, no. 12 (2011): 1094.

360. Kraut-Becher et al., "Cost-Effectiveness of Universal Screening for Chlamydia and Gonorrhea in US Jails."

Chapter 2

Poverty in America

Poverty, Health, and Neglected Tropical Diseases

In his 2001 inaugural address, President George W. Bush stated, "Americans in need are not strangers, they are citizens, not problems, but priorities, and all of us are diminished when any are helpless."[1] He challenged Americans to not just acknowledge the deep poverty that existed in the United States, but to take action to address it and exclaimed that government has "great responsibilities" for public health, public safety, civil rights, and education. He was not the first president to bring attention to poverty in America and he was not the last. Despite such statements, however, poverty remains a dark reality of millions of Americans.

An understanding of poverty in the United States—where it exists, who is most affected, why it exists, and the extent of poverty in one of the richest countries in the world—is vital because it is exactly this poverty that allows NTDs to exist. This is true throughout the globe and it is certainly the central factor here in the United States. Dr. Peter Hotez, the scientist who coined the term "Neglected Tropical Diseases," often feels like the term is misleading. In a 2018 interview with us he stated, "poverty is the overriding determinant of neglected tropical diseases, so I kind of mis-termed [it] . . . We call them tropical diseases, but they are overwhelmingly diseases of poverty."[2] That is to say that even though the diseases examined in this book are called "NTDs" they exist and are perpetuated by extreme poverty throughout the world. In an interview with Joe Rogan, Dr. Hotez further emphasized the point, stating, "I don't care where you show me poverty. Whether it's in Texas or Alabama or Nigeria or Bangladesh; I will show you these poverty-related diseases."[3]

For decades, NTDs have been largely overlooked domestically because of the belief that the conditions necessary for their existence are not present in the United States. When people think of raw sewage pooled outside doorways they think of villages in Asia, not rural communities in Alabama;

when they think of houses with no windows or cracks in the walls they think of mountain communities in Peru, not inner-city Houston; and when people think of families living on less than $2/day, they likely think of TV commercials asking them to give money to help children in Africa, not the roughly 1 million Americans for whom $2/day is their reality. We operate under the assumption that NTDs do not exist in the United States because we believe our country does not have conditions conducive to them. This assumption is false.

In this chapter, we examine poverty in America: its characteristics, distribution, and impact on the health of poor Americans. We also examine conditions that run parallel and support poverty such as income inequality and lack of upward mobility. We examine poverty broadly, so as to encompass all races, ethnicities, ages, and genders. We examine how poverty exists in the U.S.-born population as well as immigrant populations in order to paint a full picture of the conditions and social structures that give rise to American poverty and, in turn, the presence of NTDs in the United States.

POVERTY IN AMERICA

In his Pulitzer Prize winning book, *Evicted: Poverty and Profit in the American City*, Matthew Desmond states, "This degree of inequality, this withdrawal of opportunity, this cold denial of basic needs, this endorsement of pointless suffering—by no American value is this situation justified. No moral code or ethical principle, no piece of scripture or holy teaching, can be summoned to defend what we have allowed our country to become."[4] In these few short sentences, Desmond gives voice to the unacceptable degree of poverty that exists in one of the richest countries in the world. Today, close to 40 million Americans live in poverty, with 18.5 million living in what is classified as "deep poverty."[5] Deep poverty refers to those individuals living below 50 percent of the poverty threshold or, put differently, a family of four living on $12,169.50 per year. And while there are millions of Americans that officially live in deep poverty, there are millions more that hover just above the threshold.[6] As David K. Shipler aptly states, "'Poverty' is an unsatisfying term, for poverty is not a category that can be delineated merely by the government's dollar limit on annual income. In real life, it is an unmarked area along a continuum, a broader region of hardship than the society usually recognizes."[7]

Compounding the problem, the highest number of Americans living in deep poverty are children. Poverty during childhood has long-lasting consequences ranging from harm to brain development to poor health and chronic illness to a lower likelihood of graduating high school.[8] In many ways, deep poverty is passed on and becomes generational; individuals who lived in deep poverty as children are more likely to live in deep poverty as adults.[9]

In their book, *$2.00 a Day: Living on Almost Nothing in America*, Edin and Shaefer explain that roughly one out of every twenty-five families with children in America live on $2/day or less and that "the phenomenon of $2-a-day poverty among households with children had been on the rise since the nation's landmark welfare reform legislation was passed in 1996—and at a distressingly fast pace. As of 2011, the number of families in $2-a-day poverty had more than doubled in just a decade and a half."[10] The 1996 Personal Responsibility and Work Opportunity Reconciliation Act, also known as the Welfare Reform Act, signed into law by President Clinton, killed the cash welfare system and pushed over a million American families into a level of poverty unthinkable to most Americans. "Perhaps the most surprising fact, though, is how quickly the issue faded from view. A federal program in existence for sixty years, a system that had survived would-be reformers for decades—including a full-frontal attack by Ronald Reagan—was terminated by Congress and the stroke of the president's pen in the summer of 1996 without much fuss at all. Welfare, as the country knew it, was dead, and very few people seemed to care."[11]

For many it is difficult to imagine what living on less than $2/day would look like. Two dollars is less than the cost of a coffee from Starbucks. Two dollars is less than most Americans spend every day before 9 a.m. This level of poverty does exist in America, however, and the 1996 Welfare Reform all but assured its continued existence. Under the new system of welfare, poor Americans are entitled to food stamps, but most no longer receive welfare checks, meaning they are often required to sell part of their food stamps (an activity that is illegal) to get cash to buy school supplies, shoes, or clothes for their children.[12] The reality is that there are Americans living on $2/day. A lot of them. Therefore, the important question is: how did we get here?

How Poverty is Measured?

Official measures of poverty are sometimes criticized for not providing an accurate assessment of the state of poverty in the country because they only take into account pre-taxed, pre-benefit income.[13] This means that "earnings, interest, dividends, Social Security, and cash assistance" are counted as income sources, but "the federal Earned Income Tax Credit . . . also in-kind government benefits . . . such as food stamps, Medicaid, and housing and childcare assistance" are not counted.[14] The result is both inaccurate poverty statistics and an inability to effectively measure how successful in-kind programs are.

The poverty line, which plays an important role in determining which individuals can receive benefits, is set by the Census Bureau. The poverty thresholds vary by family size and composition.[15] Individuals with a "household income above 100% of their poverty threshold" are considered to be above the poverty line.[16] If a family or individual falls below 50 percent of their poverty threshold then they are considered to be in deep poverty.[17] Again, the poverty line is a pre-tax, pre-benefit assessment and it does not adjust for cost of living (i.e., the poverty line is the same in New York City as it is in College Station, Texas).

Criticisms of poverty measurements and income inequality center on these two elements. In an op-ed to the Wall Street Journal, Gramm and Early argued that public transfer payments should be included in income if we want an accurate measure of income inequality.[18] And despite other exaggerations and inaccurate assumptions in the op-ed, this core argument is logical. If income inequality is measured using the pre-taxed income of the wealthy as the high-end measurement and the pre-benefit income of the poor as the low-end measurement, the inequality gap is likely to be higher. It is important to have an accurate measure of the number of people living in poverty and the extent of income inequality.

In addition to criticism of official poverty statistics, there is a growing number of economists that believe we should measure consumption rather than income to determine poverty levels. These economists believe that measuring consumption provides a more accurate measure of poverty than does measuring income.[19] Instead, they argue, consumption is more stable than income and, therefore, provides a more accurate perception of the number of individuals living in poverty. By this measure, economists who look at poverty as a measure of consumption argue that poverty has not increased in recent years, but rather has decreased by almost 9 percent since 1980.[20] Importantly, income-based poverty gaps have increased over the past several decades while consumption-based poverty gaps have decreased.[21] Using either income or consumption poverty measurements will give you very different poverty outcomes.

When discussing the consumption poverty measure, Meyers and Sullivan (2013) state, "relying on the official poverty rate, many have concluded that we have lost the 'War on Poverty,' but improved measures of poverty show that we have actually made tremendous progress."[22] The main point of consumption poverty advocates argument is that the quality of life among people living in poverty is better than it was in previous decades because they are able to purchase more today than poor people could in the past. For example, due to stores like Walmart, items are now cheaper and, thus, more readily available to the poor. Much of this consumption ability, however, relies on in-kind government programs like food stamps. If such programs were eliminated, the United States would see a rise in consumption poverty because people would have to spend more of their small income to buy food and could not buy as many other goods.[23]

Similar to the official poverty measure or other forms of income-based poverty measures, measuring consumption poverty has its downsides. Measuring consumption rather than income can lead to inaccuracies if people are participating in consumption by borrowing money, thus incurring debt. Some consumption poverty economists also admit that obtaining an accurate measure of consumption is one of the greatest challenges with this measurement.[24]

History of Poverty and Poverty Relief in America

In his 2008 book titled, *A People's History of Poverty in America*, Stephen Pimpare writes, "Poverty and inequality have been a consistent presence in this country . . . yet we have been unwilling to acknowledge this, and instead of relieving poverty we blame poor Americans for their condition, rationalizing our neglect with disdain for their supposed lack of aspiration, their poor work ethic, their despair."[25] This quote serves to define both the history of poverty in the United States and Americans' relationship to it. As far back as the mid-1700s there were areas of concentrated poverty and by the early 1800s, cities saw the establishment of the country's first ghettos.[26] Poverty has been a mainstay of American society since the founding of the country and, more importantly, our national ideas toward poverty and anti-poverty policy has also remained remarkably unchanged. Specifically, national rhetoric throughout history has continued to view the poor as lazy and morally flawed.[27]

The historical presence of poverty does not, however, imply that there was ever an absence of relief programs. Before there were government aid programs, the poor in large cities formed their own support structures. Pimpare (2008) explains that "in big cities like New York, ethnic mutual aid societies were established early by the Scots (1756), Irish (1784), English (1786), Germans (1787), Welsh (1803), and French (1809)."[28] Ethnic communities and, later, occupations, were organizing mechanisms to provide support for the poorest in society. Religious groups or individual missionaries also became involved in poverty relief in the early 1800s with the establishment of homeless shelters, soup kitchens, and job training.[29] Even today, churches serve as a major mechanism of poor relief in states with inadequately funded programs. Additionally, throughout the 1800s, children living in extreme poverty worked as indentured servants for families that were better-off.[30] This relationship provided the children with shelter and a meager level of food security. Indeed, there were numerous examples of poverty relief prior to New Deal policies, and Pimpare (2008) emphasizes this point by stating, "the welfare state was not an innovation of the national government during the Great Depression but a creation of the first large American cities, much of it crafted by poor themselves."[31] Thus, the ingenuity and creativity of the poor has also been a consistent element of American history also.

As the nation moved into the early 1900s and experienced the economic impacts of the Second Industrial Revolution, poverty was often overlooked among the unprecedented wealth of the era.[32] As Marx (2011) describes, "The overall prosperity of the United States in the 1920s overshadowed the chronic poverty of certain vulnerable populations. These were the same populations that had always been at risk in American history: children, older Americans, minorities, female-headed families, people with disabilities, and workers with unstable or low-paying wages."[33] Put differently, Americans were now saving more than they ever had before, they were buying homes at high rates, farming was becoming increasingly productive due to advances in electricity, and these developments did not reduce poverty, they simply made it easier to overlook the poor. The prosperity of the 1920s also helped to reinforce the beliefs many Americans held that the poor only had themselves to blame.

Then, in October 1929, the stock market crashed, plunging the country into the Great Depression. When the Great Depression hit, unemployment rates jumped from 3.2 to 24.9 percent and some cities saw unemployment rates as high as 80 percent.[34] For several years, no coherent action was taken to address the problem and many upper-class Americans worried that there would be a revolution.[35] With skyrocketing rates of unemployment, so too came changes to Americans views on poverty and "by the time Franklin Roosevelt was elected in 1932, the traditional ideologies and institutions of the United States were in a state of upheaval. Americans who had grown up promoting the ideology of the 'deserving and undeserving poor' and the stigma of poor relief were now standing in line for relief."[36] This sharp increase in unemployment and Americans changing views on poverty led the federal government to eventually take responsibility for poor relief.[37]

The first relief legislation to emerge was the Federal Emergency Relief Administration (FERA) in 1933.[38] FERA provided federal relief money to states, who then distributed it to the poor.[39] One year later, in 1934, the Civil Works Administration was created and employed 4 million people per week, helping many Americans survive a harsh winter.[40] Other programs continued to be created including the Public Works Administration, the Civilian Conservation Corps, and a small food stamp program for federal workers.[41] Shortly after that, a larger-scale welfare program began to be formed. As Somers and Block (2005) describe, "the history of Federal welfare assistance in the United States begins with the 1935 Social Security Act's Aid to Dependent Children, later renamed Aid to Families with Dependent Children."[42]

Today, the Social Security Act is well-known and roughly 63 million Americans rely on their Social Security benefits to sustain them in their retirement.[43] At the time the Act was passed, however, it had a number of detractors. President Roosevelt had packaged unemployment insurance with the other elements of Social Security because unemployment insurance was too unpopular to pass on its own.[44] This packaging led to opposition in the business community, who believed the unemployed were lazy. The Act was also opposed for other reasons. Most notable of these was a fear of socialism.[45] Many politicians believed that providing large-scale poverty relief programs would eventually lead to a socialist society. There were also serious concerns about the cost of the programs and the spending deficit that was occurring as a result.[46] Lastly, some critics of the New Deal programs accused President Roosevelt of essentially buying votes by creating programs that funded the poor and unemployed.[47]

Opposition to President Roosevelt's New Deal policies extended beyond the business community and members of Congress, however. New Deal legislation suffered numerous defeats in the Supreme Court, which declared programs like the Agricultural Adjustment Act unconstitutional.[48] Shortly after his reelection in 1936, President Roosevelt proposed a bill that would increase membership on the Supreme Court as an underhanded way of overcoming the Court's opposition to many of his New Deal policies.[49] This proposal started a controversy that lasted for almost six months as the three branches of government battled for power and, in the end, created hostility toward Roosevelt among the public.[50] In the midst of all this, however, the Court began reversing their rulings on New Deal policies and siding frequently with Roosevelt on their constitutionality.[51] This reversal of beliefs on New Deal policies greatly lessened the blow when Roosevelt's proposal to expand Supreme Court membership was defeated.

The New Deal brought with it many long-lasting changes for the poor in America. Importantly, "with the New Deal, poor relief became a right of American citizens meeting certain eligibility standards, including of course, financial need."[52] And the New Deal had many successes: it increased quality of life, decreased infant mortality, and was hugely important for the Southern states, who still receive more money in support than they pay in taxes.[53] It is important to keep in mind, however, that the New Deal did not pull the country out of the Great Depression. Despite the job creation and poverty relief, it was not until World War II that the United States began to see economic recovery.

The return of economic prosperity to the United States brought with it the return of traditional beliefs about the poor. As Somers and Block discuss in their 2005 article, the return of market fundamentalism came as a surprise to many, who believed it had died off during the Great Depression. Some of the push back against anti-poverty programs was a result of many Americans' opposition to programs that benefited African Americans, but some of it was a result of changing national ideas. Specifically, "market fundamentalist views once seen as too extreme rapidly achieved mainstream status and moved the spectrum of political discourse to the right. Ideational regime change led to welfare legislation dramatically restricting the access of the poor to assistance."[54] Just as Americans' opinions regarding poverty relief were changing, however, President Lyndon B. Johnson launched his War on Poverty and the Great Society.

The War on Poverty was announced in President Johnson's State of the Union Address in 1964. At this time, approximately 20 percent of Americans lived below the poverty line and Johnson viewed this as a societal failure, not a personal moral failure of the low-income individual.[55] To emphasize this point he stated, "The cause may lie deeper in our failure to give our fellow citizens a fair chance to develop their own capacities, in a lack of education and training, in a lack of medical care and housing, in a lack of decent communities in which to live and bring up their children."[56]

Several months later in a speech at the University of Michigan, Johnson went further by laying out his agenda for the Great Society. The program sought to address poverty broadly, acknowledging many, interconnected factors that push Americans below the poverty line. The Great Society focused on educational reform—creating Head Start, providing funding for special education services, libraries, textbooks, and preschools.[57] It addressed people's living environment through the passage of the Water Quality Act of 1965, the Motor Vehicle Air Pollution Control Act of 1965, the Consumer Product Safety Commission, and the Child Safety Act.[58] The Great Society addressed issues of health with the establishment of the Medicare and Medicaid programs and it tackled issues of immigration with the passage of the Immigration and Naturalization Act of 1965.[59] These elements of the program were in addition to job training programs, loan programs for farmers, and other types of economic support programs. Arguably, the most important element of the Great Society was the Johnson Administration's focus on *all* Americans. In his 1964 State of the Union Address, President Johnson said, "Let me make one principle of this administration abundantly clear: All of these increased opportunities—in employment, in education, in housing, and in every field—must be open to Americans of every color . . . For this is not merely an economic issue, or a social, political, or international issue. It is a moral issue."[60]

President Johnson's War on Poverty was aided, if not inspired, by two influential books of the time period: John Kenneth Galbraith's 1958 book

The Affluent Society, and Michael Harrington's 1962 book *The Other America*.[61] Both books shocked and alarmed many affluent Americans, who were unaware that deep poverty still existed in America—a sentiment that is strikingly similar to today. Part of the reason poor Americans were easily overlooked in the 1950s and 1960s, was that the majority of them lived in rural areas and even more were people of color.[62] Again, not unlike today. Despite greater awareness of poverty in the United States, however, Johnson still received intense criticism for his War on Poverty.[63] The centerpiece of his Great Society program, the Economic Opportunity Act and the Office of Economic Opportunity that came along with it, were disbanded shortly after President Nixon took office.[64]

Following the end of Johnson's time as president and the dismantling of many of his Great Society programs, conventional wisdom emerged that deemed the War on Poverty a failure.[65] This perception of the War on Poverty and the Great Society programs that accompanied it is misguided, however. Recent research to reevaluate its impact show that the programs led to a 30 percent decrease in poverty.[66] Indeed, the War on Poverty did not only decrease poverty in America, but it raised the profile of the issue among average Americans, another one of Johnson's goals. "Johnson is said to have remarked to a reporter, 'I don't know if I'll pass a single law or get a single dollar appropriated, but before I'm through, no community in America will be able to ignore poverty in its midst.'"[67] Due in large part to the work of President Johnson, fewer of the people living in extreme poverty today are elderly or families with children.[68] Also notable is that, since the Great Society and the establishment of federal safety nets regardless of race (in conjunction with civil rights advancements of the last seventy years), poverty rates among African Americans has declined approximately 50 percent.[69] The great improvements made by Johnson's War on Poverty did not eliminate the problem, however. The problem of poverty in America may have lessened, but we still have a long way to go.

The Working Poor

Today, extreme poverty is concentrated in pockets of America and places like Eastern Kentucky, the poster child of Johnson's anti-poverty agenda, still struggles to escape its grips. The Personal Responsibility and Work Opportunity Act of 1996, hailed as a great piece of legislation that would fix the "broken" welfare system, reduced the number of families in Kentucky receiving welfare by 52 percent, but it did not reduce the number of families living in poverty.[70] It did not change the situation, it just removed the safety net. Kentucky, and other majority rural areas of the United States, are disproportionately impacted by high numbers of working poor.[71] In fact, the

United States is unique among wealthy countries due to the relatively high percentage of its workforce living in poverty. As Thiede et al. (2018) points out, "a recent United States (USA) government report by the Bureau of Labor Statistics estimates that 10.4 million individuals were among the working poor in 2011."[72] Importantly, poverty rates among rural workers are roughly 17 percent higher than poverty rates among urban workers.[73] As Smeeding (2006) observed in his comparative study of poverty among wealthy countries, "what seems most distinctive about the American poor, especially poor American single parents, is that they work more hours than do the resident parents in other nations while also receiving less in transfer benefits than in other nations."[74] In other words, the American working poor are working more hours, receiving lower pay, and receiving less governmental support than the working poor of other wealthy nations.

By almost all measures of poverty, the United States stands in contrast to other wealthy nations and measures of the working poor are no exception. "The United States stands out with a working poor rate of 14.5 percent (more than 2.7 s.d. above the mean), and no other country even exceeds 9.7."[75] Compared to other wealthy nations, the United States has more children living in poverty, spends less of its GDP on anti-poverty programs, and offers lower wages.[76] These factors combine to paint a stark picture. As Anglin (2002) explains, "We have yet to come to terms with popular forms of resistance and leadership, particularly in rural America. In the absence of formally organized struggles, and sometimes in their midst, we all too readily assume inertia and resignation as the response to oppressive working conditions and extreme poverty."[77]

Oppressive working conditions are nowhere more obvious than among foreign-born individuals living in the United States. Overall the number of immigrants in the United States has increased from a historic low of 4.7 percent in 1970 to almost 14 percent today.[78] This is notable because immigrants are more likely to live in poverty—particularly recently arrived immigrants—and noncitizens are more likely to work low-wage jobs.[79] Many scholars have found, however, that higher rates of poverty among immigrant populations has a nonsignificant impact on overall poverty rates in America.[80] And while any immigrant is more likely to live in poverty than U.S.-born individuals, noncitizen immigrants are also more likely than naturalized citizens to live in poverty.[81] As an additional challenge, immigrants living in poverty are increasingly moving to the suburbs.[82] As Suro et al. (2011) explains, "Traditionally, anti-poverty programs have focused on central cities, and the suburban infrastructure including local governments, nonprofits and private funders have not caught up with the new realities."[83] The increasing numbers of immigrant poor in the suburbs have an even more greatly diminished access to anti-poverty programs.

Poverty among Immigrant Populations in the United States

Undocumented immigrants face greater levels of poverty, more dangerous work environments, longer hours, and less power to negotiate their conditions, than any other members of the American workforce. As Gomberg-Muñoz (2018) argues, "U.S. laws have long cultivated sources of especially disempowered labor in these industries: first and most significantly through the system of chattel slavery, then through both domestic and international policies that have ensured a steady stream of legally disempowered workers, including African American workers in the Jim Crow south, migrant 'guest' workers, undocumented workers, incarcerated and detained workers, and those who are compelled to work in order to maintain eligibility for parole or social assistance programs."[84] In the case of undocumented workers specifically, subcontractors are used to distance large corporations from the legal violation of their hiring. In this case, "the practice of labor subcontracting in combination with pervasive use of false work eligibility documents . . . can literally erase workers from employer rolls, making their labor invisible to the state and compromising their ability to access resources and protection, as well as legal support in instances of injury and abuse."[85] This practice has many benefits for the businesses that employ undocumented workers. Shipler (2004) explains, "American government and business gain financially from your inability to legalize your presence in the country."[86] These gains come from the ability to pay lower wages and avoid insurance costs, among other financial benefits. All of these factors combined create often insurmountable obstacles for immigrants living in poverty.

"Poverty is a fact of life for a disproportionate share of first- and second-generation Mexicans residing in the United States."[87] This poverty, however, is not equally distributed. Immigrants in the South and Southwest suffer higher levels of poverty than do those in other areas of the United States largely due to the restructuring of low-wage opportunities.[88] Change in structural opportunities for immigrants has a significant impact on their ability to move out of poverty.[89] Even with structural changes taking place in areas outside the South and Southwest, 34.8 percent of Mexican immigrant families live in poverty.[90] In some border communities, like those located in Texas, general economic depression and a broad lack of opportunities help preserve the cycle of poverty by greatly limiting opportunities for the next generation.[91]

Recent Political Views on Poverty

Despite the mostly consistent national view of the poor as undeserving, elected officials of both parties have often sought to bring attention to the issues. President George W. Bush advocated for all children to have health insurance, created Medicare Part D to expand subsidizes for prescription drugs, and argued for greater federal funding for faith-based and community groups to provide aid in their local communities.[92] Even the ineffective, and arguably detrimental, No Child Left Behind policy, was created in a good faith effort to provide all children with an adequate education that could help lift them out of poverty. President Barack Obama, who succeeded President Bush in 2009, advocated continuously for raising the minimum wage as a way to fight income inequality.[93] President Obama also approached poverty with a holistic view. Steele (2009) describes this view by stating, "Obama noted, '. . . if poverty is a disease that infects an entire community in the form of unemployment and violence, failing schools and broken homes, then we can't just treat those symptoms in isolation'."[94] For President Obama, addressing poverty in America required an approach similar to President Johnson's ideals under the War on Poverty and the Great Society.

The talk of our political leaders has only managed to go so far, however. "As social-welfare analyst David Wagner has observed, it may be that our self-congratulatory rhetoric . . . obscures the less noble reality: Americans do less for the least among us than do other Western industrialized nations" and as Jimmy Carter noted, "the measure of a society is found in how they treat the weakest and most helpless citizens."[95] While the aim of President Carter's quote was decidedly outwards rather than requesting Americans to look introspectively, the sentiment remains true. In the next section, we examine the modern-day distribution of poverty in the United States to provide a fuller picture of regions and populations most impacted.

Distribution of Poverty

It would be inaccurate to say that only certain areas or certain types of Americans live in extreme poverty. All regions of the United States and all racial and ethnic groups experience poverty, but those living in the South and Appalachia experience it more deeply than many other parts of the country. In this section, we will discuss poverty in the United States by the numbers. We will delve into the racial, gender, and age dynamics of poverty to provide a detailed picture of what poverty in the United States looks like.

Although sometimes overlooked in the discussion of poverty and welfare, whites make up the largest overall number of individuals in the welfare system. In many states, the majority of individuals on the welfare rolls are white. Like poverty rates among other racial groups, however, the level of poverty among the white population varies greatly by state. The states with the highest number of white Americans living in poverty are West Virginia, Kentucky, and Arkansas with 16 percent, 14 percent, and 11 percent poverty rates, respectively.[96] Although these states lead the pack in white poverty,

Louisiana, Mississippi, Alabama, Tennessee, Idaho, New Mexico, and Oklahoma come in a close tie for fourth with poverty rates of 10 percent among the white population.[97] On the other side of the spectrum, Alaska and New Jersey lead the way with the lowest poverty rates among whites at just 4 percent and Washington, DC boasts the lowest poverty rate for whites at 3 percent.[98]

It is easy to see from the numbers that many of the states with the highest rates of poverty among the white population are located in the South. When looking at poverty rates among the African American population, the South also contains some of the highest rates of poverty, though there are large discrepancies between the poverty rates of whites in America and the poverty rates of African Americans. The states with the highest rates of poverty among African Americans include Idaho, Louisiana, Mississippi, Iowa, and West Virginia with poverty rates of 54 percent, 31 percent, 29 percent, 29 percent, and 28 percent, respectively.[99] Of those states that also had high rates of poverty among the white population—West Virginia, Louisiana, and Mississippi—the rate of poverty among African Americans is almost double the poverty rate among whites. Even the states with the lowest poverty rates for African Americans, Colorado (10%), Maryland (11%), and Connecticut (12%), the poverty rates are significantly higher than the lowest poverty rates among whites.[100]

What is most interesting, though not surprising, about the poverty rates of African Americans in the United States is that they are significantly and positively related to 1,860 slave populations.[101] States with higher concentrations of slaves in 1,860 have higher rates of African Americans living in poverty today. Additionally, "On average, the Southern black poverty rate was nearly 170 percent greater than the corresponding non-Hispanic white poverty rate,"[102] meaning that in the South, poverty rates between African Americans and whites are especially unequal.

Latinos also experience exceedingly high poverty rates as compared to America's white population. Alabama, Pennsylvania, Massachusetts, and Rhode Island have the highest rates of poverty among Latinos at 28 percent, 24 percent, 22 percent, and 22 percent, respectively.[103] These rates are lower than the highest rates of poverty found among African Americans, but most interestingly, unlike poverty of whites and African Americans, high rates of poverty among Latinos is mostly concentrated in the Northeastern United States. The states with the lowest rates of poverty among Latinos are Virginia, Maryland, and Iowa with rates of 9 percent, 9 percent, and 11 percent respectively.[104]

While poverty rates among African Americans and Latinos are notably higher than those of white Americans, poverty rates among Native American populations stand out as the highest rates of poverty among any racial/ethnic group. West Virginia is the state with the highest rate of poverty among Native Americans with 48 percent.[105] South Dakota and Mississippi follow closely behind, however, with poverty rates among Native Americans at 44 percent and 33 percent, respectively.[106] Even in states with the lowest levels of poverty among Native Americans, these rates rise above most of the highest poverty rates for whites.[107] The states with the lowest rates of poverty among Native Americans are Colorado, Kansas, Florida, and Texas with poverty rates of 9 percent, 11 percent, 13 percent, and 14 percent, respectively.[108]

The racial and ethnic differences in poverty rates can help to explain why people of color are at greater risk for NTD infection. As we have repeated throughout the book, poverty allows NTDs to survive, and in some cases to thrive. Given that levels of poverty are higher among communities of color, and specifically African Americans in the Southern states, it can explain why NTD infection rates estimates are much higher among people of color.

In addition to poverty disparities along racial and ethnic lines, there are also gender differences. Specifically, women are 38 percent more likely to live in poverty than men.[109] As of 2016, approximately 10 percent of women in the United States were living in poverty and 45 percent of these women were classified as living in extreme poverty.[110] The highest percentage of women living in poverty are Native American women at 22.8 percent, but this number is closely followed by the 21.4 percent of African American women living in poverty.[111] According to a study by the Henry J Kaiser (KFF) Family Foundation, West Virginia, Louisiana, Mississippi, and New Mexico have the highest rates of poverty among women with 18 percent, 18 percent, 17 percent, and 17 percent respectively, whereas New Mexico and West Virginia have the highest rates of poverty among men at 15 percent male poverty rates in both states.[112]

With higher rates of poverty among women, it follows that there are also high rates of poverty among children, as single mothers are more likely than any other group to live in poverty. As of 2016, there were 13.2 million children in the United States living in poverty.[113] Of these, 5.9 million children live in extreme poverty.[114] That amounts to one in twelve American children living in extreme poverty. Of even greater concern is that "Our youngest children have the highest poverty rates. In 2017, nearly 1 in 5 infants, toddlers, and preschoolers between the ages of 0 and 5 were poor at the time of greatest brain development."[115] Thus, even if child are no longer living in poverty after the age of five, the impacts will affect them for the remainder of their lives.

Poverty rates among African American children are just under 31 percent and for Latino children it is 26.6 percent.[116] That means that more than a fourth of all African American and Latino children in the United States are living in poverty. Numbers for Native American children (25.4%) and foreign-born children (25.6%) are similar.[117] For children living in female-headed households, these numbers increase even more. For example, poverty rates for children in African American female-headed households is 38.8 percent and for those in Latina female-headed households it is 40.8 percent.[118] If a child lives in a Native American female-headed household they have the greatest likelihood of living in poverty with 42.6 percent of all children in such households living under the poverty line.[119] Like other measures of poverty, white households have the lowest rates, however, even poverty rates in white-female headed households is over 30 percent.[120]

Examining the other end of the age spectrum, it can be seen that the elderly are also more likely than young or middle-aged adults to live in poverty with 7 million people over the age of sixty-five living under the poverty line.[121] These numbers mean that in 2015, roughly 2.2 percent of all households in the United States had someone over the age of sixty-five living in them and was experiencing food insecurity.[122] One of the reasons that many seniors live at or below the poverty line is that they have little income saved for retirement. A study done by the National Council of Aging found that 21 percent of married Social Security recipients and 43 percent of single recipients aged sixty-five or older depend on Social Security for more than 90 percent of their income.[123] Additionally, the study found that the median debt for senior households is $40,900. High dependence on Social Security is of even greater concern as questions about Social Security's viability have begun to swirl in recent years. Few young people today believe that Social Security will be available for them when they retire, but this perceived lack of safety net has not led to an increase in retirement savings among Americans.[124] In all likelihood, a decline of Social Security would mean millions more elderly Americans in poverty.

The final division in poverty rates is that between metropolitan and nonmetropolitan areas. Poverty rates among nonmetropolitan areas tend to be higher than those among metropolitan areas, especially in the South.[125] The disparity between metropolitan and nonmetropolitan areas is not small. As Levernier (2003) explains, "The mean poverty rate of nonmetropolitan counties is approximately 70 percent higher than that of metropolitan counties."[126] This difference in urban and rural poverty rates means that rural counties, especially those located in the South that have large African American populations, are at the greatest economic disadvantage and are the most likely to face extreme poverty.

Taken as a whole, poverty rates are highest in some of the states that make up the Deep South. As of 2017, Louisiana and Mississippi were part of a four-way tie with New Mexico and West Virginia for the highest state poverty rates in the country at 17 percent.[127] Likewise, most of the states with the lowest poverty rates are located in the North and Northeast, including

New Hampshire, with a poverty rate of 5 percent, and Maryland, with a poverty rate of 7 percent.[128] If one looks at the numbers, it is easy to discern the levels of poverty and to see that, while there is poverty everywhere in the United States, the South suffers disproportionately high numbers of low-income people. These numbers, combined with a hot, humid climate, mean that the Southern United States provides a suitable environment for the spread of NTDs.

The Link between Poverty and Health

The link between poverty and health is clear; though there is some argument about what direction the correlation goes. In a 2009 document on the right to health and international law Paola Pace wrote, "Sick people are more likely to become poor; and the poor are more vulnerable to disease and disability. Good health is central to creating the capabilities that the poor need to escape poverty."[129] To further emphasize this point, Wagstaff (2002) stated, "poor people have worse health outcomes than better-off people. This association reflects causality running in both directions: poverty breeds ill-health, and ill-health keeps poor people poor."[130] What both these scholars are documenting is that poverty does not only create worse health outcomes, but having worse health can contribute to one being stuck in poverty. The strong divide in health outcomes between those living in poverty, or near poverty, and those with more stable incomes, is important to understanding why low-income communities in the United States are at high risk for NTD infection.

Another variable that leads to negative health outcomes, health access, might be less obvious. Health access refers to both physical access and financial access. Physical access is an individual's ability to get to a health clinic or doctor's office. This can be particularly challenging in poor, rural areas because of the limited number of clinics, the low likelihood a poor individual will own a vehicle, and the lack of public transportation. Financial access is the other side of the coin, though a lack of physical and financial access often go hand-in-hand in poor, rural areas. Financial access refers to an individual's ability to pay for medical care. Many low-income individuals around the world, including here in the United States, forgo necessary medical treatment because they have no money to pay for it.[131] In fact, the United States has one of the highest disparities in the world on this particular measure. In a study done by Hero et al. (2017), the United States ranked 31st out of 32 countries on the percentage of the population that forgoes medical treatment for the lack of ability to pay, with only the Philippines scoring lower. Countries that had less disparity than the United States included Russia, South Africa, Lithuania, and Bulgaria.[132] This inability to pay means that, for many people living in poverty, they must forgo primary care entirely and often use emergency departments as their first and only access to a doctor.

Interestingly, the idea of primary care is often an afterthought in debates about health care access. The purpose of such care is to provide individuals with routine medical services and to catch medical problems early. Individuals that have access to such care are 19 percent less likely to experience premature death, but it would also save the American economy billions of dollars.[133] According to Primary Care Progress (2018), "If everyone saw a primary care provider first for their care, it would save the U.S. an estimated $67 billion every year."[134] In addition, Shi and Starfield (2000) found that the presence or absence of primary care has a larger effect on health outcomes than health insurance coverage.[135] Thus, access to primary care would make a significant macroeconomic impact, as well as improve the health of poor individuals in America.

"Poverty and low income are causally related to worse child development outcomes, particularly cognitive development and educational outcomes."[136] Some of these adverse cognitive development outcomes are a result of the chronic stress felt by many families living in poverty, and, in fact, just one year spent in poverty can lead to worse outcomes compared to children who never experienced poverty.[137] This finding shows the depth and extent of poverty's impact on development: that only one year in poverty could have lifelong impacts on children.

The United States ranks among the lowest of wealthy, industrialized countries for social mobility and child poverty when compared to countries with similar resources.[138] This is to say that for a wealthy country, the United States has unusually high rates of child poverty and unusually low rates of upward mobility. When taken as a whole, health statistics in the United States are relatively good, but these averages hide the large amount of health inequality that exists. Halfon and Newacheck (1993) found that poor families were four times as likely to use the emergency department for their usual source of care and that "poor children were hospitalized 40 percent more often and experienced longer lengths of stay," which they suggest may be accounted for by "diminished access to appropriate ambulatory health services."[139] Additionally, children from poor families have lower birth weights, higher infant mortality, and are more likely to experience malnutrition, as well as 40 percent higher rates of obesity, 30 percent higher rates of asthma, and are four times more likely to be in fair or poor health.[140] As Wagstaff (2002) wrote, "inequalities in health are almost always to the disadvantage of the poor. The poor tend to die earlier and to have higher levels of morbidity than the better-off."[141] The AAP Council went one step further by declaring, "Poverty and other adverse social determinants have a detrimental effect on child health and are root causes of child health inequity in the United States."[142]

The social dynamics of an individual's neighborhood also play an important role in health outcomes. Pickett and Pearl (2001) found that "neighbourhood [*sic*] context might affect health either directly, if simply living in a deprived neighbourhood is deleterious to health, or indirectly through such mechanisms as the availability and accessibility of health services, healthy foods or recreation facilities, environmental pollution, normative attitudes towards health, and social support."[143] The socioeconomic status of one's neighborhood may have an impact on health outcomes simply based on the availability of resources and the health of the surrounding environment.

In addition to the general health inequalities seen between the poor and the better-off, there are notable inequalities that run along the lines of race and ethnicity. In a 2015 study, Arcaya et al. wrote, "From a strictly utilitarian standpoint, the cost of health inequalities is staggering. Between 2003 and 2006 alone, the direct economic cost of health inequalities based on race or ethnicity in the United States was estimated at $230 billion. Researchers calculated that medical costs faced by African Americans, Asian Americans, and Hispanics were in excess by 30% due to racial and ethnic health inequalities."[144] Studies, including the one conducted by Arcaya et al. in 2015, consistently show that there are great disparities in infant mortality rates based on race and ethnicity with infant mortality rates for non-Hispanic blacks three times higher than those of whites.

Lastly, there are some studies that have found other factors that contribute to negative health outcomes among low-income populations. These include: the availability of unconditional cash transfers to poor families and rural residence. Regarding the availability of unconditional cash transfers, Pega et al. (2017) found that, while the cash transfers did not impact health service use, they did impact overall health outcomes.[145] The health outcomes that saw the largest impact from unconditional cash transfers were the likelihood of having an illness, the likelihood of being food insecure, the level of dietary diversity, and the likelihood of attending school.[146] With regards to rural residence, a 2019 study by Raju et al. found that both rural residence and poverty were risk factors for Chronic Obstructive Pulmonary Disease (COPD) in the United States, even among non-smokers.[147] Raju et al. (2019) wrote, "Our study shows that the greatest burden of COPD in the United States is found in rural areas, with the prevalence of COPD in rural, poor communities being nearly double that in the general population."[148] While recent research shows that rural residence has an impact on COPD risk, it can lead to other adverse outcomes, presumably because of greater difficulty accessing health care. Lastly, a study conducted by Michael Marmot found a clear association between the grade of employment for British civil servants and mortality.[149] This study clearly showed the impact of wages on health outcomes by concentrating on a specific sector of the economy.

For decades, research has shown a clear association between poverty and health, though there is still ongoing discussion as to which way the association travels. As we have shown in this section, however, regardless of directionality, those living in poverty are much more likely to experience adverse health outcomes. Individuals living in poverty are less able to take preventative measures to protect their health, often because they do not have the financial means to do so. Most notably, however, is that "in spite of high poverty rates, the United States spends a smaller proportion of gross domestic product on social safety nets, compared to other high-income nations, and the constellation of services that can help improve health and access to health care is both less comprehensive and less generous."[150] As we have noted numerous times throughout this chapter, social support systems in the United States are lacking. This is especially true when compared to other wealthy nations around the world and the health of Americans suffer as a result.

INCOME INEQUALITY

A discussion of poverty in America is incomplete without examining income inequality. Income inequality in the United States is present and growing. Kochhar and Cilluffo (2018) explains that in 2016, wealth gaps between upper income and lower and middle income are the highest in history.[151] "The income gap between Americans at the top and the bottom of the income distribution widened 27% from 1970 to 2016," meaning that not only is the gap the largest it has ever been, but it is also increasing rapidly.[152] As one may be able to guess based on the racial divisions within poverty rates, those at the lower- and middle-income levels also are not equal. "Among lower- and middle-income households, white families have four times as much wealth as black families and three times as much as Hispanic families."[153] Thus, the picture of income inequality in the United States is a division between the haves and the have nots but it is also a division among the have nots based on race and ethnicity.

But what is income inequality? In popular vernacular, many people conflate income inequality with poverty, but this is not always the case. As described by Neumayer and Plümper (2016) in their investigations, income inequality does not necessarily mean that there is a higher prevalence of poverty.[154] Instead, income inequality refers solely to the divide between the top levels of income in a country and the lower levels of income.[155] It is theoretically possible for a country to have high-income inequality but not high rates of poverty, as long as the lower levels of income do not fall into the poverty classification.

Income inequality has become a point of contention and conversation in the United States throughout the last decade, arguably reaching its peak with the Occupy Wall Street movement, which sought (with only moderate success) to draw attention to the income differences between the top 1 percent of Americans and the other 99 percent. Today, the conversation continues and can be seen most prominently in the Democratic primaries of 2019. Despite these efforts, however, "The United States exhibited disparities in most measures [of income inequality], making it unique among high-income countries."[156] This uniqueness is not a positive attribute; rather it sets the United States apart from its peers with regards to its large, and growing, unequal distribution of income. Like poverty, income inequality has important health implications, but before we explore those outcomes, let us examine how the United States came to arrive at this unfortunate uniqueness.

History of Income Inequality in the United States

In many ways, the United States has always had vast income inequalities. Take for example, the wealth of John D. Rockefeller or Andrew Carnegie juxtaposed against the meager incomes of newly freed slaves or the struggling populations of urban factory workers. Income inequality in the United States reached a peak with the top 1 percent holding 19.6 percent of the country's total income in 1928.[157] Then came the collapse. The Great Depression resulting from the collapse of the American economy inadvertently helped to create a more level playing field (though this was just a byproduct of a decimated economy not of active policy action). From the 1940s until the 1970s, the United States witnessed the lowest levels of income inequality with the top 1 percent holding only about 8 percent of the total income in the country.[158] Beginning in the late-1970s, however, this relatively low, stabilized income inequality began to change. "The share of income going to the wealthiest 10% increased from 33% of total earnings in 1978 to 50% in 2014—a level of inequality not seen since before the Great Depression. Incomes for poor and middle-income Americans have barely changed since the 1970s and, adjusted for inflation, have actually declined since 2000."[159] When income inequality began to rise, it did not stop.

Income inequality is not just coming as a result of individuals at the highest incomes amassing more and more of the country's wealth, but also from the loss of purchasing power experienced by those at the bottom. "Since 2001, annual inflation-adjusted household earnings have fallen for Americans in the bottom two-thirds of the income distribution with the largest relative losses experienced in the lower part of the income distribution."[160] Therefore, Americans at the bottom are actually making less money than they were in previous decades when their income is adjusted for inflation. As way of explanation, Gottschalk and Danziger (2005) state, "While there is still considerable uncertainty about the causes of these changes, there is broad consensus that wage rate inequality is considerably higher at the start of the 21st century than it was a quarter of a century earlier."[161]

The impact of this loss of purchasing power is far reaching and, much like the cycle of poverty itself, appears to perpetuate income inequality through generations. As a study by Bor et al. (2017) found, "income segregation across school districts in the USA increased by 15% between 1990s and 2010, and within-district segregation across schools increased by 40%. Factors contributing to rising segregation include the increasing concentration of economic growth in specific regions, the rise in housing prices during the 1990s and early 2000s, which has priced many Americans out of specific geographical housing and rental markets, and widening income inequality itself."[162] Thus, rising income inequality is creating greater segregation by income, which is having an impact on school districts across the country. With lower incomes concentrating together, there is less money to fund schools, making it more difficult for students to learn and, inherently, impacting their future earning potential.

Although income inequality and poverty are not equivalent, they often are found side-by-side and both can have serious outcomes for health. Bor et al. (2017) described this by stating, "The divergence of life expectancy for poor and middle-income Americans since 2001 reflects both changes in income distribution and a rise in gradient between income and health, with the latter a more important factor."[163] But how does income inequality in the United States compare to income inequality in other high-income nations?

Income Inequality: United States versus International Community

The United States has long stood out among high-income nations with regards to income inequality, but, like poverty measurements, it is not for positive reasons. In 2017, a report by OECD showed that the top quartile of earners in the United States held slightly over 42 percent of the country's wealth.[164] This distribution was higher than any other OECD country. Even more striking, the report showed that in 2016, the top 10 percent of earners in the United States held 79.5 percent of the country's wealth, compared to 44.9 percent in Australia, 51.1 percent in Canada, 48.3 percent in the United Kingdom, and 44.8 percent in Italy.[165] Additionally, between 2010 and 2015, there was a rate of change in wealth inequality in the United States that was more than double the next closest country.[166]

This high level of income inequality means that, while the United States has the highest level of wealth of any country, it does not have the highest median income. The average American has a median wealth of $61,667 USD, which is comparatively lower than the median wealth of adults in the United Kingdom ($97,169 USD), Japan ($103,861 USD), Canada ($106,342 USD), France ($106,827 USD), Netherlands ($114,935 USD), Belgium ($163,429 USD), and Australia ($191,453 USD).[167]

Despite the exceptionally high levels of income inequality in the United States compared to its peers across the globe, it is not unique in seeing rising inequality. A study conducted by Brian Keeley in 2015 found that "since the 1980s, income inequality has risen in most OECD countries."[168] Notably, the rise of more wealth concentrated in the top 1 percent has been most pronounced in English-speaking countries, to include the United States. The changes occurring in high-income countries is different from what is occurring in low- and middle-income countries, where income inequality is rising, but a middle class is also emerging. Interestingly, as countries across the globe take steps to reduce poverty they are experiencing growing levels of income inequality. For example, as Brazil and South Africa have made great gains in reducing poverty, their Gini points are 50 and 70, respectively.[169] OECD hypothesizes that the reduction in poverty in low- and middle-income countries is accompanied by rising income inequality largely as a result of the differences between urban and rural areas in an increasingly globalized economy.[170] Despite the changes occurring within low- and middle-income countries, the United States remains unique among high-income countries for its large, and growing, income gap.

The growth of income inequality in the United States could have important implications for overall poverty in the United States and the prevalence of NTDs. As welfare safety nets are removed and more and more Americans see their hope of wealth accumulation fade from view, one must question if we should expect increasing numbers of poor Americans and loss of purchasing power among the lower-income quartiles over the next several decades. Will jobs continue to leave rural America? Will there be no Social Security left for the young adults of today when they reach retirement? Will student loan debt make it impossible for many college graduates to build wealth? While we are not economists, and, therefore, cannot (and will not attempt to) answer these questions, they are important questions that impact growing income inequality in the United States.

Upward Mobility

An increasingly discussed element impacting the economic and social well-being of Americans is economic inequality and upward mobility. This can be more broadly defined as "The American Dream." American-born and even immigrant children are raised to believe that, in America, a person can achieve anything through hard work. In decades past, most American children, whether college educated or not, could feel some optimism that they had the potential to achieve a higher economic and social status than their parents. Increasingly, however, data is showing that this is no longer attainable and, in fact, we are coming upon the first generation that will be worse off economically than their parents.[171] Today, "one's starting position clearly predicts one's finishing rank."[172] Even more striking, a 2017 study by Chetty et al. "found that rates of absolute mobility have fallen from approximately 90 percent for children born in 1940 to 50 percent for children born in the 1980s."[173] This shows that the number of children who will achieve higher economic status than their parents has fallen by almost half.

While there are large declines in upward mobility throughout the United States, these declines are not evenly distributed. The largest declines in upward mobility are in the middle class.[174] As Markovits (2019) observed, "Absolute economic mobility is also declining—the odds that a middle-class child will out-earn his parents has fallen by more than half since mid-century—and the drop is greater among the middle class than among the poor."[175] Thus, children born to middle-class parents are the largest section of the population at risk for falling below their parents' economic level. In 2008, a study by Isaacs et al. determined that 33 percent of Americans were "downwardly mobile," meaning that they had fallen down an income bracket from the bracket their parents were in.[176] The growing disparity between the wealthy and middle-class, Markovits argues, is a result of the country's current meritocratic structure. He states, "Common usage often conflates meritocracy with equality of opportunity. But although meritocracy was embraced as the handmaiden of equality of opportunity, and did open up the elite in its early years, it now more nearly stifles than fosters social mobility . . . Middle-class families cannot afford the elaborate schooling that rich families buy, and ordinary schools lag farther and farther behind elite ones, commanding fewer resources and delivering inferior educations."[177] Quite simply, education has become the foundation of upward mobility and the middle-class cannot afford the cost of admission.

Through their extensive work, Chetty and his colleagues at Harvard University have discovered that the American Dream is fading. For young Americans today and those of the next generation, the neighborhood they grow up in has a significant impact on their outcomes in adulthood. Chetty and Hendren (2018) state, "counties with less concentrated poverty, less income inequality, better schools, a larger share of two-parent families, and lower crime rates tend to produce better outcomes for children in poor families."[178] More importantly, they have shown that moving a child from a high poverty neighborhood to a low poverty neighborhood increases their future earnings. The neighborhood a child grows up in shapes not only their future earnings but also college attendance rates and marriage patterns.[179] In this way, an individual's likelihood of living in poverty—and the level of that poverty—comes from a variety of factors including race, neighborhood demographics, and classroom size.[180]

As DeParle (2012) explains, "One reason for the mobility gap . . . may be the unusually large premiums that American employers pay for college degrees. Since children generally follow their parents' educational trajectory, that premium increases the importance of family background and stymies people with less schooling."[181] Adequate schooling does not benefit everyone equally, however. A study conducted by Zimmerman in 2019 found that male graduates from private high schools are the only ones that see a noticeable rise in mean incomes from attending elite colleges (i.e., Ivy League).[182] Women and male students from public high schools do not achieve recognizable gains in income from attending an elite college versus any other college. Part of this disparity, Zimmerman explains, may come from the tendency of male, private high school graduates to pursue careers in business following college graduation to a much greater extent than the other two sub-groups.[183] In general, however, there is a growing body of evidence linking the growing income inequality and social mobility to educational inequality. Income inequality still poses a major obstacle for the American way of life; the face of it has simply changed. "Economic inequality now distinctively concerns not poverty but wealth."[184] This is not to say that millions of Americans do not suffer in extreme poverty rather that the greatest economic inequalities today are a result of the unprecedented rise of wealth concentration and the steep decline of the middle-class.

Similar to global poverty outcomes, "the U.S. has one of the lowest rates of upward mobility in the developed world, and only a small proportion of citizens move from the class into which they were born into a higher one."[185] Predictably, even in a country that relies heavily on the idea of the American Dream, one's future opportunities are tied directly to the opportunities of their present socioeconomic class. Scott and Leonhardt (2005) emphasized this point by quoting UC Berkeley economist David Levine as saying, "being born in the elite in the U.S. gives you a constellation of privileges that very few people in the world have ever experienced. Being born poor in the U.S. gives you disadvantages unlike anything in Western Europe and Japan and Canada."[186] Put differently, if you are born wealthy, the United States is one of the best places in the world, but if you are born poor you have less opportunity than you would have if you were born in almost any other wealthy country.

Equally as important as the existing disparities, is the American public's acceptance of it. As Shariff et al. (2016) found, "people are willing to tolerate the vaulted position of the rich because they hope that they or their children may move into those ranks, and they want to maintain the advantages for their future economic station."[187] Additionally, those with more opportunity for social mobility are more accepting of income inequality than are those with less opportunity for mobility.[188] Perceptions of mobility and tolerance of inequality also vary along ideological lines. A 2015 study conducted by Chambers et al. found that people who self-identified as liberals were more likely than those that self-identified as conservatives to rate social mobility as declining.[189] In this way, conservatives are more optimistic about their own ability to move to higher economic brackets and, therefore, are more willing to tolerate economic inequality, as predicted by Shariff et al.'s (2016) study.[190] Tolerance for inequality in social mobility and income is a major contributing factor to lack of action against it.

The Link between Income Inequality and Health

Much like poverty, there is a definitive and statistically significant link between income inequality and health. This is because "health inequities are closely linked to social inequities."[191] In particular, health behaviors, healthcare, work conditions, environmental pollution, and early life conditions are vastly different at different incomes.[192] Individuals at the higher levels of income have greater access to healthcare, healthier home environments, and likely better working conditions than those individuals at lower levels of income. And like the relationship between poverty and health, the association between high rates of income inequality and greater health disparities, holds universally true.[193]

According to data collected by the World Health Organization on health outcomes and the World Bank GINI Index, people in more equitable countries live longer than individuals in less equitable countries.[194] Using data compiled from these statistics, the Institute for Policy Studies states that, "in the United States, average life expectancy is four years shorter than in some of the most equitable countries."[195] These disparities do not just impact longevity, however. Data from the World Health Organization and the Organisation for Economic Co-operation and Development (OECD) countries found that countries with lower levels of income inequality also have lower infant mortality rates than those with high levels of income inequality.[196] In fact, when looking at other high-income countries, most of which have an income inequality level that is half that of the United States, the data shows that the United States has double the infant mortality of most other high-income countries. Most starkly, the infant mortality rate in the United States is more than three times greater than the infant mortality rate in Iceland, Finland, Norway, and Sweden.[197] In other words, as income inequality increases, the population of the country with growing disparities live shorter lives and their children are more likely to die in their first year of life.

Returning focus to the United States, as income inequality has increased in recent decades those at the lowest end of the income spectrum experience greater negative health outcomes. Americans in the top 1 percent of income live an average of 10–15 years longer than individuals in the bottom 1 percent.[198] Additionally, a study conducted by Bor et al. (2017) found that life expectancy has increased for middle- and upper-income Americans, but has declined for some of the poorest Americans.[199] These findings continue to hold true at the state level as well. A study by Kennedy et al. (1998) found that "when personal characteristics are controlled for, individuals living in states with the greatest inequalities in income were 30 % more likely to report their health as fair or poor than individuals living in states with the smallest inequalities in income."[200] This disparity in health among the most unequitable U.S. states was reinforced when Shi and Starfield (2000) found that, "after controlling for individual covariates, that those living in states with less income inequality are 1.2 to 1.3 times more likely to report good/excellent health than those living in states with greater income inequality."[201]

The findings from multiple studies along with data from the World Bank and World Health Organizations demonstrate repeatedly the relationship between income inequality and health. This relationship has been shown over and over again throughout the decades, but there is yet to be policy action or a unified public health effort to address it. Hero et al. (2017) seeks to explain this by stating, "Relatively low levels of moral discomfort over income-based health care disparities despite awareness of unmet need indicate more public tolerance for health inequalities in the United States than elsewhere."[202] Americans as a whole are not that concerned with health disparities, but we should be.

CONCLUSION

"Opportunity and poverty in this country cannot be explained by either the American Myth that hard work is a panacea or by the Anti-Myth that the system imprisons the poor. Relief will come, if at all, in an amalgam that recognizes both the society's obligation through government and business, and the individual's obligation through labor and family" writes Shipler.[203] Poverty in America is multifaceted; an amalgamation of historical, social, and political determinants that often decide an American child's fate before their fifth birthday. Our inability to fully understand poverty, however, has made it difficult for the country to effectively address it. As Shipler (2004) explains, "As a culture, the United States is not quite sure about the causes of poverty, and is therefore uncertain about the solutions."[204] Therefore, even in our efforts to address the issue of poverty, we do not have a firm grasp on what would be most effective.

Additionally, despite efforts throughout American history to combat poverty, opposition to anti-poverty programs remains a stumbling block. Even among supporters of anti-poverty programs and broad social safety nets, a lack of understanding about the reality of poverty in America leads to ineffective, unrealistic, or uninformed proposals. "So it is with so many efforts to help, then and now: the good intentions of comfortable men and women, private charities, and governments is not enough, and they cannot provide meaningful assistance if they are blind to the realities of the lives they seek to improve."[205]

In the next chapter, we examine the other risk factors that contribute to the levels of NTD infection in the United States. These include an analysis of the country's water and sanitation infrastructure, inadequate housing options, food insecurity, climate change, and natural disasters. All of these elements combine with poverty and income inequality in the United States to create greater negative health outcomes for Americans and leaves many susceptible to NTDs.

NOTES

1. "Inaugural Address of George W. Bush; January 20, 2001," Yale Law School, last modified 2008, https://avalon.law.yale.edu/21st_century/gbush1.asp.
2. Hotez, personal communication, September 18, 2018.
3. Joe Rogan (Producer), "Joe Rogan Experience," Peter Hotez on Vaccines and Tropical Diseases [Podcast audio], March 23, 2019, https://podcastnotes.org/2019/03/23/hotez/.
4. Matthew Desmond, *Evicted: Poverty and Profit in the American City* (New York: Broadway Books, 2017).
5. Center for Poverty Research, "What is the Current Poverty Rate in the United States?" *University of California at Davis*. Last modified October 15, 2018, https://poverty.ucdavis.edu/faq/what-current-poverty-rate-united-states.
6. Serena Lei, "An Unwaged War on Deep Poverty," *The Urban Institute*, published December 15, 2013, https://www.urban.org/features/unwaged-war-deep-poverty.
7. David K. Shipler, *The Working Poor: Invisible in America* (New York: Borzoi Book, 2004).
8. Lei, "An Unwaged War on Deep Poverty."
9. Lei, "An Unwaged War on Deep Poverty."
10. Kathryn J. Edin and Luke H. Shaefer, *$2.00 a Day: Living on Almost Nothing in America* (New York, NY: Houghton Mifflin Harcourt Trade & Reference Publishers, 2015), 17.
11. Edin and Shaefer, *$2.00 a Day: Living on Almost Nothing in America*, 28–29.
12. Edin and Shaefer, *$2.00 a Day: Living on Almost Nothing in America.*
13. Robert Doar, "Consumption Poverty and the Official Poverty Measure," *AEIdeas*, published September 18, 2017, https://www.aei.org/economics/consumption-poverty-and-the-official-poverty-measure/.

14. Nancy K. Cauthen and Sarah Fass, "Measuring Poverty in the United States," *National Center for Children in Poverty*, published June 2008, http://www.nccp.org/publications/pub_825.html.

15. U.S. Census Bureau, "How the Census Bureau Measures Poverty," accessed December 1, 2019, https://www.census.gov/topics/income-poverty/poverty/guidance/poverty-measures.html.

16. Center for Poverty Research, "How is Poverty Measured in the United States?" *University of California at Davis*, last modified December 18, 2017, https://poverty.ucdavis.edu/faq/how-poverty-measured-united-states.

17. Center for Poverty Research, "How is Poverty Measured in the United States?"

18. Phil Gramm and John F. Early, "The Truth About Income Inequality," *The Wall Street Journal*, published November 3, 2019, https://www.wsj.com/articles/the-truth-about-income-inequality-11572813786.

19. Bruce D. Meyer and James X. Sullivan, "Winning the War: Poverty from the Great Society to the Great Recession," No. w18718, *National Bureau of Economic Research*, 2013, https://www.nber.org/papers/w18718.pdf; Jonathan Fisher, David S. Johnson, and Timothy M. Smeeding, "Inequality of Income and Consumption in the US: Measuring the Trends in Inequality from 1984 to 2011 for the Same Individuals," *Review of Income and Wealth* 61, no. 4 (2015): 630–650; Orazio P. Attanasio and Luigi Pistaferri, "Consumption Inequality," *Journal of Economic Perspectives* 30, no. 2 (2016): 3–28.

20. Meyer and Sullivan, "Winning the War: Poverty from the Great Society to the Great Recession."

21. Matthew Philips, "What's the Best Way to Measure Poverty: Income or Consumption?" *Freakonomics*, published September 14, 2011, http://freakonomics.com/2011/09/14/whats-the-best-way-to-measure-poverty-income-or-consumption/.

22. Meyer and Sullivan, "Winning the War: Poverty from the Great Society to the Great Recession."

23. Philips, "What's the Best Way to Measure Poverty: Income or Consumption?"

24. Attanasio and Pistaferri, "Consumption Inequality."

25. Stephen Pimpare, *A People's History of Poverty in America* (New York: The New Press, 2008), 195.

26. Pimpare, *A People's History of Poverty in America.*

27. Martin Gilen, *Why Americans Hate Welfare: Race, Media, and the Politics of Antipoverty Strategy* (Chicago: University of Chicago Press, 1999).

28. Pimpare, *A People's History of Poverty in America*, 29.

29. Pimpare, *A People's History of Poverty in America.*

30. Pimpare, *A People's History of Poverty in America.*

31. Pimpare, *A People's History of Poverty in America*, 30.

32. Jerry D. Marx, "American Social Policy in the Great Depression and World War II," accessed October 21, 2019, https://socialwelfare.library.vcu.edu/eras/great-depression/american-social-policy-in-the-great-depression-and-wwii/.

33. Marx, "American Social Policy in the Great Depression and World War II."

34. Marx, "American Social Policy in the Great Depression and World War II."

35. Marx, "American Social Policy in the Great Depression and World War II."

36. Marx, "American Social Policy in the Great Depression and World War II."

37. Todd C. Neumann, Price V. Fishback, and Shawn Kantor, "The Dynamics of Relief Spending and the Private Urban Labor Market during the New Deal," *The Journal of Economic History* 70, no. 1 (2010): 195–220.

38. Marx, "American Social Policy in the Great Depression and World War II"; Neumann, Fishback, and Kantor, "The Dynamics of Relief Spending and the Private Urban Labor Market during the New Deal."

39. Neumann, Fishback, and Kantor, "The Dynamics of Relief Spending and the Private Urban Labor Market during the New Deal."

40. Neumann, Fishback, and Kantor, "The Dynamics of Relief Spending and the Private Urban Labor Market during the New Deal."

41. Marx, "American Social Policy in the Great Depression and World War II."

42. Margaret R. Somers and Fred Block, "From Poverty to Perversity: Ideas, Markets, and Institutions over 200 Years of Welfare Debate," *American Sociological Review* 70, no. 2 (2005): 267.

43. Center on Budget and Policy Priorities, "Policy Basics: Top Ten Facts about Social Security," last modified August 14, 2019, https://www.cbpp.org/research/social-security/policy-basics-top-ten-facts-about-social-security#:~:targetText=Over%2063%20million%20people%2C%20or,young%20survivors%20of%20deceased%20workers.

44. Marx, "American Social Policy in the Great Depression and World War II."

45. Marx, "American Social Policy in the Great Depression and World War II."

46. Marx, "American Social Policy in the Great Depression and World War II."

47. Neumann, Fishback, and Kantor, "The Dynamics of Relief Spending and the Private Urban Labor Market during the New Deal."

48. William Leuchtenburg, "When Franklin Roosevelt Clashed with the Supreme Court–and Lost," *Smithsonian Magazine*, published May 2005, https://www.smithsonianmag.com/history/when-franklin-roosevelt-clashed-with-the-supreme-court-and-lost-78497994/.

49. William E. Leuchtenburg, "The Origins of Franklin D. Roosevelt's 'Court-Packing' Plan," *The Supreme Court Review* (1966): 347–400.

50. Leuchtenburg, "When Franklin Roosevelt Clashed with the Supreme Court–and Lost."

51. Leuchtenburg, "When Franklin Roosevelt Clashed with the Supreme Court–and Lost."

52. Marx, "American Social Policy in the Great Depression and World War II."

53. David F. Weiman, "Imagining a World without the New Deal," *The Washington Post*, published August 12, 2011, https://www.washingtonpost.com/opinions/imagining-a-world-without-the-new-deal/2011/08/03/gIQAtJoBBJ_story.html.

54. Somers and Block, "From Poverty to Perversity: Ideas, Markets, and Institutions over 200 Years of Welfare Debate," 281.

55. Aaron Cooley, "War on Poverty," *Encyclopedia Britannica*, accessed June 23, 2019, https://www.britannica.com/topic/War-on-Poverty.

56. Miller Center, "January 8, 1964: State of the Union," *University of Virginia*, accessed December 2, 2019, https://millercenter.org/the-presidency/presidential-speeches/january-8-1964-state-union.

57. History.com, "Great Society," last modified August 28, 2018, https://www.history.com/topics/1960s/great-society.

58. History.com, "Great Society."

59. History.com, "Great Society."

60. Lyndon B. Johnson, "The War on Poverty," *First State of the Union Address* (1964): 5.,http://corematerials.homestead.com/files/added_2012_2013/the_war_on_poverty_state_of_union.pdf.

61. Martha J. Bailey and Nicolas J. Duquette, "How Johnson Fought the War on Poverty: The Economics and Politics of Funding at the Office of Economic Opportunity," *The Journal of Economic History* 74, no. 2 (2014): 351–387.

62. David Torstensson, "Beyond the City: Lyndon Johnson's War on Poverty in Rural America," *Journal of Policy History* 25, no. 4 (2013): 587–613.

63. Torstensson, "Beyond the City: Lyndon Johnson's War on Poverty in Rural America."

64. Bailey and Duquette, "How Johnson Fought the War on Poverty: The Economics and Politics of Funding at the Office of Economic Opportunity."

65. Bailey and Duquette, "How Johnson Fought the War on Poverty: The Economics and Politics of Funding at the Office of Economic Opportunity"; Torstensson, "Beyond the City: Lyndon Johnson's War on Poverty in Rural America."

66. Bailey and Duquette, "How Johnson Fought the War on Poverty: The Economics and Politics of Funding at the Office of Economic Opportunity."

67. Bailey and Duquette, "How Johnson Fought the War on Poverty: The Economics and Politics of Funding at the Office of Economic Opportunity," 355.

68. Liana Fox et al., "Trends in Deep Poverty from 1968 to 2011: The Influence of Family Structure, Employment Patterns, and the Safety Net," *RSF: The Russell Sage Foundation Journal of the Social Sciences* 1, no. 1 (2015): 14–34.

69. Fox et al., "Trends in Deep Poverty from 1968 to 2011."

70. Mary K. Anglin, "Lessons from Appalachia in the 20th Century: Poverty, Power, and the 'grassroots'," *American Anthropologist* 104, no. 2 (2002): 565–582.

71. Brian C. Thiede, Daniel T. Lichter, and Tim Slack, "Working, but Poor: The Good Life in Rural America?" *Journal of Rural Studies* 59 (2018): 183–193.

72. Thiede, Lichter, and Slack, "Working, but Poor: The Good Life in Rural America," 187.

73. Thiede, Lichter, and Slack, "Working, but Poor: The Good Life in Rural America," 183–193.

74. Timothy Smeeding, "Poor People in Rich Nations: The United States in Comparative Perspective," *Journal of Economic Perspectives* 20, no. 1 (2006): 86.

75. David Brady, Andrew S. Fullerton, and Jennifer Moren Cross, "More than Just Nickels and Dimes: A Cross-National Analysis of Working Poverty in Affluent Democracies," *Social Problems* 57, no. 4 (2010): 569.

76. Smeeding, "Poor People in Rich Nations: The United States in Comparative Perspective," 86; Brady, Fullerton, and Cross, "More than Just Nickels and Dimes:

A Cross-National Analysis of Working Poverty in Affluent Democracies," 569; Ruth M. Gomberg-Muñoz, "Review Essay: Law and Migrant Labor in the 20th Century: Ghost Workers and Global Capitalism," *Loyola University Chicago, Anthropology: Faculty Publications and Other Works.* (2018), https://ecommons.luc.edu/anthropology_facpubs/21/.

77. Anglin, "Lessons from Appalachia in the 20th Century," 574.

78. Roberto Suro, Jill H. Wilson, and Audrey Singer, "Immigration and Poverty in America's Suburbs," *Metropolitan Opportunity Series at Brookings Institute* (2011); Jie Zong, Jeanne Batalova, and Jeffrey Hallock, "Frequently Requested Statistics on Immigrants and Immigration in the United States," *Migration Policy Institute* 26 (2015): 1–18.

79. Suro, Wilson, and Singer, "Immigration and Poverty in America's Suburbs"; Young et al., "More Inclusive States, Less Poverty among Immigrants? An Examination of Poverty, Citizenship Stratification, and State Immigrant Policies," *Population Research and Policy Review* 37, no. 2 (2018): 205–228.

80. Suro, Wilson, and Singer, "Immigration and Poverty in America's Suburbs"; Jeff Chapman and Jared Bernstein, "Immigration and Poverty: How are they Linked," *Monthly Lab. Rev.* 126 (2003): 10–15; Steven Raphael and Eugene Smolensky, "Immigration and Poverty in the United States," *American Economic Review* 99, no. 2 (2009): 41–44; Suro, Wilson, and Singer, "Immigration and Poverty in America's Suburbs," 13.

81. Young et al., "More Inclusive States, Less Poverty Among Immigrants?"

82. Suro, Wilson, and Singer, "Immigration and Poverty in America's Suburbs."

83. Suro, Wilson, and Singer, "Immigration and Poverty in America's Suburbs," 13.

84. Gomberg-Muñoz, "Review Essay: Law and Migrant Labor in the 20th Century," 4.

85. Gomberg-Muñoz, "Review Essay: Law and Migrant Labor in the 20th Century," 5.

86. Shipler, *The Working Poor: Invisible in America*, 114.

87. Martha Crowley, Daniel T. Lichter, and Zhenchao Qian, "Beyond Gateway Cities: Economic Restructuring and Poverty among Mexican Immigrant Families and Children," *Family Relations* 55, no. 3 (2006): 345–360.

88. Crowley, Lichter, and Qian, "Beyond Gateway Cities."

89. Frank D. Bean, Cynthia Feliciano, Jennifer Lee, and Jennifer Van Hook. "The New US Immigrants: How do They Affect Our Understanding of the African American Experience?" *The Annals of the American Academy of Political and Social Science* 621, no. 1 (2009): 202–220.

90. Steven Camarota, "Immigrants in the United States: A Profile of America's Foreign-Born Population," *Center for Immigration Studies*, published August 8, 2012, https://cis.org/Immigrants-United-States-Profile-Americas-ForeignBorn-Population.

91. Crowley, Lichter, and Qian, "Beyond Gateway Cities."

92. John J. DiIulio Jr., "The Future of Compassion: President Bush's Social Program Hasn't Yet Gotten a Chance," *Brookings Institute* (2002); Leigh Ann

Caldwell and Dan Merica, "America's Longest War," last modified January 8, 2014, https://www.cnn.com/2014/01/08/politics/war-on-poverty-50-years/index.html; Gary L. Gregg II, "George W. Bush: Domestic Affairs," *University of Virginia, Miller Center*, accessed December 2, 2019, https://millercenter.org/president/gwbush/domestic-affairs.

93. Caldwell and Merica, "America's Longest War."

94. Jennifer L. Steele, "Whatever it Takes: Geoffrey Canada's Quest to Change Harlem and America," *Harvard Educational Review* 79, no. 3 (2009).

95. Pimpare, *A People's History of Poverty in America*, 8; United Way, "Measure of Society," last modified 2016, https://www.unitedway.org/our-impact/stories/ar-measure-of-a-society.

96. Henry J Kaiser (KFF) Family Foundation, "Poverty Rate by Race/Ethnicity," last modified 2018, https://www.kff.org/other/state-indicator/poverty-rate-by-raceethnicity/?dataView=1&activeTab=map&currentTimeframe=0&selectedDistributions=total&sortModel=%7B%22colId%22:%22Location%22,%22sort%22:%22asc%22%7D.

97. Henry J Kaiser (KFF) Family Foundation, "Poverty Rate by Race/Ethnicity."

98. Henry J Kaiser (KFF) Family Foundation, "Poverty Rate by Race/Ethnicity."

99. Henry J Kaiser (KFF) Family Foundation, "Poverty Rate by Race/Ethnicity."

100. Henry J Kaiser (KFF) Family Foundation, "Poverty Rate by Race/Ethnicity."

101. Heather A. O'Connell, "The Impact of Slavery on Racial Inequality in Poverty in the Contemporary US South," *Social Forces* 90, no. 3 (2012): 713–734.

102. O'Connell, "The Impact of Slavery on Racial Inequality in Poverty in the Contemporary U.S. South."

103. Henry J Kaiser (KFF) Family Foundation, "Poverty Rate by Race/Ethnicity."

104. Henry J Kaiser (KFF) Family Foundation, "Poverty Rate by Race/Ethnicity."

105. Henry J Kaiser (KFF) Family Foundation, "Poverty Rate by Race/Ethnicity."

106. Henry J Kaiser (KFF) Family Foundation, "Poverty Rate by Race/Ethnicity."

107. Henry J Kaiser (KFF) Family Foundation, "Poverty Rate by Race/Ethnicity."

108. Henry J Kaiser (KFF) Family Foundation, "Poverty Rate by Race/Ethnicity."

109. Kayla Patrick, "National Snapshot: Poverty Among Women and Families, 2016," *National Women's Law Center*, published September 2017, https://nwlc.org/wp-content/uploads/2017/09/Poverty-Snapshot-Factsheet-2017.pdf.

110. Patrick, "National Snapshot: Poverty Among Women and Families, 2016."

111. Patrick, "National Snapshot: Poverty Among Women and Families, 2016."

112. Henry J Kaiser (KFF) Family Foundation, "Poverty Rate by Race/Ethnicity."

113. Patrick, "National Snapshot: Poverty Among Women and Families, 2016."

114. Children's Defense Fund, "Child Poverty in America 2017: National Analysis," published September 12, 2018, https://www.childrensdefense.org/wp-content/uploads/2018/09/Child-Poverty-in-America-2017-National-Fact-Sheet.pdf.

115. Children's Defense Fund, "Child Poverty in America 2017: National Analysis."

116. Patrick, "National Snapshot: Poverty Among Women and Families, 2016."

117. Patrick, "National Snapshot: Poverty Among Women and Families, 2016."

118. Patrick, "National Snapshot: Poverty Among Women and Families, 2016."

119. Patrick, "National Snapshot: Poverty Among Women and Families, 2016."

120. Patrick, "National Snapshot: Poverty Among Women and Families, 2016."

121. Juliette Cubanski et al., "How Many Seniors Live in Poverty?" *Henry J Kaiser Family Foundation*, published November 19, 2018, https://www.kff.org/medicare/issue-brief/how-many-seniors-live-in-poverty/.

122. National Council on Aging, "Economic Security for Seniors Facts," last modified 2016. https://www.ncoa.org/news/resources-for-reporters/get-the-facts/economic-security-facts/.

123. National Council on Aging, "Economic Security for Seniors Facts."

124. YiLi Chien and Paul Morris, "Many Americans Still Lack Retirement Savings," *The Regional Economist* 26, no. 1 (2018).

125. William Levernier, "An Analysis of Poverty in the American South: How are Metropolitan Areas different from Nonmetropolitan Areas?" *Contemporary Economic Policy* 21, no. 3 (2003): 372–382.

126. Levernier, "An Analysis of Poverty in the American South," 375.

127. Henry J Kaiser (KFF) Family Foundation, "Poverty Rate by Race/Ethnicity."

128. Henry J Kaiser (KFF) Family Foundation, "Poverty Rate by Race/Ethnicity."

129. Paola Pace, "Migration and the Right to Health: A Review of International Law," *International Organization for Migration.* (2009): 14, https://publications.iom.int/system/files/pdf/iml_19.pdf.

130. Adam Wagstaff, "Poverty and Health Sector Inequalities," *Bulletin of the World Health Organization* 80 (2002): 97.

131. Joachim O. Hero, Alan M. Zaslavsky, and Robert J. Blendon, "The United States Leads Other Nations in Differences by Income in Perceptions of Health and Health Care," *Health Affairs* 36, no. 6 (2017): 1032–1040.

132. Hero, Zaslavsky, and Blendon, "The United States Leads Other Nations in Differences by Income in Perceptions of Health and Health Care."

133. Primary Care Progress, "The Case of Primary Care," accessed September 14, 2018, https://www.primarycareprogress.org/primary-care-case/.

134. Primary Care Progress, "The Case of Primary Care."

135. Leiyu Shi and Barbara Starfield, "Primary Care, Income Inequality, and Self-Rated Health in the United States: A Mixed-Level Analysis," *International Journal of Health Services* 30, no. 3 (2000): 541–555.

136. Ajay Chaudry and Christopher Wimer, "Poverty is Not Just an Indicator: The Relationship between Income, Poverty, and Child Well-Being," *Academic Pediatrics* 16, no. 3 (2016): S23.

137. Chaudry and Wimer, "Poverty is Not Just an Indicator: The Relationship between Income, Poverty, and Child Well-Being," S23.

138. AAP Council on Community Pediatrics, "Poverty and Child Health in the United States," *Pediatrics* 137, no. 4 (2016): e20160339.

139. Neal Halfon and Paul W. Newacheck, "Childhood Asthma and Poverty: Differential Impacts and Utilization of Health Services," *Pediatrics* 91, no. 1 (1993): 59.

140. Michael Marmot, "The Influence of Income On Health: Views of an Epidemiologist," *Health Affairs* 21, no. 2 (2002): 31–46; David Wood, "Effect of

Child and Family Poverty on Child Health in the United States," *Pediatrics* 112, no. 3 (2003): 707–711; Chaudry and Wimer, "Poverty is Not Just an Indicator: The Relationship between Income, Poverty, and Child Well-Being," S23.

141. Wagstaff, "Poverty and Health Sector Inequalities," 98.

142. AAP Council on Community Pediatrics, "Poverty and Child Health in the United States."

143. Kate E. Pickett and Michelle Pearl, "Multilevel Analyses of Neighbourhood Socioeconomic Context and Health Outcomes: A Critical Review," *Journal of Epidemiology & Community Health* 55, no. 2 (2001): 120.

144. Mariana C. Arcaya, Alyssa L. Arcaya, and S. V. Subramanian, "Inequalities in Health: Definitions, Concepts, and Theories," *Global Health Action* 8, no. 1 (2015): 27106.

145. Frank Pega et al., "Unconditional Cash Transfers for Reducing Poverty and Vulnerabilities: Effect On Use of Health Services and Health Outcomes in Low-and Middle-Income Countries," *Cochrane Database of Systematic Reviews* 11 (2017).

146. Pega et al., "Unconditional Cash Transfers for Reducing Poverty and Vulnerabilities."

147. Sarath Raju et al., "Rural Residence and Poverty are Independent Risk Factors for Chronic Obstructive Pulmonary Disease in the United States," *American Journal of Respiratory and Critical Care Medicine* 199, no. 8 (2019): 964.

148. Raju et al., "Rural Residence and Poverty are Independent Risk Factors for Chronic Obstructive Pulmonary Disease in the United States," 964.

149. Michael G. Marmot et al., "Health Inequalities among British Civil Servants: The Whitehall II Study," *The Lancet* 337, no. 8754 (1991): 1387–1393.

150. Hero, Zaslavsky, and Blendon, "The United States Leads Other Nations in Differences by Income in Perceptions of Health and Health Care," 1037.

151. Kochhar, Rakesh, and Anthony Cilluffo, "Income Inequality in the US is Rising Most RAPIDLY AMONG ASIANS," *Pew Research Center* (2018), https://www.pewsocialtrends.org/2018/07/12/income-inequality-in-the-u-s-is-rising-most-rapidly-among-asians/.

152. Kochhar and Cilluffo, "Income Inequality in the US is Rising Most Rapidly Among Asians."

153. Kochhar and Cilluffo, "Income Inequality in the US is Rising Most Rapidly Among Asians."

154. Eric Neumayer and Thomas Plümper, "Inequalities of Income and Inequalities of Longevity: A Cross-Country Study," *American Journal of Public Health* 106, no. 1 (2016): 160–165.

155. Neumayer and Plümper, "Inequalities of Income and Inequalities of Longevity."

156. Hero, Zaslavsky, and Blendon, "The United States Leads Other Nations in Differences by Income in Perceptions of Health and Health Care," 1035.

157. Matthew Johnston, "A Brief History of Income Inequality in the United States," *Investopedia*, last modified June 25, 2019, https://www.investopedia.com/articles/investing/110215/brief-history-income-inequality-united-states.asp.

158. Johnston, "A Brief History of Income Inequality in the United States."

159. Jacob Bor, Gregory H. Cohen, and Sandro Galea, "Population Health in an Era of Rising Income Inequality: USA, 1980–2015," *The Lancet* 389, no. 10077 (2017): 1475.

160. Bor, Cohen, and Galea, "Population Health in an Era of Rising Income Inequality: USA, 1980–2015," 1477.

161. Peter Gottschalk and Sheldon Danziger, "Inequality of Wage Rates, Earnings and Family Income in the United States, 1975–2002," *Review of Income and Wealth* 51, no. 2 (2005): 231.

162. Bor, Cohen, and Galea, "Population Health in an Era of Rising Income Inequality: USA, 1980–2015," 1486.

163. Bor, Cohen, and Galea, "Population Health in an Era of Rising Income Inequality: USA, 1980–2015," 1480.

164. Carlotta Balestra and Richard Tonkin, "Inequalities in Household Wealth Across OECD Countries: Evidence from the OECD Wealth Distribution Database," *OECD Working Paper No. 88*. (2018), http://www.oecd.org/officialdocuments/publicdisplaydocumentpdf/?cote=SDD/DOC(2018)1&docLanguage=En.

165. Balestra and Tonkin, "Inequalities in Household Wealth Across OECD Countries."

166. OECD Wealth Distribution Database, "Wealth," last modified January 2018, https://stats.oecd.org/Index.aspx?DataSetCode=WEALTH.

167. OECD Wealth Distribution Database, "Wealth."

168. Brian Keeley, "What's Happening to Income Inequality?" *Income Inequality: The Gap between Rich and Poor* (Paris: OECD Publishing, 2015), 32.

169. Keeley, "What's Happening to Income Inequality?"

170. Keeley, "What's Happening to Income Inequality?"

171. Raj Chetty et al., "The Fading American Dream: Trends in Absolute Income Mobility since 1940," *Science* 356, no. 6336 (2017): 398–406.

172. John R. Chambers, Lawton K. Swan, and Martin Heesacker, "Perceptions of US Social Mobility Are Divided (And Distorted) Along Ideological Lines," *Psychological Science* 26, no. 4 (2015): 413.

173. Chetty et al., "The Fading American Dream: Trends in Absolute Income Mobility since 1940."

174. Chetty et al., "The Fading American Dream: Trends in Absolute Income Mobility since 1940."

175. Daniel Markovits, *The Meritocracy Trap: How America's Foundational Myth Feed Inequality, Dismantles the Middle Class, and Devours the Elite* (New York: Penguin Press, 2019).

176. Julia B. Isaacs, Isabel V. Sawhill, and Ron Haskins, "Getting Ahead or Losing Ground: Economic Mobility in America," *The Brookings Institute* (2008), https://www.brookings.edu/wp-content/uploads/2016/06/02_economic_mobility_sawhill.pdf.

177. Markovits, *The Meritocracy Trap: How America's Foundational Myth Feed Inequality, Dismantles the Middle Class, and Devours the Elite*, 14.

178. Raj Chetty and Nathaniel Hendren, "The Impacts of Neighborhoods on Intergenerational Mobility II: County-Level Estimates," *The Quarterly Journal of Economics* 133, no. 3 (2018): 1163.

179. Raj Chetty and Nathaniel Hendren, "The Impacts of Neighborhoods on Intergenerational Mobility I: Childhood Exposure Effects," *The Quarterly Journal of Economics* 133, no. 3 (2018): 1107–1162.

180. Raj Chetty et al., "How Does Your Kindergarten Classroom Affect Your Earnings? Evidence from Project STAR," *The Quarterly Journal of Economics* 126, no. 4 (2011): 1593–1660.

181. Jason DeParle, "Harder for Americans to Rise from Lower Rungs," *The New York Times*, published January 4, 2012, https://www.nytimes.com/2012/01/05/us/harder-for-americans-to-rise-from-lower-rungs.html.

182. Seth D. Zimmerman, "Elite Colleges and Upward Mobility To Top Jobs and Top Incomes," *American Economic Review* 109, no. 1 (2019): 1–47.

183. Zimmerman, "Elite Colleges and Upward Mobility To Top Jobs and Top Incomes."

184. Markovits, *The Meritocracy Trap: How America's Foundational Myth Feed Inequality, Dismantles the Middle Class, and Devours the Elite.*

185. Reid Ewing et al., "Does Urban Sprawl Hold Down Upward Mobility?" *Landscape and Urban Planning* 148 (2016): 81.

186. Janny Scott and David Leonhardt, "Shadowy Lines that Still Divide," *The New York Times* (2005), https://www.nytimes.com/2005/05/15/us/class/shadowy-lines-that-still-divide.html.

187. Azim F. Shariff, Dylan Wiwad, and Lara B. Aknin, "Income Mobility Breeds Tolerance for Income Inequality: Cross-National and Experimental Evidence," *Perspectives on Psychological Science* 11, no. 3 (2016): 378.

188. Shariff, Wiwad, and Aknin, "Income Mobility Breeds Tolerance for Income Inequality: Cross-National and Experimental Evidence," 378.

189. Chamber, Swan, and Heesacker, "Perceptions of US Social Mobility are Divided (And Distorted) Along Ideological Lines."

190. Shariff, Wiwad, and Aknin, "Income Mobility Breeds Tolerance for Income Inequality: Cross-National and Experimental Evidence."

191. Gopal K. Singh et al., "Social Determinants of Health in the United States: Addressing Major Health Inequality Trends for the Nation, 1935–2016," *International Journal of MCH and AIDS* 6, no. 2 (2017): 139–164.

192. Singh et al., "Social Determinants of Health in the United States."

193. Bruce P. Kennedy et al., "Income Distribution, Socioeconomic Status, and Self Rated Health in the United States: Multilevel Analysis," *BMJ* 317, no. 7163 (1998): 917–921.

194. Institute for Policy Studies, "Inequality and Health," Accessed December 1, 2019, https://inequality.org/facts/inequality-and-health/.

195. Institute for Policy Studies, "Inequality and Health."

196. Institute for Policy Studies, "Inequality and Health."

197. Institute for Policy Studies, "Inequality and Health"; World Health Organization, "Probability of Dying per 1000 Live Births: Data by Country," last modified October 14, 2019, http://apps.who.int/gho/data/node.main.525?lang=en; OECD Wealth Distribution Database, "Income inequality," last modified 2020, https://data.oecd.org/inequality/income-inequality.htm.

198. Raj Chetty et al., "The Association between Income and Life Expectancy in the United States, 2001–2014," *JAMA* 315, no. 16 (2016): 1750–1766.

199. Bor, Cohen, and Galea, "Population Health in an Era of Rising Income Inequality: USA, 1980–2015."

200. Kennedy et al., "Income Distribution, Socioeconomic Status, and Self Rated Health in the United States: Multilevel Analysis."

201. Shi and Starfield, "Primary Care, Income Inequality, and Self-Rated Health in the United States: A Mixed-Level Analysis," 547.

202. Hero, Zaslavsky, and Blendon, "The United States Leads Other Nations in Differences by Income in Perceptions of Health and Health Care," 1032.

203. Shipler, *The Working Poor: Invisible in America*, 300.

204. Shipler, *The Working Poor: Invisible in America*, 4.

205. Pimpare, *A People's History of Poverty in America*, 3.

Chapter 3

Forgotten but not Gone

Neglected Tropical Disease Risk Factors

In chapter 1, we reviewed some of the NTDs that are currently prevalent in the United States, such as Chagas disease, hookworm, toxocariasis, ascariasis, and trichomoniasis. Whether they were spread through sewage, insect, or sex, the overarching characteristic that all of these diseases have in common is their disproportionately high impact on those living in poverty. In chapter 2, we discussed what poverty in the United States looks like, with the poor living among the rich. In this chapter, we delve into how many low-income Americans live in conditions similar to those typically associated with poverty in low-income countries. Basic human rights such as equal access to adequate sanitation, housing, healthcare, education, and even food are routinely denied to the poorest and most vulnerable Americans. Many of those impacted by the policies and laws that shaped their lives in the last centuries are so far entrapped in the cycle of poverty that they are unable to escape. For this reason, although NTDs have been mostly forgotten, we cannot assume that the conditions that cause them to thrive do not exist. They did not disappear with the modernization and industrialization.

This chapter breaks down some of the risk factors associated with NTDs and examines them in the context of poverty in the United States. Some of these risk factors are more closely associated with NTDs than others. For instance, there is an obvious association between stray animals and the soil-transmitted helminths. However, the relationship between a centuries-old tradition of eating dirt and disease prevention or prevalence may be less obvious. Although the topics of sanitation, housing, education, employment, health access, climate change, natural disasters, and geophagy may not immediately appear related, they each represent a unique facet within the cycle of poverty that leaves millions of Americans vulnerable to NTDs.

SANITATION OVERVIEW

Each November 19th, the world celebrates a peculiar holiday—World Toilet Day. This event, established in 2001, seeks to bring awareness to the global sanitation crisis and the 4.2 billion people without access to safely managed sanitation.[1] The World Health Organization defines sanitation as the provision of facilities and services for the safe management of human excreta from the toilet to containment and storage and treatment on-site or conveyance, with more broad definitions including the disposal of animal waste as well.[2] The United Nations Sustainable Development Goals dedicate an entire goal to improving sanitation and access to drinking water, particularly in low-income countries in sub-Saharan Africa, Central Asia, Southern Asia, Eastern Asia, and Southeastern Asia.[3] Yet, wealthy countries like the United States still struggle to provide this basic human right and essential service to its most isolated and low-income residents. This struggle of marginalized populations is hardly a new occurrence. They have long grappled with those with power to enact changes for the provision of basic sanitation services.

As of 2014, an estimated half million households in the United States did not have access to complete plumbing facilities such as hot and cold running water, a flushing toilet, and a shower or bathtub.[4] A statement by Professor Philip Alston, United Nations Special Rapporteur on Extreme Poverty and Human Rights highlighted some of these issues, which he encountered on his visit to the United States in 2017. He stated that the United States ranks thirty-sixth in the world for water and sanitation, and recalled encounters with, "sewage filled yards in states where governments don't consider sanitation facilities to be their responsibility."[5] Additionally, a study conducted in central Appalachia found poor sanitation to be a community health risk in rural areas where the dispersal of untreated sewage into watersheds is associated with high fecal contamination levels.[6] This is an important reminder that simply having the ability to flush waste down the toilet does not make the problem disappear.[7] The presence of sewage in places where people walk, play, and live each day is a significant risk factor for many diseases, including NTDs. In fact, the primary method of transmission for hookworm and roundworm is through contaminated soil associated with sanitary facilities.[8]

Bacterial infections, such as *Campylobacter, Escherichia coli*, *Leptospira*, *Salmonella*, *Shigella*, *Yersinia enterocolitica*, can spread through contact with sewage or sewage contaminated water. All of these bacteria cause diarrheal illness and a range of other symptoms.[9] Hepatitis A and Polio are two viruses that spread through sewage. Even viruses spread through vectors can experience increased proliferation due to the presence of sewage. Both St. Louis Encephalitis and West Nile Virus Encephalitis are transmitted by *Culex* mosquitoes, who seek out polluted and foul water to lay their eggs. Parasites like *Necator americanus*, *Giardia intestinalis*, and *Cryptosporidium parvum* also thrive in sewage. Additionally, inadequate garbage disposal or collection services create breeding sites for some of the vectors that spread NTDs. Once exposed to the environment, the diseases mentioned above have varying life expectancies. Protozoa can potentially last for days, viruses and bacteria for months, and helminths for years.[10] Contaminated sewage can spread to waterways and local wells that individuals may rely on for drinking water if they are unable to pay for the installation of lines that connect to the municipal water system. If they are even aware of the contamination, they are often forced to make a decision between drinking contaminated water, consuming water substitutes such as sugary beverages, or buying more expensive bottled water.[11] Successful programs that provide adequate access to quality sanitation and water can decrease the association between poverty and disease.[12]

Although water and sanitation systems are integral to the prevention of disease and overall public health, these systems have become a neglected investment. The intended operational life of existing equipment is nearing its end in many areas, creating a severe need for system repairs.[13] Millions of dollars are lost due to damage caused by thousands of water pipes bursting each year as a result of this neglect. Meanwhile, the expansion of these services is out of reach for other areas altogether. This is especially true for those not connected to municipal water-treatment plants in regions such as Appalachia and the Black Belt of the Southern United States.

Historically, sanitation systems were managed primarily on a local basis. This changed when the Great Depression led to infrastructural investments as a way to revitalize the economy and provide additional employment opportunities.[14] The establishment of the Public Works Administration, along with its accompanying $3.3 billion in financing, resulted in the massive expansion of new sewage system construction projects and upgrades.[15] Population shifts toward suburban areas following World War II placed increasing strains on the abilities of municipalities to provide services, and septic systems were utilized to fill the gap. Additionally, growing concern over environmental pollution led to the 1948 Federal Water Pollution Control Act, which allocated $22.5 million each year over a five-year period to states for the purpose of constructing wastewater treatment facilities.[16] Amendments later doubled the amount of funding available for this purpose and created regulations such as the Federal Water Pollution Control Administration, which is now known as the Federal Water Quality Administration.

From 1965 to 1983, the Water Resources Council was the entity "charged with the responsibility of assessing the nation's water supplies, coordinating plans for larger programs, weighing the costs and benefits of project plans, making policy recommendations, and allocating money to states for planning grants."[17] Then in 1972, the Clean Water Act and its subsequent amendments provided unprecedented levels of federal funding for the construction of wastewater treatment infrastructure. Shortly afterward in 1974, the passage of the Safe Drinking Water Act established the first regulatory program for the cooperation of federal, state, and local levels to manage water systems.[18] Although the Environmental Protection Agency established the national drinking water standards at the federal level, it would be up to each state to determine their own regulation methods to enforce these standards. The 1980s saw a shift toward military funding in lieu of federal investment in infrastructure. As construction grants were replaced by the State Revolving Fund, funding for water and sanitation infrastructure has continuously lessened over time.[19] Additionally, existing wastewater management rules and regulations often lack effective enforcement mechanisms. Oftentimes, the responsibility is divided among multiple state or local government agencies. Many of these agencies lack the resource capacity to monitor individual septic systems or those in rural or isolated areas.[20] The regulation and enforcement activity that does occur is typically focused on the initial planning or construction of the system, compounding the overall lack of accountability for ensuring that these systems are sustainable in the long-term.

Today, over three-quarters of Americans are served by municipal water-treatment plants, which utilize a network of pipes to carry wastewater to the treatment plants.[21] This waste undergoes primary treatment as the liquid and solid wastes are separated, and secondary treatment when bacteria breaks down contaminants before being killed off by chlorine. At this stage, other contaminants are optionally removed as well, utilizing a variety of specialized processes. Finally, if it meets federal regulatory standards, the treated waste is released to a nearby body of water. If standards are not met, the untreated waste may be released to surface water, causing potentially serious problems in the surrounding environment. Additionally, malfunctions in both private and public sewage lines can result in structural failure, blockages, and overflows. The Environmental Protection Agency (EPA) estimates that 23,000 to 75,000 of these overflows occur each year.[22]

The remaining 23 percent of Americans utilize septic tank systems buried underground on their property.[23] Similar to water-treatment plants, waste that is flushed into a septic tank is also separated into liquid and solid layers. While the solids form a sludge that must be routinely removed, the liquids flow into a drain field in the soil. There, microbes are tasked with the consumption of bacteria, viruses, and nutrients. A properly designed and maintained septic tank will prevent this waste from entering surface or groundwater sources. However, the soil type the septic tank operates in can play a major role in its ability to carry out these functions properly.

Soil is formed from mixtures of clay, silt, and sand. The dominant soil type in the Southeastern United States is ultisols, which are characterized by low native fertility, subsurface clay accumulations, and their reddish appearance due to iron oxides.[24] This soil type is typically located in humid tropical and subtropical climates, as found in the Southern United States. Although these soil conditions are ideal for agricultural cotton production, the high clay content of soils in the South is highly detrimental for sanitation. This is due to the fact that clay soils are not able to absorb the water and liquid waste emitted by the septic tank. As such, the drain field of the septic tank often becomes backed up and can cause flooding back into the resident's bathtub or sink or the pooling of sewage in their yards. These conditions are exacerbated by seasonal weather conditions, such as heavy rainfall from thunderstorms and tropical storms.[25] Rural areas that are not within close proximity to municipal sewages rely on septic tanks that frequently do not maintain proper function when placed in soils with a high clay content.

Lowndes County, mentioned earlier for the discovery of hookworm infections among its residents, is a place where conditions such as these are a harsh reality. Despite a publication by the Alabama Department of Public Health denying the existence of hookworm, another study conducted in 1993 found similar results. This study was a survey of children living in nearby Wilcox County and it found that approximately one-third of those under the age of ten tested positive for at least one kind of helminth infection.[26] As such, sewage and soil contamination has the potential to impact many residents. The Natural Resources Conservation Service's Soil Limitations Rating System categorizes Lowndes County as "very limited" in terms of septic tank absorption fields.[27] The Alabama Department of Public Health estimates that "between 40 to 90 percent of homes have either inadequate or no septic system . . . and half of the septic systems that have been installed aren't working properly."[28] This problem is worsened by the criminalization of these leaky sewage systems. For instance, residents in Alabama have been prosecuted by the state for failing to comply with health codes related to sewage disposal.

While the Alabama Department of Public Health regulates on-site sewage systems, many of the residents that experience these problems live in unincorporated areas of the county. These areas are less wealthy than more urbanized cities and counties, and typically are unable to build up the necessary tax base that would make connecting these areas to municipal systems financially manageable for local governments. In cases where management entities experienced problems regulating their sanitation system, health code violations were addressed through an administrative process rather than criminal charges. In contrast, individual residents facing similar problems were subject to fines, criminal charges for a Class C misdemeanor, arrest, or serving jail time.[29] In 2002, the Lowndes County Health Department found that thirty-seven families were threatened with jail time because their dwellings were in violation of state health code due to lack of properly working septic systems.[30] Frequently, the residents were unable to pay a fine due to the same income shortage that led to their inability to pay for an adequate septic tank or repairs to begin with.

Furthermore, when some residents were able to obtain the funds to pay for a septic tank, they were told that only septic systems specifically designed for individual properties would be deemed acceptable by the health department.[31] In one instance, even when a resident did pay to have an engineer design and install a system, it was deemed "makeshift" and "bootleg."[32] Whether residents struggle to resolve failures to meet health code standards or continue without effort toward the issue, the resulting outcome of fines is often the same. In some cases, arrests resulted from the inability to pay fines, which in turn detract from the funds residents have available to work toward fixing the problem. This cycle is a direct outcome of the "criminalization of poverty."[33] When these efforts failed to yield results, some residents who were unable to install engineer-designed septic systems faced the possibility of eviction or removal from their own properties.

Because of the fear generated by outcomes such as this, residents may distrust health officials and fail to report issues with their sanitation system. At one point, the state health department in Alabama had cited approximately 700 people within a year.[34] Although they serve as a regulatory agency by issuing citations when residents fail to apply with health code standards, local and state health departments often lack the resources to make improvements. They are able to provide residents with lists of engineers and installers to work on their septic systems, and suggestions for where to apply for grants such as the U.S. Department of Agriculture's rural development program.[35] However, the paperwork to qualify is extensive. Some programs require documents such as a current driver's license and home insurance information, which can be difficult for some low-income or elderly individuals to provide.[36] Typically, those who understand their community needs best, such as nonprofits and individuals, are ineligible to apply for federal funding for sanitation infrastructural improvements.[37] Despite this, these individual property and homeowners are primarily responsible for the costly burden of sanitation, even when the conditions and costs surpass the abilities and capacity of their own local and state governments.[38] In terms of enforcement, health departments rely on local police enforcement and the judicial system to carry out the criminal process of punishing those who fail to comply.

Despite the threat of prosecution, some refuse to pay for a failing septic system when they feel like it is the responsibility of their local and state government to expand services to their area. As an example, Bishop Ira McCloud, pastor of the Jesus Christ Church of God the Bibleway of the Apostolic Faith in Pike County, Alabama, was arrested after an adjoining property owner complained to the health department that the church's newly purchased septic tank failed and began flooding his property.[39] This occurred despite the fact that the church was within close proximity of municipal sewer lines. Once his case was thrown out due to a corporate loophole, Bishop McCloud successfully sued the city in order to have the church connected to the municipal system. With connections to municipal systems often unavailable, and the unreliability and costly nature of septic systems, some residents resort to straight piping their waste. Straight piping utilizes a network of pipes to route waste from indoor toilets to disposal areas outdoors, where it remains "untreated and uncontained, accessible by animals and people."[40] Despite the fact that straight piping is illegal, the use of such systems is widespread among poor, rural communities in Appalachia and Southeastern United States.[41]

Although several urban and rural areas of the United States struggle from lack of access and affordability of sanitation, there is insufficient demographic data available, with the last national census data on sanitation collected three decades ago.[42] While it is difficult to grasp the full extent of this problem throughout the entirety of the American South, the Alabama Center for Rural Enterprise has made significant strides in finding ways to identify and address these issues. In 2013, the nonprofit utilized funding from the FY '02 Appropriations Act in conjunction with the EPA's National Decentralized Wastewater Demonstration Project to conduct house-to-house surveys. Later in 2015, they collaborated with students, faculty, and staff from Duke University to revise these survey questions and gain a more accurate picture of household perceptions of water infrastructure and their communication with local government and nongovernment officials regarding these concerns. The survey found that approximately half of the respondents in Hayneville considered raw sewage a severe community issue, and about a quarter lived on a property with a malfunctioning septic tank.[43]

RACE AND SANITATION

Historically, race has impacted the accessibility of sanitation. Native American, Alaskan Native, black, and Latino households are all at increased risk of experiencing "plumbing poverty" in clusters and regions of the United States.[44] Households with incomplete plumbing are often found in clusters with other households facing similar problems.[45] In areas where wastewater infrastructure is generally thought to be sufficient, individuals without plumbing may not be visible enough to render attention from regulation authorities. Policies fail to account for the role of race and systemic barriers to overcoming these problems, such as substandard housing, lack of healthcare access, limited access to high-quality educational opportunities, and barriers to employment. Instead, individuals are isolated, punished, and even criminalized for their inability to meet the standard living conditions.[46] In the case of Lowndes County, African Americans have historically been expected to overcome such barriers despite the fact that they were often only permitted to live on the worst land in the county. While, historically, whites owned land for cotton production at higher elevations with better drainage, African Americans were typically only able to acquire land in lowland areas that were less productive and flooded more frequently.[47]

Throughout history, marginalized communities are often excluded from sewer infrastructure and the economic development that accompanies it. In America, it seems as though the accessibility of water and sanitation revolves around economic incentives even more so than social divisions. Areas without preexisting connections to water and sanitation services are poor candidates for attracting new businesses. Because of this, these rural, low-income areas remain stagnant due to limited employment opportunities and growth within their community. These areas also lose out on tax revenues contingent on the presence of businesses and large populations. Consequently, the areas continue to lack the revenue to formulate a tax base necessary to fund such infrastructural improvements. Sales and property taxes are regressive, and deduct a greater percentage of income from individuals with low socioeconomic status. Direct charges, which are often used for sewers and sanitation services, are even more regressive because the charge does not adjust depending on the home's value.[48]

The Unique Challenge of Sanitation in Colonias

While some experience extreme difficulties managing their septic tanks, others lack this basic infrastructure entirely. An example of where these conditions are common are American colonias, which often do not have access to septic or sewage systems, drinking water, electricity, or adequate housing. Colonias describes the residential area of a town in Mexican Spanish, and is the term used for more than 2,000 communities that are primarily located in Texas.[49] Many colonia residents, measured at 35 percent by 2014, were born in another country before migrating to the United States. Rather than moving farther north, these migrants settled near the border in order to stay closer to relatives, remain in a community accepting of Latino culture and language, and because they often lacked pre-established connections such as relatives or friends in the United States that would provide a support network.[50] Forty percent of colonia residents live below the poverty line, while another 20 percent live precisely at or slightly above it.[51] Although efforts have been made to improve colonias in recent years, there were still 337 of these communities without basic infrastructure by 2014.[52]

Colonia communities consist of a mixture of trailers, small traditionally built homes, and makeshift shacks. Oftentimes roads are unpaved and garbage is discarded and burned outdoors.[53] These low standards of living result in poorer health outcomes for colonia residents. For example, a study of data tracked by the Texas Department of State Health Services found that counties containing colonias had a higher risk of hospitalization for infectious diseases than those that did not. These infectious diseases include Amebiasis, Brucellosis, Candidiasis, Chickenpox, Coccidioidomycosis, ill-defined intestinal infections, intestinal infections due to other organisms, bacterial food poisoning, rickettsioses, salmonella infections, typhus, viral exanthemata, pulmonary tuberculosis, septicemia, shigellosis, disease due to coxsackie virus, typhoid and paratyphoid fevers, and Whooping cough.[54]

Those in positions of political power have few incentives to prioritize the needs of colonia residents, as many are unable to vote. As such, the Texas state government allowed these areas to remain largely unregulated. This land was often sold to low-income Latinos by developers, who charged interest rates as high as 25 percent and refused to relinquish the property title until it was paid for in full.[55] If a payment was missed, the purchaser risked losing their land, house, and the money they had already put down toward the property. As many of the purchasers were agricultural workers, settling down in rural lands that are close to widely available jobs made property in the colonias seemed to be an affordable option compared to other housing opportunities.

However, the developers did nothing to provide basic services to these properties, which were under high demand although they lacked access to water, electricity, or sewage systems. It took until 1989 for the Texas legislature to request that state agencies develop rules that require new residential developments to have access to water and sewer services.[56] Still, residents now struggle to meet the requirements of local building codes in order to be connected to these municipal water and sewage systems. Additionally, the cost of installing water and sewers in homes sometimes exceeds the value of the residence itself, making such improvements impractical.[57]

One example of this is in Elgin, where the Elgin Bank of Texas bought 150 acres in Travis County in the 1990s with the intention of subdividing it without first getting the county's approval of a plat, or plot blueprints.[58] Travis County officials argued that local code indicated that developers needed permission from the county before subdividing an area was allowed. However, Elgin Bank selected other parts from the local government code that stated a plat was only necessary if the land was intended for public use and for the establishment of new roads. Although the judge first ruled in favor of Travis County, the courts later overturned this ruling "in support of the developers' interest and age-old Texas property rights."[59] This decision enabled developers to sell properties under horrible conditions. For example, the lack of adequate access to roads on these properties made it difficult for county fire and emergency respondents to reach residences. Although legislators and lobbyists have worked over time to remedy situations such as the one created by Elgin Bank, the problem of development occurring before infrastructure is in place remains a difficult issue to solve. One solution, offered by the Texas Water Development Board, enables counties that adhere to their Model Subdivision Rules eligible for state-funded grants through the Economically Distressed Area Program.[60] However, developers complain that these rules cause extensive financial strain to fulfill these regulations before the land has even sold. Cases such as this present a clear idea of just how complicated and politically charged these issues can be for communities in states that have historically favored land rights.

What's Next?

State and local officials and leaders will need to secure funding for wastewater projects, particularly those that provide grants to nonprofits and individuals for the purpose of helping homeowners make improvements to their wastewater infrastructure. Policy-makers should also allocate more funding to programs such as the Clean Water State Revolving Fund, Water Pollution Control Grant, and ARC Community Infrastructure Grants to improve publicly available wastewater infrastructure. To improve the longevity of these systems, increased funding will also be needed to give state and local agencies the resources they need to effectively monitor and regulate the systems within their jurisdiction.[61] Short-term solutions for residents to reduce the spread of NTDs despite inadequate sanitation infrastructure includes removing or covering places where water collects outdoors to reduce the number of breeding sites where mosquitoes can proliferate near homes. Gutters, drains, discarded tires, trash, or rain buckets that allow for standing water create perfect breeding ground for mosquitoes. Environmentally friendly mosquito dunks can offer an affordable solution to sources of water that are unable to be drained, such as small pools, ponds, or ditches.[62] In the next section, we will discuss how other inadequate housing factors can contribute to a greater risk of NTD infection.

HOUSING

Dengue, chikungunya, Zika, yellow fever, Chagas, and leishmaniasis are all spread by vectors, or insects that carry parasites and viruses that can make people sick. Screening on windows, doors, and eaves can reduce the likelihood that *Aedes*, *Anopheles*, and *Culex* mosquitoes, sand flies, or triatomines are able to infiltrate homes.[63] Additionally, the condition of the exterior and interior of the house is important to prevent insects from entering residences. Reducing the number of cracks in the walls, floors, and ceilings will reduce the number of entry points available to mosquitoes, triatomines, sandflies, and other pests. When implemented alongside other vector-control management strategies, housing improvements have perhaps the greatest chance at reducing the impact of NTDs that are vector-borne.[64]

Although NTD interventions that prevent vectors from proliferating near and inside homes through housing improvements can be highly effective in managing vectors, the cost of the interventions and the lack of substantial clinical evidence supporting the epidemiological impact of such interventions has led to the role of housing in vector management to be trivialized throughout history.[65] While some of the interventions listed are easy to implement, others are much harder for struggling, low-income individuals and families. Oftentimes, housing can be the largest expense of a household's budget.[66] A study of urban mothers who were reliant on welfare found that the mothers made paying for housing and food a priority before using what was left, typically an insufficient amount, to pay other bills.[67] Another study of low-income populations of color in the Southern United States found that renters and households in urban areas had more options for adequate housing in comparison to rural areas.[68] Although NTDs often impact those living in low-income rural areas, there are some NTDs that present a health threat to those living in low-income urban areas as well.[69]

Subsidized housing, or sharing housing with family or roommates, can reduce the burden of this expense, but the overall burden of the cost of housing as a proportion of the earned wages of a low-income individual or family can be daunting. A national report found that over one-third of households experiencing low levels of food security had to choose between paying their rent or mortgage and purchasing food, while over half of those experiencing very low food security had to face the same decision.[70] Aside from the cost of paying rent or the mortgage, occupants also have to pay for water, electricity, and other services depending on their availability. Even this portion of the cost of housing can be a substantial burden. The same study found that nearly half of those with low food security had to choose between paying for utilities and food, with an even larger percentage of families with very low food security caught in the same dilemma.[71] For these reasons, even low-cost interventions to improve the conditions of housing are financially out of reach for some. Housing codes are a mechanism to enforce the requirement of screens in residences, however lessons from sanitation enforcement discussed in the previous section shows that such requirements often serve to further marginalize, and possibly criminalize, those who are already facing substantial financial difficulties.[72]

The Elements of Adequate Housing

According to the United Nations Human Rights Office of the High Commissioner, "the human right to adequate housing is more than just four walls and a roof. It is the right of every woman, man, youth and child to gain and sustain a safe and secure home and community in which to live in peace and dignity."[73] Their *Right to Adequate Housing Toolkit* lays out the several elements that make up the components of adequate housing.[74] The first is legal security of tenure, in which the occupants have legal protection to prevent forced eviction or threats that force the occupants to become displaced. Perhaps the elements of housing adequacy that are most visible detractions for the current housing accessible to low-income individuals are the affordability, habitability, accessibility, and location of housing.

Accessibility refers to adequate measures in place to prevent discrimination against marginalized and disadvantaged individuals.[75] Today, housing opportunities available to marginalized populations are molded by several factors, including "(1) federal housing policies, (2) institutional and individual discrimination in housing markets, (3) geographic changes that have taken place in the nation's urban centers, and (4) limited incomes."[76] Historically, racial discrimination has been a major cause of the disparities that currently exist in housing availability and quality. The Federal Housing Administration exacerbated the effects of segregation by providing subsidies to builders who constructed subdivisions that specifically prohibited African Americans from living in them, while simultaneously refusing to insure mortgages around neighborhoods where African Americans lived.[77] The Fair Housing Act, passed in 1968, outlawed housing discrimination on the basis of race, color, religion, sex, familial status, national origin, or disability.[78] Yet, marginalized populations in the Southern United States continue to face difficulty accessing housing due to a number of factors, including higher levels of worst-case needs renters. Worst-case needs renters are those with low incomes that are less than half the median income of their area of residence, the cost of their rent is more than half of their income, or live in substandard or inadequate housing.[79] Worst-case needs renters are more prevalent in the West and Southern United States, especially in urban suburbs where housing assistance is more unavailable. Among those with worst-case needs, 45.5 percent are non-Hispanic white renters, 23.5 percent are Hispanic renters, and 21.7 percent were non-Hispanic black renters.[80] However, when compared to the demographics of the population, non-Hispanic blacks and Hispanic renters are over-represented.[81] Many of the communities of color that were impacted by policies fueled by discrimination have remained trapped in the same low-income areas decades later. Others have been pushed out by gentrification, as the rising cost of rent and property values makes it impossible for the original occupants to rent and homeowners to afford. Much of the housing that does remain available to those living in poverty is in poor condition.

The element of habitability means that spacing should be sufficient, and that protection from the elements such as the cold, damp, heat, rain, and disease vectors, is offered.[82] The American Housing Survey measures physical adequacy of a housing unit based off of whether or not the unit contains hot and cold running water, a bathtub or shower, flushing toilets, plumbing facilities, electricity, heating, exposed wiring, water leaks, holes in the floor, wide cracks, large areas of peeling paint, and rodent infestation.[83] However, if the maintenance costs exceed what occupants are able to pay in order to fix these conditions, occupants may be forced to abandon the unit, or landlords may upgrade the unit to charge an increased price that the current occupants are no longer able to afford.[84] One survey found that 15 percent of low-income renter housing has moderate to severe physical inadequacies.[85]

The availability of services, materials, facilities, and infrastructure is an element requiring that occupants are provided with access to safe drinking water, sanitation, and utilities such as electricity to cook, heat, and light the housing.[86] As discussed in the previous sections, lack of sanitation and plumbing is clearly a burden on many households in the Southern United States and Appalachia. The accessibility and affordability of clean water is also a barrier. As discussed with sanitation, rural and isolated areas are often not connected to municipal lines. Even when households are connected to the municipal water supply, this does not guarantee they are provided with clean water. More than one-tenth of households in the United States are unable to afford the price of their water bills.[87] Because many of these households are often clustered together, utility companies may face difficulties when large proportions of their customers are unable to afford their services. Utilities and electricity are absent in many homes for varying lengths of time. Almost a third of households in the United States report that they have faced hardship in order to pay their utility bill, with higher percentages of Latinos and racial minorities experiencing similar difficulties.[88] In 2018, over 900,000 households in Texas had their utilities cut off due to unpaid bills.[89] A study aimed at identifying predictors of hardships in affording utilities found that compared to changes in income and household composition, a household member becoming ill was the strongest indication that the household would have difficulty.[90] Although the federal Low-Income Home Energy Assistance Program and other state programs were created to reduce the burden of utilities among low-income households, less than one-fifth of eligible households participate in LIHEAP.[91] The high rates of households without electricity, clean water, and sanitation means that many households in the United States fall short of meeting the availability of services element.

Lastly, the element of location means that the housing must be within range of employment opportunities, schools, and healthcare facilities.[92] The accessibility of education, employment, and healthcare will be discussed later in this chapter. However, another important aspect of housing is that the housing should not be in an area that exposes occupants to pollution sites. Low-income communities and communities with higher concentrations of people of color are at greater risk for exposure to air pollution. Even when the air quality is considered acceptable by federal health standards, fine particulate matter created by sources such as diesel engines, power plants, and refineries, is still a health concern.[93] Soot, as it is commonly referred to, and other air pollutants can cause a range of negative health outcomes such as asthma, cardiovascular problems, lung disease, cancer, and low birth weights.[94] A study conducted in the United States found that although white individuals consume and generate more pollution than African Americans and Latinos, they breathe approximately 17 percent less pollution than they cause.[95] In contrast, African American and Latino individuals breathe in air with over 50 percent more pollution than they cause. Additionally, the use of pesticides by the agriculture industry in rural areas of the Southern United States has raised concerns that poor communities with high concentrations of African American residents are disproportionately exposed to these chemicals. This can be seen extensively throughout the Mississippi Delta.[96] Pesticides that are sprayed from elevated heights often drift away from their intended target and toward nearby homes and schools. Pesticide drift has been proven to cause a vast array of negative health outcomes, especially for children.[97] The chemicals are known to cause "dermatological, gastrointestinal, neurological, carcinogenic, respiratory, reproductive, and endocrine effects."[98]

Even worse, some low-income communities are intentionally polluted for profit. A small community in Jefferson County, Alabama, named West Jefferson, became a literal dumping ground for human feces.[99] A nearby landfill named Big Sky Environmental, one of Alabama's 173 operational landfills, was the destination for the transportation of waste from New York and New Jersey. For residents of West Jefferson, the smell of the waste was unbearable. The odor became so bad that residents had difficulty breathing and began having headaches. Although heavy protests from the residents halted further shipments of waste, many poor, rural communities with large proportions of residents who are people of color remain dumping grounds. Cheap land surrounding low-income communities with little political clout have never been high on the political agenda, and waste management companies have capitalized on these communities' invisibility. If they are able, residents surrounding the landfill property are often forced to abandon their homes due to the living conditions brought about by the landfills, while those who remain are pressured into selling their devalued lands so that landfills can continue to expand. Although the residents of these areas are predominately people of color, previous rulings by the EPA have refused to take accountability for the role of discrimination in these occurrences. Environmental injustices such as these cause negative health outcomes for low-income populations and minorities, and contribute to a lack of housing that meets the requirements for the location element of adequate housing.

CONCLUSION

Many Americans in the Southern United States are unable to afford and access adequate housing. A great deal of the housing that is available to low-income households is often of poor quality. Many households struggle to afford basic utilities such as electricity, water, and sanitation. This makes most housing interventions that would reduce the impact of vector-borne NTDs unattainable. Because of this, these communities remain vulnerable to disease, in addition to other negative health outcomes that result from living in inadequate housing. Lastly, it is important to note that one facet of poverty and housing has greatly been overlooked in existing literature in relation to NTD research. Research regarding the impacts of homelessness on vulnerability to NTD infections in the United States is largely absent. This is a large void of information, given that over 500,000 Americans are homeless.[100] As of 2018, over 40 percent of the homeless population consists of African Americans, while 21 percent consists of Latinos.[101] The housing crisis in the Western United States has created a boom of homelessness in several cities, where even moderately well-employed residents are unable to afford housing.[102] Still, even more Americans living in poverty are at risk of homelessness. Because homeless individuals are the most vulnerable populations to disease, it will be important to address this gap moving forward.

FOOD INSECURITY

In the previous section, we discussed how low-income families often grapple with food insecurity as they struggle to afford expenses such as housing. As of 2016, over 40 million Americans lived in households lacking food security.[103] This figure closely resembles the number of individuals in the United States living in poverty. However, rates of food insecurity are not equally distributed across the geography of the United States. Although food insecurity impacts many areas, rates are particularly high in the Appalachia, Mississippi Delta, and along the Texas-Mexico border.[104] Southern states have the highest rates of food insecurity, especially in rural areas.[105] Food insecurity is defined by the USDA as "a household-level economic and social condition of limited or uncertain access to adequate food."[106] While food insecurity does not directly cause infection with NTDs, it acts as a risk factor that exacerbates the effects of the infection and leaves the individual more vulnerable to malnourishment.

NTDs, specifically parasitic and bacterial infections, are often in direct competition with the human body for nutrition.[107] Of these, soil-transmitted helminths are most closely tied to undernutrition.[108] In the United States, *Ascaris lumbricoides* and *Necator americanus*, the worms responsible for ascariasis and hookworm infection, are the most likely culprits of undernutrition. Even in individuals who are well-fed, infection with intestinal worms can lead to malnutrition as nutrients are drained through diarrhea and intestinal bleeding, which causes anemia.[109] For individuals and families who already struggle to afford or access food, these infections undermine the value and utility of what little nutrition they are able to absorb from the resources they do have. Because of this, food insecurity is a significant risk factor in both an individual's vulnerability to NTDs, as well as the severity of resulting health outcomes from the infection.

A vicious cycle is created where an infected individual's body increases its metabolic rate in an attempt to defend against the infection, burning nutrients and energy more quickly in the process.[110] The body's ability to absorb nutrients is inhibited, leading to further undernutrition, which only makes the body even more vulnerable to diseases. Deficiencies in macronutrients such as protein, as well as micronutrients, such as iron, zinc, and vitamins, cause the body to be increasingly susceptible to infection.[111] Zinc deficiency in particular inhibits the ability of the body to heal from wounds, which diminishes the integrity of the skin to act as a barrier to infection.[112] Undernourished individuals also experience greater severity when affected by other illnesses.[113] Because of this dilemma, the role of nutrition in NTD infections creates a chicken and egg question. Did lack of access to nutritional foods and impoverished conditions cause the infection, or did the infection itself cause undernourishment?[114] Oftentimes, the answer is both. Many NTDs worsen undernutrition by increasing the number of calories the body needs to function, while simultaneously draining the body of nutrients.[115]

Causes and Severity of Food Insecurity

Educational attainment, wages, the accessibility of public transportation, and a variety of other socioeconomic factors influence food insecurity. Although food insecurity is strongly associated with poverty, it is not limited to those of low socioeconomic status.[116] There are many other causes and factors that facilitate food insecurity in the United States. Geographical location and social isolation can make accessing food on a regular basis a difficult task, especially for the elderly and disabled. Inability to access nutritious food in particular may lead to individuals settling for cheaper or more accessible fast food options instead.[117] The negative health outcomes resulting in undernutrition, such as chronic illnesses or disabilities, may make it even more difficult for individuals to seek out healthy foods. Additionally, many individuals who are food insecure also lack access to health insurance to seek treatment for medical problems associated with undernutrition.[118] This makes seeking affordable healthcare for food-insecurity related illnesses extremely difficult.

Another cause of food insecurity are the "food deserts" created by diminishing numbers of grocery stores as local stores are replaced by large supermarket chains.[119] This is particularly true for rural areas. Food deserts leave individuals unable to access affordable and quality food options.[120] Especially for those lacking transportation, traveling to the grocery store to buy fresh food can be an unattainable.[121] Sometimes, chains like Dollar Generals are the only businesses aside from convenience stores where residents are able to buy food.[122] Although these stores offer some cheaper options, it can also result in local businesses closing up shop. Rural residents are hit particularly hard by the impact of food deserts, especially given that rural communities often do not have local programs and support that are available in urban areas, such as food banks and soup kitchens.[123] Oftentimes, the stores that are available carry primarily processed foods and lack options to purchase healthy, fresh fruits, vegetables, and whole-grain products. Although an individual may be food insecure, they might not necessarily be hungry. Poverty is associated with the intake of affordable, energy dense foods, which in turn may lead to an excess in caloric consumption and weight gain.[124] One study found that low-income, food-insecure households had a higher prevalence of children who were overweight in comparison with high-income, food-secure households.[125] Obesity is highly prevalent in the United States, and the costs of childhood obesity in particular are especially disturbing, with consequential increases in both morbidity and premature mortality.[126]

There are varying degrees of severity for food security, as determined by the U.S. Department of Agriculture's Guide to Measuring Food Security.[127] Four main categories are used to determine where households fall in terms of food insecurity severity. If a household is considered food secure, it means that there is insufficient evidence that the household is food insecure. Food insecure without hunger defines households where there is evidence that the food supply is inadequate or is of reduced quality, as well as the presence of unusual coping patterns. However, in this classification minimal reduction in food intake occurs. Households that are moderately food insecure with hunger are defined by the household's adults reducing their nutritional intake to the degree that they regularly experience hunger. This is raised to the most severe category when the children of the household are also forced to reduce food intake to the degree that they regularly experience hunger. While this does not account for all of the dimensions of food insecurity, it provides a measurable scale.

Programs Targeting Food Insecurity

The contributions of food banks, soup kitchens, grocery stores, restaurants, and shelters play a major role in reducing food insecurity at a local level.[128] Aside from the many private food assistance networks and programs that combat food insecurity across America, there are also various federal programs in the United States aimed at reducing food insecurity. The most expansive program is the Supplemental Nutrition Assistance Program, or SNAP. Although established by the Food Stamp Act of 1964, SNAP did not become a national program until a decade later. The program is targeted toward low-income families and to be eligible a household's gross income must be under 130 percent of the poverty line, net income cannot exceed the household-size specific poverty line, and its total assets must not exceed $2,000, or $3,000 if there is a senior or disabled individual.[129] SNAP allows beneficiaries to purchase food from authorized retail food outlets. However, 54 percent of SNAP-recipient households, and over 25 percent of households just above the eligibility requirements, are still food insecure.[130] Despite the obvious benefits of SNAP, many who are eligible do not apply. SNAP requires that individuals recertify their eligibility, and the cost of transportation or taking time off from work to travel to the office are often infeasible for low-income individuals. Additionally, individuals may fear the stigmatization they receive as a result of redeeming SNAP benefits.

Other programs are targeted specifically toward mothers and children. One such program is the Special Supplemental Nutrition Program for Women, Infants, and Children (WIC). In addition to receiving food tailored to fit the nutritional requirements of pregnant and new mothers, infants, and young children, WIC has additional benefits such as nutritional counseling.[131] Additional programs such as the National School Lunch Program and the School Breakfast Program offer free or reduced-price meals to children attending public and nonprofit schools. These programs, however, exclude children who dropped out of school or are homeschooled. When school is not in session during the summer, food insecurity increases, which points to evidence that the programs make an impact on food security.[132] When schools are able to continue serving meals during the summer, food insecurity decreases.[133] Programs such as these have made a notable dent in food insecurity, but because the socioeconomic conditions impacting food insecurity continue to prevail, millions remain food insecure despite these efforts.

Food Insecurity and Child Development

Children are especially harmed by food insecurity, as developmental problems and negative health outcomes that result from lack of nutrients could have consequences that last a lifetime. It is important to note that the food insecurity rate of households with children are much higher than those without.[134] The impact of undernutrition can begin as early as while the child is in utero, where growth may be restricted if the mother is not taking in adequate nutrients. This can result in the low birth weights of infants, as well as poor development such as "lower cognition scores, decreased activity and expressiveness, poor language development, and behavioural [*sic*] difficulties."[135] During the early life of the child, severe lack of nutrition can cause stunted growth. Decreased stunting rates are associated with an adequate income and socioeconomic position.[136] Stunting that occurs before the child reaches the age of two or three has been associated with cognitive deficits throughout the child's lifetime, as well as specific outcomes such as poor school achievement and an increased likeliness that the child will drop out of school.[137] Among children ages six to twelve, food insecurity was "associated with poorer mathematic scores, grade repetition, absenteeism, tardiness, visits to a psychologist, anxiety, aggression, psychosocial dysfunction, and difficulty getting along with other children."[138] Among adolescents ages fifteen to sixteen, food insecurity can also result in mental health problems such as depression and suicide symptoms.[139] These negative health outcomes of food insecurity reduce the labor productivity and earning potential of millions of children and adults, further contributing to the cycle of poverty and perpetuating the conditions that leave them vulnerable to disease.[140] In the next section, the negative impacts of poverty on education and unemployment are further discussed.

Perpetuating the Cycle: Education and Employment

Disparities in the quality of education received by low-income communities and people of color result in children being denied access from opportunities and support during the most critical development stages of their lives. Not only do these children approach the starting line of life at a distinct disadvantage compared to their wealthier peers, but they continuously face more barriers through struggles such as food insecurity, housing inadequacy, and poorer health outcomes that make healthy mental, physical, and emotional growth more difficult. Over time, these factors snowball and the overall level of educational attainment is often diminished. Lower educational attainment results in limited employment opportunities for these individuals in the future. Often all that is available are low-wage jobs that deprive employees of living wages and further feed the cycle of poverty. Low wages and lack of access to jobs providing insurance coverage means that healthcare is often unaffordable. As such, lack of prevention and early treatment can result in severe health consequences such as disability and increased morbidity and mortality. NTDs likely present a portion of the disease burden that goes unrecognized among these populations.

Aside from linkages between certain NTDs and low levels of education and poverty, not much is discussed in the literature about the role of education and NTDs. This topic takes place within a much larger discussion about the impact of education and poverty on health. Although there are many causal factors of poverty, the importance of the role of education cannot be overstated. Six aspects of poverty in particular have strong negative influences on child development and education, including the state of poverty, the severity of poverty, the duration of poverty, the timing of poverty in relation to the child's age, community characteristics, and the impact of poverty on those whom the child has relationships with.[141]

Although over half of a century has passed since *Brown v Board of Education*, racial disparities continue to play a role in the quality of education available for African American and Latino students. Research has shown that one of the strongest predictors of racial gaps in educational achievement is whether the child attends school with a high proportion of low-income students.[142] An analysis conducted in 2011 found that seventeen states have a majority of public school students that are eligible for free and reduced-price meals. Of those states with the majority of students living in poverty, most of them reached across the South, Southwest, and West Coast.[143] Within states that have large disparities in educational expenditures, many of them are people of color or low-income students living in either urban districts that have the worst fiscal expenditures, or rural districts that represent the greatest fiscal inequality.[144] Although the federal government does provide approximately 10 percent of funding for public schools, state and local governments cover the remainder.[145] A study by the Department of Education reported that 45 percent of schools with high concentrations of poverty receive less state and local funding than other schools in their district.[146] For local governments, the amount they are able to invest in schools is often derived from property taxes. Because property values are low in areas where low-income populations are concentrated, there are less resources available to fund schools.

This results in diminished opportunities, such as fewer course offerings and fewer classes with advanced coursework such as Advanced Placement or International Baccalaureate, which provide students with chances to earn college credit.[147] Poorer school districts are often unable to provide the electives, field trips, new textbooks or library books, and enrichment programs that wealthier school districts can.[148] Additionally, schools with greater proportions of students of color and low-income students are more likely to have less experienced teachers as their instructors because the low wages provided to teachers at these schools do not attract experienced teachers.[149] Additionally, a report by the Center for American Progress found that many districts have teacher assignment practices that directly assign the least experienced teachers to schools with high proportions of students of color and those living in poverty.[150] In high-needs schools such as these, teacher retention rates are dismal as many feel the conditions are insurmountable.[151]

Poor, rural districts face unique problems, such as the availability and affordability of broadband access for schools, or hot spots for their students to take home when they live in areas that are too isolated for companies to provide coverage.[152] When internet access is unavailable, parents lose access to portals to view their child's progress, and students lack a valuable tool for completing assignments, online classroom discussions, research, and college applications. Schools play a critical role in providing resources and an environment that encourages achievement.[153] When academic growth curves are compared between low socioeconomic status and high, the gap suggests that the school environment, and lack thereof during the summer, likely has a strong role in providing support.[154] For reasons such as these, improving the quality and equity of education would prove valuable in mitigating the effects of poverty and providing children with a support system, resources, and skill set that they otherwise may not get at home. Schools in low-income areas often struggle to compensate for the lack of social capital that students living in poverty are exposed to in comparison to their peers of higher socioeconomic status.[155] This includes being surrounded by or having contact with others who have experienced success which can create networks that provide support to the student as they seek their first jobs, internships, and scholarships. Those not exposed to this support system are likely unaware of the opportunities available to them.

Education is also a critical component of promoting more positive health outcomes. It is the process by which children develop the capacity for learning, critical thinking, and problem solving that individuals continue to build on throughout their lifetime.[156] Education centered on improving public health often takes place in schools, as do many public health interventions such as testing children's hearing and eyesight, improving sex education, and instilling the importance of handwashing.[157] Physical education classes teach students about their bodies and making healthy choices, while also requiring students to partake in physical activity, which can also improve academic performance.[158] Many chronic illnesses such as circulatory diseases, diabetes, liver disease, and some psychological conditions are associated with adults that have lower levels of educational attainment.[159] In short, the quality of education an individual receives will have a lifelong impact on their health.

There is also a direct link between poverty, education, and employment opportunities. An example of the coming problems many states may soon face is in Dallas, Texas, where the city is struggling as companies have started relocating to areas with better prospects of a skilled workforce. The relocation is leaving behind communities with fewer employment opportunities. Higher levels of educational attainment have a causal relationship with wage increases. Over the decades, the overall educational attainment in the South has increased, although the educational attainment of the South's labor force is plagued by inequalities for minorities and those living in rural areas.[160] Those living in rural areas are more likely to be underemployed, mostly due to the limited employment opportunities in most rural areas.

However, the current economic strategy dominant in many Southern states, in which states offered tax incentives and union-free workplaces that appeal to industries, results in the creation of low-paying jobs.[161] The lack of available jobs that pay a living wage further perpetuates the cycle of poverty throughout right-to-work states. Additionally, Southern and Midwestern states were greatly impacted by reductions in the manufacturing industry since 1998, when blue-collar manufacturing jobs once provided a large bulk of middle-income jobs.[162] Wages earned by these workers today no longer affords them a middle-class lifestyle.[163] Worse, remaining manufacturing jobs are increasingly turned over to temporary staffing agencies, whose workers are paid even less. While the service sector's growth has provided a wide range of jobs in the food industry, retail, and other industries, many of these jobs are low-paying as well. Wages and income are closely related to health outcomes because, in addition to serving as the deciding factor on healthcare affordability, they both impact other health-related resources like food, housing, and environment.[164] One study found that workers in states where minimum wage levels were lower had higher rates of reporting unmet medical needs.[165]

Oftentimes, low-wage earners without medical benefits prefer to not seek medical care because they fear that they will find out about a health issue they are unable to afford treatment for. This creates a culture of avoidance in terms of healthcare, rather than encouraging the less expensive option of early detection and treatment. Because of this, common chronic conditions are allowed to worsen and impede individuals' quality of life on a regular basis. This, coupled with the lack of knowledge of NTDs among healthcare providers and patients, means the prospects for early diagnosis and treatment of an NTD infection are grim. In terms of vulnerabilities to NTDs, there is a direct relationship with employment for individuals that work in professions that require employees to be outdoors a great deal of time, such as the agricultural industry, as they are more likely to be exposed to NTDs compared to other types of employment.[166] More broadly, however, employment and the wage-earning status of individuals is the most closely related factor to whether or not the individual will live in poverty, and, as such, suffer from poor health outcomes and vulnerability to NTD infections.

Healthcare Accessibility

The previous sections have all discussed the links between various risk factors and health, particularly as it pertains to NTDs. Keeping in mind that NTDs often have the greatest impact on the most isolated and low-income individuals, it is important to address the unique challenges of healthcare accessibility in terms of seeking healthcare in rural areas, where over 51 million Americans live.[167] The accessibility of health services is determined by the "availability; accessibility; affordability; accommodation (relations between providers and patients); and acceptability (patients accept providers or providers accept patients)" of healthcare.[168] Although rural hospitals experience less vacancies, just one such vacancy is incredibly costly, and may inhibit the hospital from continuing to provide the service.[169] One method used to determine such inadequacies is the health manpower shortage area (HMSA), which designates areas where healthcare professionals are "over-utilized, excessively distant, or inaccessible to the population."[170] Another label used to designate an area with insufficient healthcare is a medically underserved area, which includes high infant mortality rates, high poverty rates, and where a high proportion of the population is elderly in addition to fulfilling the criteria of HMSA.[171]

In the 1970s, the National Health Service Corps volunteered to serve as healthcare professionals in areas where shortages existed, such as low-income rural and urban areas. Throughout the 1980s, trends leaning toward deregulation and competitive markets resulted in scaling back on government interventions in rural health. A Graduate Medical Education National Advisory Committee report predicted that a large surplus in physicians would result in an improved dispersal of healthcare professionals in areas that previously did not have a competitive advantage for attracting physicians, such as rural areas.[172] However, vast disparities remained between the number of physicians between urban and rural areas.

Today, those in rural areas face a number of unique challenges depending on the diverse characteristics of the communities in which they live. One of the most prevalent issues continues to be the limited number of physicians, specialists, and long-term care options. Additionally, concerns over the quality of the healthcare are increased due to "difficulty getting accurate diagnoses, lack of trust in health care providers, physicians' perceived lack of interest in patients, difficulty scheduling an appointment, and/or long waiting times at such appointments."[173] Another problem many face in rural areas is securing adequate transportation to access medical care. For those unable to afford a car or gas, public transportation is limited or non-existent. For those driving, something as simple as a lack of road markings could make it more difficult for those traveling to navigate the area.[174] Although recent digital services seem to provide an alternative method of seeking treatment through telemedicine, this form of healthcare would still be difficult to access for those isolated in areas where internet connection is not available.

Social isolation also plays a role in how healthcare is perceived and practiced. Residents of communities with various facilities or programs spread out thinly may not be aware of existing resources in order to take advantage of them.[175] As a result of this, they may have formed habits of self-reliance, and might be reluctant to seek treatment or may rely on forms of alternative medicine. Additionally, as discussed earlier, some may avoid seeking treatment altogether out of fear that they may have a health condition they may be financially ill-equipped to treat. Other barriers to health include language and cultural differences, such as those experienced by immigrants. Latino immigrant populations in particular may find healthcare difficult to access, as many employers do not cover the cost of health insurance and much of the employment is offered only on a seasonal basis.[176] The colonias, where many immigrants reside, sometimes establish community centers where residents can partake in health education and screenings. However, many choose to travel to Mexico to seek health care and dentistry services, as well as pharmaceuticals for a more affordable price.

The affordability of pharmaceuticals and health care is a significant problem, especially for those without health insurance. A study found that in comparison to older residents, younger residents had worse access to service in terms of having a regular source of care and health insurance.[177] It acknowledged the vital role Medicare and Medicaid holds as improving access to healthcare for older adults, and noted how younger populations were less likely to receive private health insurance through their work. This highlights the need for the expansion of programs such as Medicaid to provide for those who currently do not qualify, but still have a financial need for more affordable healthcare. Although many Southern states have opposed the Affordable Care Act, Kentucky chose to embrace Medicaid expansions to cover over 300,000 additional state residents.[178] This expansion primarily benefited those too poor to purchase private insurance, but who are ineligible to qualify for Medicaid under normal circumstances because of a slightly higher income.[179] Although the cost of insuring new enrollees is high, the policy aims to offset this by saving on the current cost of uncompensated care. Tennessee, which has its own history with Medicaid expansion when its 1990s efforts resulted in insurmountable costs and cutbacks, chose not to follow suit.[180] Today, the impact of these decisions can be seen by comparing the two neighboring states. In terms of lower-income populations, Kentucky's rate of those who are uninsured is 6 percent versus the uninsured rate in Tennessee, which increased to roughly 10 percent in 2019.[181] Other states that did not expand Medicaid have also fallen further behind states that did in the proportion of the population that is insured.[182] Even when individuals are able to secure insurance, there are discrepancies of provider reimbursement rates among public and private insurance. In some cases this serves to disincentivize scheduling appointments and performing costly services for those with public insurance, which may result in a bias against more low-income patients.[183] This is just one example of how communities and states that may appear similar geographically, culturally, and politically have diverse health policies that compound the lack of homogeneity among rural populations. This can make assessing the needs of these isolated populations difficult.

One such population are those with disabilities living in rural areas. This is particularly important in the context of NTDs because these infections often produce chronic, debilitating symptoms. A disability is defined by the Americans with Disabilities Act as "a physical or mental impairment that substantially limits one or more major life activities of an individual, a record of such an impairment, or being regarded as having such an impairment."[184] Disabilities are prevalent in rural communities, but there is little data available to document the unique healthcare needs of those with various disabilities in such areas.[185] Although there are a higher proportion of disabilities among rural children living in poverty in comparison to those not living in poverty or in urban environments, we do know these children are less capable of accessing pediatric care, and must travel greater distances to reach healthcare providers.[186] Because existing health services for those living in rural areas with disabilities are insufficient, other methods have been used such as outreach workers, regional specialized care centers, and mobile units.[187] Interventions such as these will continue to provide options for those with disabilities, who are often among the most underserved members of their community. For this reason, coupled with the fact that NTDs cause a wide range of chronic disabilities, future interventions and research will be necessary to determine the true burden of disease among these populations as related to NTDs. Overall, improving the accessibility and affordability of healthcare, prioritizing preventative care, and reducing the impoverished conditions that cause negative health outcomes will be necessary to reduce the impact of NTDs and other chronic diseases. Next, we will discuss the role of environmental changes and natural disasters as a risk of NTD infection.

CLIMATE CHANGE AND NATURAL DISASTERS

In the United States, the Gulf Coast in particular represents a "perfect storm," where natural disasters, climate change, high rates of poverty, and migration create a favorable habitat for the proliferation of NTDs.[188] In the Gulf Coast states of Texas, Louisiana, Mississippi, Alabama, and Florida, approximately 10 million people live below the poverty line.[189] Among those living in these states, an estimated 5–6 percent of the overall population are infected with at least one NTD.[190] Tropical and subtropical regions, or those around the equator, receive more direct light in comparison to regions further from the equator.[191] This results in increased plant survival, and, therefore, more biodiversity.[192] This includes greater numbers and species of parasites and vectors than found in other regions of the world. Because of this, humans dwelling in these regions have historically faced greater exposure to parasitic diseases, which has created the foundation for a cycle of poverty through inhibited development.[193] Gulf Coast states are vulnerable to a range of parasitic and vector-borne diseases such as Chagas, toxocariasis, ascariasis, hookworm, neurocysticercosis, trichomoniasis, West Nile, Zika, Dengue, and chikungunya. The petrochemical and shipping industries in the Gulf Coast are an important component of the American economy, and the health of the populations residing in this area must be safeguarded accordingly.[194] As such, the detection, prevention, and treatment of NTDs will be essential as climate change will likely result in an increasing disease burden of NTDs and the migration of NTD vectors into areas where they have not been previously endemic.[195] The prevalence of some of these diseases is largely dependent on environmental conditions. Throughout the twentieth and twenty-first centuries, unprecedented levels of climate change due to human activity, such as greenhouse gas emissions, has been associated with increasing temperatures.[196] As temperatures become warmer, precipitation will continue to become more extreme, and storms increasingly more violent. These factors are compounded by deforestation and environmental degradation to create conditions more favorable to parasites and their vectors.[197]

Climate Change and Vector-borne Diseases

Some of these NTD parasites and vectors include triatomines, mosquitoes, and soil-transmitted helminths such as those causing hookworm infection, toxocariasis, and ascariasis. Triatomines, the vector responsible for spreading the *Trypanosoma cruzi* parasite responsible for Chagas disease, is also impacted by changes in climate. Increased temperatures are associated with geographical shifts in the distribution of triatomines, as the bugs are capable of moving further north where temperatures have become relatively warmer.[198] Temperatures above 30°C, when combined with low humidity, can result in exceeding feeding rates among triatomines in an effort to avoid dehydration.[199] It is possible that this could lead to a significant increase in Chagas infection rates, as the disease is transmitted through the site of the bite wound that occurs during the insect's meals. Additionally, high temperatures can increase the development of the *T. cruzi* parasite within the vector.

Warmer temperatures also mean that the geographical range of mosquitoes will continue to grow.[200] As temperatures increase, areas with winters that were previously uninhabitable due to freezing temperatures, will now provide year-round breeding grounds.[201] As temperatures increase, areas where mosquitoes already breed year-round will experience faster breeding rates, increased hatch rates, increased developmental rates, increased reproduction rates, and the ability for mosquitoes to begin laying eggs at a younger age.[202] As such, the entire reproductive cycle of the mosquito will be altered by these changes, and their numbers and ability to spread can be expected to increase exponentially.[203] Additionally, female mosquitoes feed more often when temperatures are warmer, which increases the frequency of the event that exposes humans to disease.[204]

Lastly, climate change is associated with changes in the biological development of soil-transmitted helminths.[205] Higher temperatures cause hookworms to develop more quickly, which in turn reduces the amount of time it takes for them to become infective. *A. lumbricoides*, the roundworm causing ascariasis, experiences faster development within their eggs as temperatures increase. Up to a certain point, increased precipitation and relative humidity is beneficial to all soil-transmitted helminths by improving egg and larvae development by preventing them from losing moisture. Hookworms have increased larval survival rates when humidity is increased, while all other soil-transmitted helminths experience increased larval survival as humidity decreases. Put differently, changes in climate are creating more hospitable habits for many types of NTDs.

The Impact of the World's Changing Climate on Natural Disasters

As discussed in the previous section, heavy rainfall events are likely to cause an increase in vector-borne disease transmission, especially if it occurs early in the transmission season.[206] This is particularly alarming because of the Gulf Coast's long history of natural disasters such as hurricanes and flooding. Natural disasters such as Hurricanes Ima, Maria, Harvey, Matthew, Sandy, Katrina, Rita, Ivan, Frances, Charley, and Tropical Storm Allison have pummeled the Gulf Coast in the last 20 years alone. Adverse weather events such as these are likely to continue, especially given the threat posed by climate change. Increased risk of extreme weather events such as heavy rainfall, flooding, and hurricanes are associated with human-induced global warming.[207] Sunny-day flooding, or tidal flooding that occurs along the East and Gulf Coast of the United States, has increased in frequency throughout the last two decades and will continue to cause damage to streets and wastewater infrastructure.[208]

Poor residents of the Gulf Coast remain particularly vulnerable to flooding and natural disasters. Decades of "racial injustice, economic inequality, and short-term, profit-driven development practices" with inadequate flood-control mechanisms have resulted in the most disadvantaged populations dwelling in the areas most vulnerable to flooding.[209] These low-income populations are the same people most at risk of exposure to NTDs. Many health and social issues, and the socioeconomic and racial disparities that fuel them, persist long after the floodwaters have receded.[210] As climate change continues to threaten the Gulf Coast with natural disasters of increasing quantity and intensity, it will be more important than ever to understand the social issues that have resulted in increased vulnerability to natural disasters and disease spread.

Disasters result in a wide range of negative health outcomes.[211] There are cases of disability and injury that are attributed to events related directly to a natural disaster, such as infrastructural damage or road accidents. After the event, there is an increased risk of infectious diseases spread by vectors or contaminated water and food. Flooding, heavy rains, and hurricanes can all cause the release of contaminants ranging from household cleaners to sewage into the environment. Pathogenic organisms from the raw sewage can cause infections in humans due to drinking or cooking with contaminated water, entering the bloodstream through an open wound, contact with contaminated household items that were submerged in flood waters, or even eating seafood extracted from polluted water.[212] This can result in surges of flesh-eating bacteria, antibiotic-resistant staph infections, diarrheal disease from noroviruses, and respiratory infections and diseases.[213] Following Hurricane Harvey in 2017, the destruction of wastewater infrastructure caused the release of sewage into environmental waters, which ultimately resulted in high levels of human fecal contamination in waterways that drain into the Gulf of Mexico.[214]

Additionally, preexisting chronic diseases can be exacerbated by the disaster as medications may become more inaccessible and individuals experience greater levels of stress. Medical facilities are often destroyed or put under increased strain as they absorb displaced populations.[215] These facilities face difficulty when providing displaced patients with even routine health needs, such as kidney dialysis.[216] Hurricanes and natural disasters disrupt hospitals and clinics that are already running at maximum capacity on a daily basis. For example, Hurricane Katrina caused the number of available clinics in

New Orleans to decrease from 90 to 16, and the number of physicians went from approximately 4,486 to a mere 1,200.[217] In such circumstances, it can be expected that those remaining physicians would be put under enormous pressure in overcrowded clinics. Their focus would be more likely to shift toward acute symptoms, and attention would likely be diverted away from chronic illnesses.

Mental health is also impacted by natural disasters due to trauma associated with the event or insecurity caused by loss of social capital such as housing or possessions. Individuals of low socioeconomic status are often more likely to report emotional problems following a disaster.[218] People who work hourly wage jobs, such as service-oriented jobs, are often not paid during disasters or their aftermath.[219] In contrast, middle- and high-income individuals who are salaried often continue to receive a paycheck. These individuals are able to recover from loss more easily and quickly because they often benefit from insurance, social safety nets, and entitlement programs.[220] Women are often at an even greater disadvantage due to lower wages than men, as well as childcare responsibilities. However, the influence of poverty in the scale of devastation brought about by a natural disaster does not stop there. Overall vulnerability to natural disasters is heavily based on socioeconomic status. Rather than wiping out landscapes indiscriminately and smoothing out differences, natural disasters, "deepen and erode the rut of social differences they encounter."[221] While this has been an issue in the Gulf Coast throughout the history of the United States, perhaps at no time was it more apparent than when Hurricane Katrina struck Louisiana, Mississippi, and Alabama in 2005.

Prior to Katrina, the budget of the New Orleans Corps of Engineers had been slashed by 80 percent, which greatly reduced resources available for pumping and levee improvements.[222] In the decades leading up to Katrina, racial segregation resulted in the geographic distribution of African Americans in the central areas of New Orleans, which were at highest risk of flooding.[223] The middle- and upper-income whites resided in the suburbs outside the city or on higher ground. Although only 12 percent of whites were living in poverty in New Orleans, 35 percent of African Americans were living in poverty.[224] In total, over a quarter of residents in New Orleans lived below the federal poverty line. One of the consequences of the socioeconomic disparities that persist in New Orleans was an increase in adverse health outcomes among low-income individuals.

In comparison to whites, African Americans experience higher rates of chronic health conditions such as heart disease, asthma, diabetes, cancer, and HIV/AIDS.[225] To make matters worse, a large portion of this population lacked health insurance to access affordable medical care for their illnesses, and instead relied on the public hospital system.[226] During a natural disaster, these chronic conditions can become increasingly life threatening. Periods of time when food or clean water are unavailable pose a particularly deadly threat to diabetics.[227] Those with compromised immune systems due to HIV/AIDS infections are more vulnerable to pathogens found in contaminated floodwaters.

Socioeconomic status is a significant determinant of the degree to which an individual is impacted by a natural disaster. Those living in poverty have a higher probability of dying or sustaining an injury as a result of a natural disaster, have proportionately greater material losses, and face more barriers to responding, recovering, and reconstructing following the storm.[228] Socioeconomic status also played a major role in whether or not individuals were capable of evacuating from Hurricane Katrina. Although only 17 percent of low-income whites did not have access to a car, almost 60 percent of low-income African Americans lacked access to a car.[229] Additionally, the elderly may have difficulty obtaining transportation due to mobility constraints.[230]

In the aftermath of a natural disaster, government agencies and local volunteers are often faced with a difficult conundrum. In many of the dwellings struck by the disaster, it can be difficult to distinguish whether the property's dismal conditions are caused by the storm, or if the damage was due to the poor condition of the housing prior to the storm.[231] In the case of Hurricane Hugo, church volunteers and government relief workers working to rebuild the communities after the storm often stopped when they had dealt with all of the problems associated directly with the storm's damage.[232] Recovery agents and programs are most frequently only interested in the immediate impact of the storm, rather than the conditions that made residences vulnerable to begin with.[233] Even after a disaster, many of those impacted continued to suffer because of the lack of obtainable living wage jobs. Although reconstruction contracts after Hurricane Katrina were awarded to firms that promised to pay their workers living wages, the Davis-Bacon Act was repealed within days.[234] This legislation required those awarded federal contracts to pay their workers a wage amount equal to that of the prevailing area, but instead the wage floor reduction resulted in more low-paying jobs. The cycle of poverty responsible for the living conditions and vulnerabilities that amplified the impact of Hurricane Katrina for low-income families still persists today.

The racial and socioeconomic divides that persist in the Gulf Coast and the United States as a whole will continue to leave those most vulnerable to natural disasters to face an equally disturbing fate. The everyday living conditions and health disparities of low-income families result in tragedies that may not be considered as newsworthy as a Category 5 hurricane, but they exist nonetheless. Although cloaked in the invisibility of decades of marginalization, the loss of life, loss of productivity due to disability, and the loss of quality of life for thousands of Americans is an "unnatural disaster" in its own right. The impact of these disasters will continue to worsen in the future due to climate change, so it is imperative to address these challenges now. Another factor that influences the prevalence of NTDs in the environment is the presence of stray animal populations.

Stray or Sheltered Animal Populations and Pet Care

As discussed previously in relation to soil-transmitted helminths, cats and dogs exposed to parasitic diseases serve as a reservoir for some of the parasites that cause NTD infection in humans. Infection with soil-transmitted helminths is not uncommon if the animal does not receive preventative treatment and is exposed to a contaminated environment. The roundworm, *Ascaris lumbricoides*, which causes the disease ascariasis in humans is spread by both dogs and cats that are infected with the parasite. *Toxocara canis* and *Toxocara cati* infect dogs and cats respectively. Dogs and cats digest the eggs of the parasites when coming into contact with infected soil or eating infected prey.[235] Either the eggs pass through the animal's system through excrement, or the worms reproduce inside their bodies, and eggs are later dispersed through the animal's excrement. Several anthelmintic drugs are available to treat infected dogs and cats. Additionally, monthly preventatives can protect dogs from becoming infected with *A. lumbricoides* and *T. canis*, as well as many other parasites. By reducing the prevalence of worm infections in dogs and cats in communities, fewer eggs will contaminate the environment and cause human infection.

In addition to the diseases mentioned above, dogs and cats can both serve as reservoirs for the parasite *Trypanosoma cruzi*, which causes Chagas disease in infected humans. Symptoms rarely manifest in cats, but dogs initially display signs of the disease ranging from fever, anorexia, lethargy, lymphadenopathy, hepatomegaly, splenomegaly, cardiac conduction abnormalities or arrhythmias, and later during the chronic phase can experience congestive heart failure, dilated cardiomyopathy, and arrhythmias.[236] Dogs that are exposed to triatomines while outdoors in areas where the vector is endemic are most at risk of becoming infected with the disease. Because of this, stray dogs are often vulnerable to infection. A study of dogs at an animal shelter in Southern Louisiana found that almost 16 percent of the dogs tested PCR-positive for infection.[237] Even among the well-cared for dogs employed by the U.S. government to work along the Texas-Mexico border, a study found that *T. cruzi* infection was widespread despite regular veterinary care, high-quality food and shelter, and the status of the dogs as highly valued by their handlers and the government.[238] Although experiments have been conducted in an attempt to produce a treatment for Chagas infection in dogs, no effective treatment is currently available.[239] Drugs such as Fluralaner are currently undergoing trials to produce a preventative for dogs that would kill the triatomines that blood feed on the dogs.[240] Additionally, a successful vaccine has yet to be developed. Preventative measures can be taken to limit the exposure of the dogs to the triatomines that carry the parasite. These include preventing dogs from eating insects or small animals that may be infected with the disease, and providing the dog with shelter indoors.[241] Although infected dogs cannot directly infect humans with Chagas through direct disease transmission, reducing the prevalence of Chagas in dogs would lessen the reservoir available for triatomines endemic to the area to become infected with the disease by feeding on infected dogs.

The United States has an estimated population of more than 78 million dogs and 85.8 million cats that are owned by people in the United States.[242] While there are no definitive figures for the total number of stray dogs and cats living in the United States, approximately 3.3 million dogs and 3.2 million cats are taken to animal shelters each year.[243] Stray dogs and cats are especially vulnerable to parasites, as they have little shelter from exposure and receive no preventative care or treatment. For domestic dogs and cats, their vulnerability to parasitic diseases is often determined by the level of care provided by their owner. Low-income families and individuals are often unable to afford preventative care or treatment for their animals. The lives of people and their pets are closely tied.[244] When people struggle with affording food, healthcare, and adequate housing, their pets often suffer as well. In the case of NTDs, poor health outcomes and the vulnerabilities of one population are inextricably linked to the other. The next section will discuss another environmental risk factor that relates to soil-transmitted helminths.

Geophagy

Although geophagy, or eating dirt, has been practiced globally across ethnic, social, and economic boundaries, in America it is a cultural custom associated largely with African American populations in the Southern United States.[245] The practice has likely been passed down for generations beginning with slaves who brought the custom with them from Africa, where geophagy was common among children and adults.[246] Eating dirt was used for medicinal purposes such as a treatment for diarrhea and to provide nutrients to pregnant or lactating women. A study conducted on dirt sold for consumption at a market in Ghana was found to contain minerals such as phosphorus, potassium, calcium, magnesium, copper, zinc, manganese, and iron.[247] Historically, the clay was taken from its source and baked on a stove or in an oven prior to consumption.[248] Because of this, parasites like soil-transmitted helminths would not survive the baking process and would be unable to infect individuals through the consumption of clay.

A study published in 1942 discusses geophagy as being a widespread practice in Mississippi among African American populations.[249] The reasons some gave for the habit was that it tasted good, it was thought to be healthy, and was believed to be especially beneficial for pregnant women. The clay these individuals seek is thought to vary in quality based on the location it is found. For example, the dirt from the Delta region was seen as being of poor quality. The study poses possible reasoning from where the cultural practice may have originated from. The first proposal was that it may have been related to hookworm, as those who were infected were said to crave dirt. This theory was discredited, largely because the county health officer had stated that hookworm was not prevalent in the area due to the soil type, but we know today that hookworms are likely prevalent in the region. Second, eating dirt was thought to address nutritional deficiencies, such as iron. This may explain why the dirt was particularly popular among pregnant women.

Geophagy is still practiced today in the United States. A study that compiled the National Health and Nutrition Examination Survey from years 1971–1975 to 1976–1980 determined that between 1 and 2.5 percent of the population ingests soil or another type of non-food substance.[250] The prevalence of this trait was higher among African Americans than whites, and among those of lower socioeconomic status compared to those of higher socioeconomic status. A short film about geophagy in the South, *Eat White Dirt*, was produced by Adam Forrester and aired in 2017.[251] The film discusses the white dirt market, known as the "kaolin belt" in Georgia, where customers can purchase dirt to eat at the closest convenience store. Kaolin is a chalky white clay used in the production of porcelain, paper, and paint.[252] But, it is also a very popular snack for some residents of the Southern United States. One of the reasons the film was made was to destigmatize those who choose to eat dirt, as generations before them have done.[253] Although geophagy as prepared and consumed in this context is not a risk factor for becoming infected with an NTD, folklore of the practice among those infected with hookworm adds an interesting piece to the puzzle of NTD prevalence in the Southern United States.

CONCLUSION

In this chapter, we demonstrated the intersections between the various risk factors of NTDs and how they are interconnected with the cycle of poverty, marginalization, and isolation both physically and socially. Social determinants of health such as education, employment, housing, healthcare accessibility, and geophagy will determine an individual's level of vulnerability to NTDs. Additionally, natural disasters and climate change will continue to have an impact on the sanitation infrastructure and spread of soil-transmitted helminths and vector-borne diseases throughout the United States, especially when considering the presence of stray and domestic animals serving as reservoirs and sources of disease transmission. In the next chapter we provided a detailed explanation of the poverty and other risk factors that exist in the five communities we worked with over the course of our study. The descriptions of each community addressed in the next chapter were constructed through focus group interviews, one-on-one interviews, and numerous conversations during visits. We have attempted to capture the vibrant nature of each community, along with their challenges and concerns. We aimed to convey the complexity of the challenges facing these communities and help Americans not from these communities gain a better understanding of the realities. It is not simply a problem of healthcare access or inadequate education, or a lack of proper sanitation. The poverty, inequality, and NTD issue in the United States exists because numerous systems are failing and there are limited or no resources to fix the problem.

NOTES

1. UN Water, "World Toilet Day 2019," accessed August 15, 2019, https://www.worldtoiletday.info/.
2. World Health Organization, "Sanitation," accessed August 15, 2019, http://www.who.int/topics/sanitation/en/.
3. United Nations Sustainable Development Goals, "Water and Sanitation," accessed August 15, 2019, https://www.un.org/sustainabledevelopment/water-and-sanitation/.
4. Brian Byrne, "A Shocking Number of Americans Don't Have a Toilet," *The Week*, published November 24, 2015, https://theweek.com/articles/590312/shocking-number-americans-dont-have-toilet.
5. Philip Alston, "Statement on Visit to the USA, by Professor Philip Alston, United Nations Special Rapporteur on Extreme Poverty and Human Rights," *New York: United Nations Office of The High Commissioner for Human Rights*, published December 15, 2017, www.ohchr.og/EN/NewsEvents/Pages/DisplayNews.aspx.
6. Jacob Cantor et al., "Tracking the Downstream Impacts of Inadequate Sanitation in Central Appalachia," *Journal of Water and Health* 15, no. 4 (2017): 580–590.
7. Jamie Bartram and Sandy Cairncross, "Hygiene, Sanitation, and Water: Forgotten Foundations of Health," *PLoS Med* 7, no. 11 (2010): e1000367.
8. Ross Pink, "Child Rights, Right to Water and Sanitation, and Human Security," *Health and Human Rights* 14 (2012): E78–E87.
9. Indiana State Department of Health, "Diseases Involving Sewage," accessed August 15, 2019, https://www.in.gov/isdh/22963.htm.
10. Charles P. Gerba and James E. Smith, "Sources of Pathogenic Microorganisms and Their Fate During Land Application of Wastes," *Journal of Environmental Quality*

34, no. 1 (2005): 42–48; Robert H. Wayland III and E. T. Oppelt, "Onsite Wastewater Treatment Systems Manual," *Environmental Protection Agency* (2002): 367.

11. Erin Arcipowski et al., "Clean Water, Clean Life: Promoting Healthier, Accessible Water in Rural Appalachia," *Journal of Contemporary Water Research & Education* 161, no. 1 (2017): 1–18; Tim K. Mackey et al., "Emerging and Reemerging Neglected Tropical Diseases: A Review of Key Characteristics, Risk Factors, and the Policy and Innovation Environment," *Clinical Microbiology Reviews* 27, no. 4 (2014): 949–979.

12. Bernd Genser et al., "Impact of a City-wide Sanitation Intervention in a Large Urban Centre on Social, Environmental and Behavioural Determinants of Childhood Diarrhoea: Analysis of Two Cohort Studies," *International Journal of Epidemiology* 37, no. 4 (2008): 831–840.

13. Keith Miller, Kristina Costa, and Donna Cooper, "How to Upgrade and Maintain Our Nation's Wastewater and Drinking-water Infrastructure," *Washington: Center for American Progress* (2012): 31.

14. Jennifer S. Carrera and Catherine Coleman Flowers, "Sanitation Inequity and the Cumulative Effects of Racism in Colorblind Public Health Policies," *American Journal of Economics and Sociology* 77, no. 3–4 (2018): 941–966.

15. Jennifer Carrera, "Sanitation and Social Power in the United States," PhD Dissertation, University of Illinois at Urbana-Champaign (2014): 81.

16. Carrera, "Sanitation and Social Power in the United States," 78–86.

17. Carrera, "Sanitation and Social Power in the United States," 79.

18. Carrera, "Sanitation and Social Power in the United States," 81.

19. Carrera, "Sanitation and Social Power in the United States," 85–86.

20. Amanda Stoner, "Regulatory Deficiencies in Wastewater Infrastructure in Rural Appalachia," *Sustainable Dev. L. & Pol'y* 18 (2017): 30.

21. Mary Anna Evans, "Flushing the Toilet Has Never Been Riskier," *The Atlantic*, published September 17, 2015, https://www.theatlantic.com/technology/archive/2015/09/americas-sewage-crisis-public-health/405541/.

22. Evans, "Flushing the Toilet Has Never Been Riskier."

23. Evans, "Flushing the Toilet Has Never Been Riskier."

24. Andrielle N. Swaby, Mark D. Lucas, and Robert M. Ross, *The Teacher-Friendly Guide to The Earth Science of The Southeastern US*, 2nd ed. (Ithaca, New York, Paleontological Research Institution, 2016): 272–27.

25. Emily Meza, "Examining Wastewater Treatment Struggles in Lowndes County, AL," Duke University Library, published April 27, 2018, https://dukespace.lib.duke.edu/dspace/bitstream/handle/10161/16516/MP_2018_04_20_FinalDraft.pdf?sequence=1.

26. A. L. Badham (1993, June), Wilcox County Alabama: Needs Assessment. *University of Alabama at Birmingham, School of Public Health.* Master's Thesis.

27. Meza, "Examining Wastewater Treatment Struggles in Lowndes County, AL."

28. Flowers, "A County Where the Sewer Is Your Lawn."

29. Carrera, "Sanitation and Social Power in the United States," 137.

30. Carrera and Flowers, "Sanitation Inequity and the Cumulative Effects of Racism in Colorblind Public Health Policies," 941–966.

31. Carrera, "Sanitation and Social Power in the United States," 111.

32. Carrera, "Sanitation and Social Power in the United States," 106.

33. Carrera, "Sanitation and Social Power in the United States," 129.

34. Sabrina Tavernise, "A Toilet, But No Proper Plumbing: A Reality in 500,000 U.S. Homes," *The New York Times*, published September 27, 2016, https://www.nytimes.com/2016/09/27/health/plumbing-united-states-poverty.html.

35. Logan Scott, Interview With Corresponding Author, unpublished, 2009.

36. Maxwell Izenberg et al., "Nocturnal Convenience: The Problem of Securing Universal Sanitation Access in Alabama's Black Belt," *Environmental Justice* 6, no. 6 (2013): 200–205.

37. The Alabama Department of Environmental Management, "State Revolving Fund (SRF)," last modified 2019, http://www.adem.state.al.us/programs/water/srf.cnt.

38. Catherine C. Flowers, JoAnn K. Ward, and Inga Winkler, "Flushed and Forgotten Sanitation and Wastewater in Rural Communities in the United States," The Alabama Center for Rural Enterprise (ACRE), The Columbia Law School Human Rights Clinic, The Institute for the Study of Human Rights at Columbia University, published May 2019, https://www.humanrightscolumbia.org/sites/default/files/Flushed%20and%20Forgotten%20-%20FINAL%20%281%29.pdf.

39. Tracy Rysavy, "What Does Sewage Have to Do With It?" *Green America*, accessed September 20, 2019, https://greenamerica.org/drinking-water-risk/what-does-sewage-have-do-it.

40. Izenberg et al., "Nocturnal Convenience: The Problem of Securing Universal Sanitation Access in Alabama's Black Belt."

41. Mark Elliot et al., "Surface Discharge of Raw Wastewater Among Unsewered Homes in Central Alabama," *AGUFM* 2017 (2017): PA24A–06.

42. E. Riggs, J. Hughes, D. Irvin, and K. Leopard, "An Overview of Clean Water Access Challenges in the United States," *Global Water Challenge and The Environmental Finance Center, School of Government, University of North Carolina: Chapel Hill, NC, USA* (2017).

43. Erika Weinthal, Elizabeth Albright, Catherine C. Flowers, and Emily Stewart, "Solution-Centered Collaborative Research in Rural Alabama," Social Science Research Council, published March 6, 2018, https://items.ssrc.org/insights/solution-centered-collaborative-research-in-rural-alabama/.

44. Shiloh Deitz and Katie Meehan, "Plumbing Poverty: Mapping Hot Spots of Racial and Geographic Inequality in US Household Water Insecurity," *Annals of the American Association of Geographers* 109, no. 4 (2019): 1092–1109.

45. Stephen P. Gasteyer et al., "Basics Inequality: Race and Access to Complete Plumbing Facilities in the United States," *Du Bois Review: Social Science Research on Race* 13, no. 2 (2016): 305–325.

46. Carrera and Flowers, "Sanitation Inequity and the Cumulative Effects of Racism in Colorblind Public Health Policies," 941–966.

47. Carrera and Flowers, "Sanitation Inequity and the Cumulative Effects of Racism in Colorblind Public Health Policies," 941–966.

48. Leah Platt Boustan et al., "Income Inequality and Local Government in the United States, 1970–2000." No. w16299. *National Bureau of Economic Research* (2010): 7.

49. Chris McGreal, "America's Poorest Border Town: No Immigration Papers, No American Dream," *The Guardian*, published November 19, 2015, https://www.theguardian.com/us-news/2015/nov/19/americas-poorest-border-town-no-immigration-papers-no-american-dream.

50. Pia M. Orrenius, Madeline Zavodny, and Leslie Lukens, *Why Stop There?: Mexican Migration to The US Border Region*, No. 0803. Federal Reserve Bank of Dallas, 2008.

51. Deyanira Nevárez Martinez, María G. Rendón, and Diego Arroyo, "Los Olvidados/The Forgotten: Reconceptualizing Colonias as Viable Communities," *Progress in Planning* (2019): 100450; J. Barton et al., "Las Colonias in the 21st Century: Progress Along the Texas-Mexico Border," *Federal Reserve Bank of Dallas Community Development*, published April 2015, https://www.dallasfed.org/~/media/documents/cd/pubs/lascolonias.pdf.

52. Alana Semuels, "The American Neighborhoods Without Water, Sewers, or Building Codes," *The Atlantic*, published March 3, 2016, https://www.theatlantic.com/business/archive/2016/03/the-americans-without-running-water/471909/.

53. Gaby Galvin, "An Inside Look Into America's Third World," *US News & World Report*, published May 16, 2018, https://www.usnews.com/news/healthiest-communities/articles/2018-05-16/americas-third-world-border-colonias-in-texas-struggle-to-attain-services.

54. Brian Russell Knab, "Infectious Disease and the South Texas Colonias," PhD Diss., *University of Texas Libraries* 2016, HYPERLINK "https://repositories.lib.utexas.edu/handle/2152/44560" https://repositories.lib.utexas.edu/handle/2152/44560.

55. McGreal, "America's Poorest Border Town: No Immigration Papers, No American Dream."

56. Ken Paxton, Office of the Attorney General of Texas, "Colonias Prevention Laws," accessed September 15, 2019, https://www.texasattorneygeneral.gov/divisions/colonias-prevention/colonias-prevention-laws.

57. Gaby, "An Inside Look Into America's Third World."

58. Brad Rollins, "A Sprawling Slum in San Marcos' Shadow," *San Marcos Mercury*, published November 14, 2011, http://smmercury.com/2011/11/14/a-sprawling-slum-in-san-marcos-shadow/.

59. Rollins, "A Sprawling Slum in San Marcos' Shadow."

60. Rollins, "A Sprawling Slum in San Marcos' Shadow."

61. Stoner, "Regulatory Deficiencies in Wastewater Infrastructure in Rural Appalachia," 30.

62. City of College Station, "Mosquito Abatement Program," accessed August 1, 2019, https://www.cstx.gov/departments___city_hall/neighborhood/mosquito.

63. World Health Organization, "Keeping the Vector Out: Housing Improvements for Vector Control and Sustainable Development," published 2017, https://www.who.int/social_determinants/publications/keeping-the-vector-out/en/.

64. Gonzalo M. Vazquez-Prokopec, Audrey Lenhart, and Pablo Manrique-Saide, "Housing Improvement: A Novel Paradigm for Urban Vector-Borne Disease Control?" (2016): 567–569.

65. Vazquez-Prokopec, Lenhart, and Manrique-Saide, "Housing Improvement: A Novel Paradigm for Urban Vector-borne Disease Control?"

66. Sheila Mammen, Jean W. Bauer, and Leslie Richards, "Understanding Persistent Food Insecurity: A Paradox of Place and Circumstance," *Social Indicators Research* 92, no. 1 (2009): 151.

67. Kathryn Edin and Laura Lein, *Making Ends Meet: How Single Mothers Survive Welfare and Low-Wage Work* (Russell Sage Foundation, 1997).

68. Sung-jin Lee, Kathleen R. Parrott, and Mira Ahn, "Exploring Housing Challenges of Low-Income Minority Populations in the Southern United States," *Cityscape* (2012): 73–98.

69. Peter J. Hotez, "Global Urbanization and the Neglected Tropical Diseases," *PLoS Neglected Tropical Diseases* 11, no. 2 (2017): e0005308.

70. Myoung Kim, Jim Ohls, and Rhoda Cohen, *Hunger in America: 2001 National Report Prepared for America's Second Harvest*, No. d27650c180224c58bb7776dbb9283d15 (Mathematica Policy Research, 2001).

71. Cohen, Kim, and Ohls, *Hunger in America: National Report Prepared for America's Second Harvest.*

72. Vazquez-Prokopec, Lenhart, and Manrique-Saide, "Housing Improvement: A Novel Paradigm for Urban Vector-borne Disease Control?"

73. The United Nations Human Rights Office of the High Commissioner, "Fact Sheet on the Right to Adequate Housing Toolkit," accessed November 1, 2019, https://www.ohchr.org/EN/Issues/Housing/toolkit/Pages/RighttoAdequateHousingToolkit.aspx.

74. The United Nations Human Rights Office of the High Commissioner, "Fact Sheet on the Right to Adequate Housing Toolkit."

75. National Housing Law Project, "Fair Housing & Housing for People With Disabilities," accessed November 1, 2019, https://www.nhlp.org/initiatives/fair-housing-housing-for-people-with-disabilities/.

76. R. D. Bullard, *Dumping in Dixie: Race, Class, and Environmental Quality* (Boulder, CO: Westview, 1990), http://www.ciesin.org/docs/010-278/010-278chpt1.html.

77. Terry Gross, "A 'Forgotten History' of How the U.S. Government Segregated America," *NPR*, published May 3, 2017, https://www.npr.org/2017/05/03/526655831/a-forgotten-history-of-how-the-u-s-government-segregated-america.

78. National Housing Law Project, "Fair Housing & Housing for People With Disabilities."

79. Matthew Doherty, "Worst Case Housing Needs Have Gotten . . . Worse," *United States Interagency Council on Homelessness (USICH)*, published September 28, 2017, https://www.usich.gov/news/worst-case-housing-needs-have-gotten-worse/.

80. Doherty, "Worst Case Housing Needs Have Gotten . . . Worse."

81. Doherty, "Worst Case Housing Needs Have Gotten . . . Worse."

82. National Housing Law Project, "Fair Housing & Housing for People With Disabilities."

83. Frederick Eggers and Fouad Moumen, "American Housing Survey: Housing Adequacy and Quality as Measured by the AHS," available at SSRN 2284174 (2013).

84. Lance Freeman, "America's Affordable Housing Crisis: A Contract Unfulfilled," *American Journal of Public Health* 92, no. 5 (2002): 709–712.

85. "Strategic Plan FY2000–FY2006," Washington, DC: U.S. Dept of Housing and Urban Development (2000).

86. National Housing Law Project, "Fair Housing & Housing for People With Disabilities."

87. Elizabeth A. Mack and Sarah Wrase, "A Burgeoning Crisis? A Nationwide Assessment of the Geography of Water Affordability in the United States," *PloS One* 12, no. 1 (2017): e0169488.

88. Sasha Ingher, "31 Percent of U.S. Households Have Trouble Paying Energy Bills," *NPR*, published September 19, 2018, https://www.npr.org/2018/09/19/649633468/31-percent-of-u-s-households-have-trouble-paying-energy-bills.

89. Jim Polson, "More Americans Are Getting Their Electricity Cut Off," *Bloomberg.com*, published October 13, 2017, https://www.bloomberg.com/news/articles/2017-10-13/in-great-american-blackout-millions-go-dark-due-to-unpaid-bills.

90. Ryan Finnigan and Kelsey D. Meagher, "Past Due: Combinations of Utility and Housing Hardship in the United States," *Sociological Perspectives* 62, no. 1 (2019): 96–119.

91. US Department of Health and Human Services, "LIHEAP Home Energy Notebook for Fiscal Year 2011" (2014).

92. National Housing Law Project, "Fair Housing & Housing for People With Disabilities."

93. Cheryl Katz, "People in Poor Neighborhoods Breathe More Hazardous Particles," *Scientific American*, published November 1, 2012, https://www.scientificamerican.com/article/people-poor-neighborhoods-breate-more-hazardous-particles/.

94. Junji Cao et al., "Fine Particulate Matter Constituents and Cardiopulmonary Mortality in a Heavily Polluted Chinese City," *Environmental Health Perspectives* 120, no. 3 (2012): 373–378.

95. Christopher Tessum et al., "Inequity in Consumption of Goods and Services Adds to Racial–ethnic Disparities in Air Pollution Exposure," *Proceedings of the National Academy of Sciences* 116, no. 13 (2019): 6001–6006.

96. Brian Williams, "'That We May Live': Pesticides, Plantations, and Environmental Racism in the United States South," *Environment and Planning E: Nature and Space* 1, nos. 1–2 (2018): 243–267.

97. Nicole Kehoe, "How Dangerous Is Pesticide Drift?" *Scientific American*, published September 17, 2012, https://www.scientificamerican.com/article/pesticide-drift/.

98. Polyxeni Nicolopoulou-Stamati et al., "Chemical Pesticides and Human Health: The Urgent Need for a New Concept in Agriculture," *Frontiers in Public Health* 4 (2016): 148; B. Alewu, and C. Nosiri, "Pesticides and Human Health," *Pesticides in the Modern World–Effects of Pesticides Exposure. InTech* (2011): 231–250; World Health Organization, *Public Health Impact of Pesticides Used in Agriculture*, 1990; Margaret Sanborn, "Non-cancer Health Effects of Pesticides: Systematic Review and Implications for Family Doctors," *Canadian Family*

Physician 53, no. 10 (2007): 1712–1720; Wissem Mnif, "Effect of Endocrine Disruptor Pesticides: A Review," *International Journal of Environmental Research and Public Health* 8, no. 6 (2011): 2265–2303; Karen M. Semchuk, Edgar J. Love, and Robert G. Lee, "Parkinson's Disease and Exposure to Agricultural Work and Pesticide Chemicals," *Neurology* 42, no. 7 (1992): 1328–1328; Catharina Wesseling et al., "Agricultural Pesticide Use in Developing Countries: Health Effects and Research Needs," *International Journal of Health Services* 27, no. 2 (1997): 273–308; Brenda Eskenazi, Asa Bradman, and Rosemary Castorina, "Exposures of Children to Organophosphate Pesticides and Their Potential Adverse Health Effects," *Environmental Health Perspectives* 107, no. Suppl 3 (1999): 409–419; James W. Jaeger, Ian H. Carlson, and Warren P. Porter, "Endocrine, Immune, and Behavioral Effects of Aldicarb (carbamate), Atrazine (triazine) and Nitrate (fertilizer) Mixtures at Groundwater Concentrations," *Toxicology and Industrial Health* 15, nos. 1–2 (1999): 133–151; Ana M. Garcia, "Pesticide Exposure and Women's Health," *American Journal of Industrial Medicine* 44, no. 6 (2003): 584–594; Pascale Salameh et al., "Respiratory Diseases and Pesticide Exposure: A Case-Control Study in Lebanon," *Journal of Epidemiology & Community Health* 60, no. 3 (2006): 256–261; Dennis D. Weisenburger, "Human Health Effects of Agrichemical Use," *Human Pathology* 24, no. 6 (1993): 571–576; Sally M. Bradberry, Alex T. Proudfoot, and J. Allister Vale, "Glyphosate Poisoning," *Toxicological Reviews* 23, no. 3 (2004): 159–167; Reini W. Bretveld et al., "Pesticide Exposure: The Hormonal Function of the Female Reproductive System Disrupted?" *Reproductive Biology and Endocrinology* 4, no. 1 (2006): 30; Kate L. Bassil et al., "Cancer Health Effects of Pesticides: Systematic Review," *Canadian Family Physician* 53, no. 10 (2007): 1704–1711; Jane A. Hoppin et al., "Pesticides and Atopic and Nonatopic Asthma Among Farm Women in the Agricultural Health Study," *American Journal of Respiratory and Critical Care Medicine* 177, no. 1 (2008): 11–18; Marina Bjørling-Poulsen, Helle Raun Andersen, and Philippe Grandjean, "Potential Developmental Neurotoxicity of Pesticides Used in Europe," *Environmental Health* 7, no. 1 (2008): 50; Nel Roeleveld and Reini Bretveld, "The Impact of Pesticides on Male Fertility," *Current Opinion in Obstetrics and Gynecology* 20, no. 3 (2008): 229–233; K. A. Osman and M. Stoytcheva, *Pesticides in The Modern World–Effects of Pesticides Exposure* (2011); Sara Mostafalou and Mohammad Abdollahi, "Pesticides and Human Chronic Diseases: Evidences, Mechanisms, and Perspectives," *Toxicology and Applied Pharmacology* 268, no. 2 (2013): 157–177; Gilles-Eric Séralini et al., "Republished Study: Long-term Toxicity of a Roundup Herbicide and a Roundup-tolerantgenetically Modified Maize," *Environmental Sciences Europe* 26, no. 1 (2014): 14; Darshana Sudip Thakur et al., "Glyphosate Poisoning With Acute Pulmonary Edema," *Toxicology International* 21, no. 3 (2014): 328.

99. Oliver Milman, "'We're Not a Dump' – Poor Alabama Towns Struggle Under the Stench of Toxic Landfills," *The Guardian*, published April 15, 2019, https://www.theguardian.com/us-news/2019/apr/15/were-not-a-dump-poor-alabama-towns-struggle-under-the-stench-of-toxic-landfills.

100. National Alliance to End Homelessness, "State of Homelessness," accessed December 1, 2019, https://endhomelessness.org/homelessness-in-america/homeless ness-statistics/state-of-homelessness-report/.

101. National Alliance to End Homelessness, "Racial Disparities in Homelessness in the United States," published June 6, 2018, https://endhomelessness.org/resource/ racial-disparities-homelessness-united-states/.

102. Alastair Gee, "America's Homeless Population Rises for the First Time Since the Great Recession," *The Guardian*, published December 6, 2017, https://www. theguardian.com/us-news/2017/dec/05/america-homeless-population-2017-official-count-crisis.

103. Alisha Coleman-Jensen et al., "Statistical Supplement to Household Food Security in the United States in 2017." No. 2238-2019-2890 (2018).

104. Craig Gundersen and James P. Ziliak, "Food Insecurity Research in the United States: Where we Have Been and Where We Need to Go," *Applied Economic Perspectives and Policy* 40, no. 1 (2018): 119–135.

105. Joy Rayanne Piontak and Michael D. Schulman, "Food Insecurity in Rural America," *Contexts* 13, no. 3 (2014): 75–77.

106. Alicia Coleman-Jensen, Christian A. Gregory, and Matthew P. Rabbitt, "Definitions of Food Security," *United States Department of Agriculture Economic Research Service*, last modified September 4, 2019, https://www.ers.usda.gov/ topics/food-nutrition-assistance/food-security-in-the-us/definitions-of-food-sec urity.aspx.

107. Duong, "What Do Neglected Tropical Diseases Have to Do With Nutrition?," *Global Citizen*, August 15, 2018, https://www.globalcitizen.org/en/content/neglected -tropical-diseases-ntds-nutrition/.

108. Rolf Klemm et al., "Linking Undernutrition and Selected Neglected Tropical Diseases" (2015).

109. Eileen Stillwaggon, "The Ecology of Poverty: Nutrition, Parasites, and Vulnerability to HIV/AIDS," *AIDS, Poverty and Hunger: Challenges and Responses. International Food Policy Research Institute*, Washington (2006): 167–180.

110. Duong, "What Do Neglected Tropical Diseases Have to Do With Nutrition?"

111. Stillwaggon, "The Ecology of Poverty: Nutrition, Parasites, and Vulnerability to HIV/AIDS."

112. Ranjit Kumar Chandra, "Nutrition and the Immune System: An Introduction," *The American Journal of Clinical Nutrition* 66, no. 2 (1997): 460S–463S.

113. Craig Gunderson, Brent Kreider, and John Pepper, "The Economics of Food Insecurity in the United States," *Applied Economic Perspectives and Policy* 33, no. 3 (2011): 281–303.

114. Duong, "What Do Neglected Tropical Diseases Have to Do With Nutrition?"

115. Stillwaggon, "The Ecology of Poverty: Nutrition, Parasites, and Vulnerability to HIV/AIDS."

116. Gundersen and Ziliak, "Food Insecurity Research in the United States: Where We Have Been and Where We Need to Go."

117. "Fast Facts About Food Insecurity," *Case Management Monthly* 16(9): 2–3 (2019), http://search.ebscohost.com.srv-proxy2.library.tamu.edu/login.aspx?direct=true&db=ccm&AN=138447865&site=eds-live.

118. Gundersen and Ziliak, "Food Insecurity Research in the United States: Where We Have Been and Where We Need to Go."

119. Piontak and Schulman, "Food Insecurity in Rural America."

120. Centers for Disease Control and Prevention, "Understanding Food Deserts," last modified July 1, 2020, https://www.cdc.gov/Features/FoodDeserts/.

121. Piontak and Schulman, "Food Insecurity in Rural America."

122. Chris McGreal, "Where Even Walmart Won't Go: How Dollar General Took Over Rural America," *The Guardian*, published August 13, 2018, https://www.theguardian.com/business/2018/aug/13/dollar-general-walmart-buhler-haven-kansas.

123. Piontak and Schulman, "Food Insecurity in Rural America."

124. Adam Drewnowski and Stephen E. Specter, "Poverty and Obesity: The Role of Energy Density and Energy Costs," *The American Journal of Clinical Nutrition* 79, no. 1 (2004): 6–16; Nicole Darmon, Elaine Ferguson, and André Briend, "Do Economic Constraints Encourage the Selection of Energy Dense Diets?" *Appetite* 41, no. 3 (2003): 315–322.

125. Patrick H. Casey et al., "Children in Food-insufficient, Low-income Families: Prevalence, Health, and Nutrition Status," *Archives of Pediatrics & Adolescent Medicine* 155, no. 4 (2001): 508–514.

126. John J. Reilly, J. Kelly, and D. C. Wilson, "Accuracy of Simple Clinical and Epidemiological Definitions of Childhood Obesity: Systematic Review and Evidence Appraisal," *Obesity Reviews* 11, no. 9 (2010): 645–655.

127. Gary Bickel et al., "Guide to Measuring Household Food Security" (2000).

128. Gundersen and Ziliak, "Food Insecurity Research in the United States: Where We Have Been and Where We Need to Go."

129. Gundersen and Ziliak, "Food Insecurity Research in the United States: Where We Have Been and Where We Need to Go"; Judith Bartfeld et al., *SNAP Matters: How Food Stamps Affect Health and Well-being* (Stanford University Press, 2015).

130. Craig Gunderson, Brent Kreider, and John V. Pepper, "Reconstructing the Supplemental Nutrition Assistance Program to More Effectively Alleviate Food Insecurity in the United States," *RSF: The Russell Sage Foundation Journal of The Social Sciences* 4, no. 2 (2018): 113–130; J. Ziliak, "Modernizing SNAP Benefits," The Hamilton Project, Policy Proposal 2016–06, https://www.hamiltonproject.org/assets/files/ziliak_modernizing_snap_benefits.pdf.

131. Angie Hunt, "For Food Security, SNAP and WIC Aren't Redundant," *Futurity*, published June 13, 2019, https://www.futurity.org/food-security-families-2082362-2/.

132. Jay Bhattacharya and Janet Currie, "Youths at Nutrition Risk: Malnourished or Misnourished?," In *Risky Behavior Among Youths: An Economic Analysis* (University of Chicago Press, 2001), 483–522; Mark Nord and Kathleen Romig, "Hunger in the Summer: Seasonal Food Insecurity and the National School Lunch and Summer Food Service Programs," *Journal of Children and Poverty* 12, no. 2 (2006): 141–158.

133. Daniel P. Miller, "Accessibility of Summer Meals and the Food Insecurity of Low-income Households With Children," *Public Health Nutrition* 19, no. 11 (2016): 2079–2089.

134. Gundersen and Ziliak, "Food Insecurity Research in the United States: Where We Have Been and Where We Need to Go."

135. Mariana Chilton, Michelle Chyatte, and Jennifer Breaux, "The Negative Effects of Poverty & Food Insecurity on Child Development," *Indian Journal of Medical Research* 126, no. 4 (2007): 262.

136. Mercedes De Onis et al., "The WHO Multicentre Growth Reference Study: Planning, Study Design, and Methodology," *Food and Nutrition Bulletin* 25, no. 1_suppl_1 (2004): S15–S26.

137. Cesar G. Victora et al., "The Pelotas Birth Cohort Study, Rio Grande do Sul, Brazil, 1982–2001," *Cadernos de Saude Publica* 19, no. 5 (2003): 1241–1256.

138. Diana F. Jyoti, Edward A. Frongillo, and Sonya J. Jones, "Food Insecurity Affects School Children's Academic Performance, Weight Gain, and Social Skills," *The Journal of Nutrition* 135, no. 12 (2005): 2831–2839; Ronald E. Kleinman et al., "Hunger in Children in the United States: Potential Behavioral and Emotional Correlates," *Pediatrics* 101, no. 1 (1998): e3–e3; Michael J. Murphy et al., "Relationship Between Hunger and Psychosocial Functioning in Low-income American Children," *Journal of The American Academy of Child & Adolescent Psychiatry* 37, no. 2 (1998): 163–170; Katherine Alaimo, Christine M. Olson, and Edward A. Frongillo, "Food Insufficiency and American School-aged Children's Cognitive, Academic, and Psychosocial Development," *Pediatrics* 108, no. 1 (2001): 44–53.

139. Jyoti, Frongillo, and Jones, "Food Insecurity Affects School Children's Academic Performance, Weight Gain, and Social Skills"; Katherine Alaimo, Christine M. Olson, and Edward A. Frongillo, "Family Food Insufficiency, But Not Low Family Income, is Positively Associated With Dysthymia and Suicide Symptoms in Adolescents," *The Journal of Nutrition* 132, no. 4 (2002): 719–725.

140. Bapu Vaitla, Stephen Devereux, and Samuel Hauenstein Swan, "Seasonal Hunger: A Neglected Problem With Proven Solutions," *PLoS Med* 6, no. 6 (2009): e1000101.

141. H. Bruce Ferguson, Sarah Bovaird, and Michael P. Mueller, "The Impact of Poverty on Educational Outcomes for Children," *Paediatrics & Child Health* 12, no. 8 (2007): 701–706.

142. Sean F. Reardon, Joseph P. Robinson, and Ericka S. Weathers, "Patterns and Trends in Racial/ethnic and Socioeconomic Academic Achievement Gaps," *Handbook of Research in Education Finance and Policy* (2008): 497–516.

143. S. D. Sparks, "New Student Majority in South and West: Poor Children," *Education Week* 33, no. 9 (2013): 6.

144. Linda Darling-Hammond, "Unequal Opportunity: Race and Education," *Brookings*, published March 1, 1998, https://www.brookings.edu/articles/unequal-opportunity-race-and-education/.

145. Chris Duncombe, "Unequal Opportunities: Fewer Resources, Worse Outcomes for Students in Schools With Concentrated Poverty," *The Commonwealth*

Institute, published October 26, 2017, https://www.thecommonwealthinstitute.org/2017/10/26/unequal-opportunities-fewer-resources-worse-outcomes-for-students-in-schools-with-concentrated-poverty/.

146. U.S. Department of Education, "Equity of Opportunity," accessed October 15, 2019, https://www.ed.gov/equity.

147. Duncombe, "Unequal Opportunities."

148. Alana Semuels, "Good School, Rich School; Bad School, Poor School," *The Atlantic*, published August 25, 2016, https://www.theatlantic.com/business/archive/2016/08/property-taxes-and-unequal-schools/497333/.

149. Ary Spatig-Amerikaner, "Unequal Education: Federal Loophole Enables Lower Spending on Students of Color," *Center for American Progress* (2012).

150. Spatig-Amerikaner, "Unequal Education."

151. Paul Barnwell, "Why Teachers Quit: It's Not About Money (or Low-Pay)," *The Atlantic*, published May 27, 2015, https://www.theatlantic.com/education/archive/2015/05/the-ongoing-struggle-of-teacher-retention/394211/.

152. Marie Bjerede, "Rural Districts Face Challenges and Opportunities With Technology Access," *Technology Solutions That Drive Education*, published January 2, 2018, https://edtechmagazine.com/k12/article/2018/01/rural-districts-face-challenges-and-opportunities-technology-access.

153. H. Bruce Ferguson, Sarah Bovaird, and Michael P. Mueller, "The Impact of Poverty on Educational Outcomes for Children," *Paediatrics & Child Health* 12, no. 8 (2007): 701–706.

154. Karl L. Alexander, Doris R. Entwisle, and Linda S. Olson, "Schools, Achievement, and Inequality: A Seasonal Perspective," *Educational Evaluation and Policy Analysis* 23, no. 2 (2001): 171–191.

155. Semuels, "Good School, Rich School; Bad School, Poor School."

156. Catherine E. Ross and Chia-ling Wu, "The Links Between Education and Health," *American Sociological Review* (1995): 719–745.

157. Louk W. H. Peters et al., "Effective Elements of School Health Promotion Across Behavioral Domains: A Systematic Review of Reviews," *BMC Public Health* 9, no. 1 (2009): 182.

158. Catherine N. Rasberry et al., "The Association Between School-based Physical Activity, Including Physical Education, and Academic Performance: A Systematic Review of the Literature," *Preventive Medicine* 52 (2011): S10–S20.

159. Jeannine S. Schiller, Jacqueline W. Lucas, and Jennifer A. Peregoy, "Summary Health Statistics for US Adults: National Health Interview Survey, 2011" (2012).

160. Leif Jensen, Jill L. Findeis, and Qiuyan Wang, "Labor Supply and Underemployment in the Southern United States," *Journal of Rural Social Sciences* 16, no. 1 (2000): 5.

161. Chris Kromm, "The South's Economic Crisis," *Facing South*, published October 18, 2011, https://www.facingsouth.org/2011/10/the-souths-economic-crisis.html.

162. Robert Scott, "The Manufacturing Footprint and the Importance of U.S. Manufacturing Jobs," *Economic Policy Institute*, published January 22, 2015,

https://www.epi.org/publication/the-manufacturing-footprint-and-the-importance-of-u-s-manufacturing-jobs/.

163. Ken Jacobs et al., "Producing Poverty: The Public Cost of Low-Wage Production Jobs in Manufacturing," *UC Berkely Center for Labor Research and Education*, published May 10, 2016, http://laborcenter.berkeley.edu/producing-poverty-the-public-cost-of-low-wage-production-jobs-in-manufacturing/.

164. Robert A. Hahn and Benedict I. Truman, "Education Improves Public Health and Promotes Health Equity," *International Journal of Health Services* 45, no. 4 (2015): 657–678.

165. Kelly McCarrier et al., "Associations Between Minimum Wage Policy and Access to Health Care: Evidence From the Behavioral Risk Factor Surveillance System, 1996–2007," *American Journal of Public Health* 101, no. 2 (2011): 359–367.

166. Eridan M. Coutinho et al., "Factors Involved in Schistosoma Mansoni Infection, in Rural Areas of Northeast Brazil," *Memórias do Instituto Oswaldo Cruz* 92 (1997): 707–715.

167. N. Douthit et al., "Exposing Some Important Barriers to Health Care Access in the Rural USA," *Public Health* 129, no. 6 (2015): 611–620.

168. Ping Zhang, Guoyu Tao, and Lynda A. Anderson, "Differences in Access to Health Care Services Among Adults in Rural America by Rural Classification Categories and Age," *Australian Journal of Rural Health* 11, no. 2 (2003): 64–72.

169. Lanis L. Hicks, "Availability and Accessibility of Rural Health Care," *The Journal of Rural Health* 6, no. 4 (1990): 485–506.

170. "Title 42 CFR Parts 1-60," Federal Register, (1988).

171. Hicks, "Availability and Accessibility of Rural Health Care."

172. John Wills, Louis Garrison, and Itzhak Jacoby, *Report of The Graduate Medical Education National Advisory Committee to The Secretary, Department of Health and Human Services: Modeling, Research, and Data Technical Panel* (U.S. Department of Health and Human Services, Public Health Service, Health Resources Administration, Office of Graduate Medical Education, 1981).

173. R. Turner Goins et al., "Perceived Barriers to Health Care Access Among Rural Older Adults: A Qualitative Study," *The Journal of Rural Health* 21, no. 3 (2005): 206–213.

174. Goins et al., "Perceived Barriers to Health Care Access Among Rural Older Adults: A Qualitative Study."

175. Goins et al., "Perceived Barriers to Health Care Access Among Rural Older Adults: A Qualitative Study."

176. Larry Ortiz, Lydia Arizmendi, and Llewellyn J. Cornelius, "Access to Health Care Among Latinos of Mexican Descent in Colonias in Two Texas Counties," *The Journal of Rural Health* 20, no. 3 (2004): 246–252.

177. Zhang, Tao, and Anderson, "Differences in Access to Health Care Services Among Adults in Rural America by Rural Classification Categories and Age."

178. Tom Wilemon, "TN, KY Are Miles Apart on Medicaid," *The Tennessean*, published July 22, 2013, https://passportmedia.wordpress.com/2013/07/22/tn-ky-are-miles-apart-on-medicaid/.

179. Rachel Garfield et al., "The Coverage Gap: Uninsured Poor Adults in States That do Not Expand Medicaid–an Update," Menlo Park, CA: Kaiser Family Foundation (2016).

180. Wilemon, "TN, KY Are Miles Apart on Medicaid."

181. KFF, "Health Insurance Coverage of the Total Population," accessed November 15, 2019, https://www.kff.org/other/state-indicator/total-population/?currentTimeframe=0&selectedRows=%7B%22states%22:%7B%22kentucky%22:%7B%7D%7D%7D&sortModel=%7B%22colId%22:%22Location%22,%22sort%22:%22asc%22%7D; Brett Kelman, "Tennessee Suffered Third-largest Increase of Uninsured People in the Nation, Census Reports," *Tennessean*, published September 11, 2019, https://www.tennessean.com/story/news/health/2019/09/11/tennessee-uninsured-residents-tenncare-census-report/2276127001/.

182. State Health Access Data Assistance Center, "Study of the Impact of the ACA Implementation in Kentucky," *Foundation for a Healthy Kentucky*, published 2016, http://files.constantcontact.com/1b4946a6001/7cc9e76b-04fa-45d3-8ac3-6ef33d321d13.pdf.

183. John Loftus et al., "Rural-urban Differences in Access to Preventive Health Care Among Publicly Insured Minnesotans," *The Journal of Rural Health* 34 (2018): s48–s55; Xinxin Han et al., "Reports of Insurance-based Discrimination in Health Care and Its Association With Access to Care," *American Journal of Public Health* 105, no. S3 (2015): S517–S525.

184. "Americans With Disabilities Act of 1990, Pub. L. No. 101–336, 104 Stat. 328." Americans With Disabilities Act (ADA) (1990).

185. Denise M. Lishner et al., "Access to Primary Health Care Among Persons With Disabilities in Rural Areas: A Summary of the Literature," *The Journal of Rural Health* 12, no. 1 (1996): 45–53.

186. Linda M. Levey, James P. Curry, and Samuel Levey, "Rural-urban Differences in Access to Iowa Child Health Services," *The Journal of Rural Health* 4, no. 2 (1988): 59–72.

187. Lishner et al., "Access to Primary Health Care Among Persons With Disabilities in Rural Areas," 45–53.

188. Elisaveta P. Petkova et al., "Climate Change and Health on the US Gulf Coast: Public Health Adaptation is Needed to Address Future Risks," *International Journal of Environmental Research and Public Health* 12, no. 8 (2015): 9342–9356.

189. Petkova et al., "Climate Change and Health on the US Gulf Coast."

190. Peter J. Hotez and Sheila Jackson Lee, "US Gulf Coast States: The Rise of Neglected Tropical Diseases in 'Flyover Nation'," *PLOS Neglected Tropical Diseases* 11, no. 11 (2017): e0005744.

191. Charles Warren Thornthwaite, "An Approach Toward a Rational Classification of Climate," *Geographical Review* 38, no. 1 (1948): 55–94.

192. R. B. Waide et al., "The Relationship Between Productivity and Species Richness," *Annual Review of Ecology and Systematics* 30, no. 1 (1999): 257–300.

193. Felicia Keesing et al., "Impacts of Biodiversity on the Emergence and Transmission of Infectious Diseases," *Nature* 468, no. 7324 (2010): 647–652.

194. Peter J. Hotez, Kristy O. Murray, and Pierre Buekens, "The Gulf Coast: A New American Underbelly of Tropical Diseases and Poverty," *PLoS Neglected Tropical Diseases* 8, no. 5 (2014): e2760.

195. Vanina Guernier, Michael E. Hochberg, and Jean-François Guégan, "Ecology Drives the Worldwide Distribution of Human Diseases," *PLoS Biol* 2, no. 6 (2004): e141.

196. Rebecca E. Hirsch, *Climate Migrants: On the Move in a Warming World* (Twenty-First Century Books, 2016), 8–10.

197. Jennifer Leaning and Debarati Guha-Sapir, "Natural Disasters, Armed Conflict, and Public Health," *New England Journal of Medicine* 369, no. 19 (2013): 1836–1842; Mackey et al., "Emerging and Reemerging Neglected Tropical Diseases: A Review of Key Characteristics, Risk Factors, and the Policy and Innovation Environment," 949–979.

198. Guernier, Hochberg, and Guégan, "Ecology Drives the Worldwide Distribution of Human Diseases."

199. Rodolfo U. Carcavallo and Susana Curto de Casas, "Some Health Impacts of Global Warming in South America: Vector-borne Diseases," *Journal of Epidemiology* 6, no. 4 supp (1996): 153–157.

200. Peggy Deichstetter, "The Effect of Climate Change on Mosquito-Borne Diseases," *The American Biology Teacher* 79, no. 3 (2017): 169–173.

201. David Andrew Ewing et al., "Modelling the Effect of Temperature on the Seasonal Population Dynamics of Temperate Mosquitoes," *Journal of Theoretical Biology* 400 (2016): 65–79.

202. Barry W. Alto and Steven A. Juliano, "Temperature Effects on the Dynamics of Aedes Albopictus (Diptera: Culicidae) Populations in the Laboratory," *Journal of Medical Entomology* 38, no. 4 (2001): 548–556; R. S. Kovats et al., "Early Effects of Climate Change: Do They Include Changes in Vector-borne Disease?" *Philosophical Transactions of The Royal Society of London: Series B: Biological Sciences* 356, no. 1411 (2001): 1057–1068.

203. Jan C. Semenza et al., "Mapping Climate Change Vulnerabilities to Infectious Diseases in Europe," *Environmental Health Perspectives* 120, no. 3 (2012): 385–392.

204. Su Hyun Lee et al., "The Effects of Climate Change and Globalization on Mosquito Vectors: Evidence From Jeju Island, South Korea on the Potential for Asian Tiger Mosquito (Aedes Albopictus) Influxes and Survival From Vietnam Rather Than Japan," *PloS One* 8, no. 7 (2013): e68512.

205. Haylee J. Weaver, John M. Hawdon, and Eric P. Hoberg, "Soil-transmitted Helminthiases: Implications of Climate Change and Human Behavior," *Trends in Parasitology* 26, no. 12 (2010): 574–581.

206. Gerardo Chowell et al., "Assessing the Potential Impact of Vector-borne Disease Transmission Following Heavy Rainfall Events: A Mathematical Framework," *Philosophical Transactions of The Royal Society B* 374, no. 1775 (2019): 20180272.

207. Dim Coumou and Stefan Rahmstorf, "A Decade of Weather Extremes," *Nature Climate Change* 2, no. 7 (2012): 491–496.

208. Carolyn Gramling, "'Sunny Day' High Tide Floods Are on the Rise Along U.S. Coasts," published July 15, 2019, https://www.sciencenews.org/article/sunny-day-high-tide-floods-are-rise-along-us-coasts.

209. Alexis Madrigal, "Why the Gulf Coast Is Uniquely Vulnerable to Disasters," *The Atlantic*, published August 29, 2017, https://www.theatlantic.com/technology/archive/2017/08/why-the-gulf-coast-is-uniquely-vulnerable-to-disasters-hurricane-harvey/538374/.

210. Angus Cook et al., "10th Anniversary Review: Natural Disasters and Their Long-term Impacts on the Health of Communities," *Journal of Environmental Monitoring* 10, no. 2 (2008): 167–175.

211. Cook et al., "10th Anniversary Review: Natural Disasters and Their Long-term Impacts on the Health of Communities."

212. Environment Texas Research & Policy Center, "Raw Sewage Released by Hurricane Harvey," published September 20, 2017, https://environmenttexascenter.org/reports/txe/raw-sewage-released-hurricane-harvey.

213. Wudan Yan, "Grappling With the Health Consequences of Floods: Hurricanes, Monsoons, and Heavy Rains Have Researchers Studying How to Prevent the Diseases That Often Follow," *IEEE Pulse* 9, no. 2 (2018): 26–30.

214. Vikram Kapoor et al., "Real-time Quantitative PCR Measurements of Fecal Indicator Bacteria and Human-associated Source Tracking Markers in a Texas River Following Hurricane Harvey," *Environmental Science & Technology Letters* 5, no. 6 (2018): 322–328.

215. Gregg P. Greenough and Thomas D. Kirsch, "Hurricane Katrina. Public Health Response–Assessing Needs," *New England Journal of Medicine* 353, no. 15 (2005): 1544–1546.

216. Cook et al., "10th Anniversary Review: Natural Disasters and Their Long-term Impacts on the Health of Communities."

217. Judy Stone, "Hurricanes, Poverty, and Neglected Infections," *Scientific American Blog Network*, published August 30, 2012, https://blogs.scientificamerican.com/molecules-to-medicine/hurricane-katrina-poverty-and-neglected-infections/.

218. Robert C. Bolin, "Disaster Impact and Recovery: A Comparison of Black and White Victims," *International Journal of Mass Emergencies and Disasters* 4, no. 1 (1986): 35–50.

219. Alice Fothergill and Lori A. Peek, "Poverty and Disasters in the United States: A Review of Recent Sociological Findings," *Natural Hazards* 32, no. 1 (2004): 89–110.

220. Michel Masozera, Melissa Bailey, and Charles Kerchner, "Distribution of Impacts of Natural Disasters Across Income Groups: A Case Study of New Orleans," *Ecological Economics* 63, nos. 2–3 (2007): 299–306.

221. Neil Smith, "There's no Such Thing as a Natural Disaster: Understanding Katrina," *SSRC Perspectives From The Social Sciences* (2006).

222. Sidney Blumenthal, "Katrina Comes Home to Roost," *The Guardian*, published September 2, 2005, https://www.theguardian.com/world/2005/sep/02/hurricanekatrina.usa10.

223. Camilla Stivers, "'So Poor and so Black': Hurricane Katrina, Public Administration, and the Issue of Race," *Public Administration Review* 67 (2007): 48–56.

224. The Urban Institute, "Katrina: Demographics of a Disaster," published September 9, 2005, https://www.urban.org/sites/default/files/publication/52091/900835-katrina-demographics-of-a-disaster_0.pdf.

225. U.S. Department of Health and Human Services Office of Minority Health, "Profile: Black/African Americans," accessed December 2019, https://minorityhealth.hhs.gov/omh/browse.aspx?lvl=3&lvlid=61.

226. Stephen Zuckerman and Teresa Coughlin, "Initial Health Policy Responses to Hurricane Katrina and Possible Next Steps" (2006).

227. Leah J. Tulin, "Poverty and Chronic Conditions During Natural Disasters: A Glimpse at Health, Healing, and Hurricane Katrina," *Geo. J. on Poverty L. & Pol'y* 14 (2007): 115.

228. Fothergill and Peek, "Poverty and Disasters in the United States," 89–110.

229. Kristen Lavelle and Joe Feagin, "Hurricane Katrina: The Race and Class Debate," *Monthly Review* 58, no. 3 (2006): 52.

230. Masozera, Bailey, and Kerchner, "Distribution of Impacts of Natural Disasters Across Income Groups."

231. Fothergill and Peek, "Poverty and Disasters in the United States: A Review of Recent Sociological Findings."

232. Catherine Simile and Kristen S. Miller, "They Could See Stars From Their Beds: The Plight of the Rural Poor in the Aftermath of Hurricane Hugo" (1992).

233. T. B. Edsall, "Bush Suspends Pay Act in Areas Hit by Storm," *Washington Post*, *9*, D3, published September 9, 2005, https://www.washingtonpost.com/wp-dyn/content/article/2005/09/08/AR2005090802037.html.

234. Masozera, Bailey, and Kerchner, "Distribution of Impacts of Natural Disasters Across Income Groups."

235. Parsons, "Ascarid Infections of Cats and Dogs," 1307–1339.

236. Rachel Curtis et al., "Chagas Disease in Texas Information for Veterinary Professionals With Canine Patients," *Texas A&M University School of Veterinary Medicine and Biomedical Sciences*, accessed August 2019, https://kissingbug.tamu.edu/files/canine-chagas-disease-2.pdf.

237. Ardem Elmaya et al., "High Prevalence of Trypanosoma Cruzi Infection in Shelter Dogs From Southern Louisiana, USA," *Parasites & Vectors* 12. no. 1 (2019): 322.

238. Alyssa C. Meyers, Marvin Meinders, and Sarah A. Hamer, "Widespread Trypanosoma Cruzi Infection in Government Working Dogs Along the Texas-Mexico Border: Discordant Serology, Parasite Genotyping and Associated Vectors," *PLoS Neglected Tropical Diseases* 11, no. 8 (2017): e0005819.

239. Eleonora Lima Alves Cunha et al., "Benznidazole, Itraconazole and Their Combination in the Treatment of Acute Experimental Chagas Disease in Dogs," *Experimental Parasitology* 204 (2019): 107711.

240. M. A. Laiño et al., "An Oral Dose of Fluralaner Administered to Dogs Kills Pyrethroid-Resistant and Susceptible Chagas Disease Vectors for at Least Four Months," *Veterinary Parasitology* 268 (2019): 98–104.

241. Curtis et al., "Chagas Disease in Texas Information for Veterinary Professionals With Canine Patients."

242. Pet Leadership Council, "2015–2016 APPA National Pet Owners Survey – Generational Report," accessed August 19, 2019, https://www.google.com/url?rct=j&sa=t&url=http://www.americanpetproducts.org/pubs_generationalreport.asp&ct=ga&cd=CAIyGjMyOWZlN2U4NmFkZjU2M2E6Y29tOmVuOlVT&usg=AFQjCNGzc1w9n3jhBk5rW-wRiuk6JFhh8Q.

243. American Society for the Prevention of Cruelty to Animals, "Pet Statistics," accessed August 19, 2019, https://www.aspca.org/animal-homelessness/shelter-intake-and-surrender/pet-statistics.

244. Matt Bershadker, "Acting on the Critical Link Between Pets, People, and Poverty," American Society for the Prevention of Cruelty to Animals, published February 26, 2019, https://www.aspca.org/blog/acting-critical-link-between-pets-people-and-poverty.

245. Donald E. Vermeer and Dennis A. Frate, "Geophagy in a Mississippi County," *Annals of the Association of American Geographers* 65, no. 3 (1975): 414–424.

246. John M. Hunter, "Geophagy in Africa and in the United States: A Culture-Nutrition Hypothesis," *Geographical Review* (1973): 170–195.

247. Hunter, "Geophagy in Africa and in the United States: A Culture-Nutrition Hypothesis."

248. Vermeer and DFrate, "Geophagy in a Mississippi County."

249. Dorothy Dickins and Robert N. Ford, "Geophagy (dirt Eating) Among Mississippi Negro School Children," *American Sociological Review* 7, no. 1 (1942): 59–65.

250. Naida Gavrelis et al., "An Analysis of the Proportion of the US Population That Ingests Soil or Other Non-food Substances," *Human and Ecological Risk Assessment: An International Journal* 17, no. 4 (2011): 996–1012.

251. Emelyn Rude, "The American South Is Still Eating White Dirt," *Vice*, published June 5, 2015, https://www.vice.com/en_us/article/pgxwvk/the-american-south-is-still-eating-white-dirt.

252. P. Wallace, *Eat White Dirt*, Directed by Forrester A., United States: Public Broadcasting Service, 2015; Linda Chen, "The Old and Mysterious Practice of Eating Dirt, Revealed," *NPR*, published April 2, 2014, https://www.npr.org/sections/thesalt/2014/04/02/297881388/the-old-and-mysterious-practice-of-eating-dirt-revealed.

253. Rude, "The American South Is Still Eating White Dirt."

Chapter 4

The People's Voice

Poverty and NTDs in the Modern-Day South

NTDs are diseases of extreme poverty. Scientists around the world understand them biologically and methods exist to prevent individuals from becoming infected with these chronic, and often deadly, diseases. Additionally, screening methods and treatments exist for the majority of the diseases that fall within the classification of NTDs. Given the extensive knowledge of these diseases, how they spread, and how they are treated, it is vital that attention is paid to NTDs in the United States. They exist as a direct result of social, political, and economic elements, not because we lack prevention methods. As Dr. Peter Hotez explained, "poverty is the overriding determinant of Neglected Tropical Diseases . . . it's the social determinants that are driving these diseases."[1] That is to say, poverty, and the social elements in the United States that allow extreme poverty to persist, are the driving cause of NTD infection.

While nowhere in the United States is exempt from poverty, the South has a long history of social inequality and political and economic oppression, which created and maintains much of the extreme poverty that still persists in the region. The social and political structures of slavery and the Jim Crow era contributed directly to the legacy of poverty that many African Americans in the South still fight to escape. As Nelson Mandela stated, "Like slavery and apartheid, poverty is not natural. It is man-made and can be overcome and eradicated by the actions of human beings."[2] The disproportionate levels of poverty among people of color, largely due to structural inequalities, is a main reason that NTD infection rates are higher among African Americans and Latinos. But to say the story of NTDs is tied only to the legacy of slavery would be inaccurate. As a white, female resident in her late twenties, who had lived in one of the communities in this study for years, put it: "poverty has no race." People of every race and ethnicity live in poverty in the United States.

This extreme poverty persists throughout a wealthy country like the United States because, "poverty is not simply a lack of resources but also of political capital/voice."[3] Any place in which people are politically and economically marginalized, regardless of race, may struggle with poverty.

The diversity of poverty is as important to keep in mind as the historical and current social and political structures that allow for extreme poverty to exist. This book focuses on extreme poverty in rural communities because rural communities face different challenges than do communities of urban poverty. Many of the rural communities we visited are isolated, which makes it easier for their fellow Americans to remain ignorant of the challenges these community residents face. In most of the communities we visited, poverty promotes poverty. A lack of resources and political power creates almost insurmountable obstacles for even the most motivated individuals. These are communities of tremendous need, but also communities of tremendous strength. Many residents believed that things would get better and were actively working to improve the community. The best way to describe the individuals that participated in this study is: resilient and giving. All the communities we worked with had many of their residents unemployed and 30 percent or more living below the poverty line. All the communities we worked with struggled to provide their children with a decent education. Many had inadequate housing, water, sanitation or all three. Some struggled to put food on the table, but all spoke passionately about their visions for their community's future. Many of the communities still struggled with racism and political oppression, which helped to hold them firmly in the grips of poverty, and all were realistic about the challenges they faced in bringing in jobs, improving schools, and reducing negative health outcomes.

It is easy for middle-class or upper-class Americans to forget that these communities exist. They are not on TV and they are not in the newspapers. They struggle in silence and isolation. They are in counties and states with limited resources as it is, which makes it that much more difficult for health departments and politicians to find the funding and personnel to look at public health issues, let alone the existence of NTDs. In other words, it is easier to *not* look at the problem than to look at it and find solutions. There are no villains in this story, just individuals facing different sets of seemingly impossible challenges.

It is the blame-oriented narrative of poverty that allows many Americans to turn a blind eye to the struggles of the communities in this study and the hundreds of others like them throughout the country. Over the course of 14 months we held focus groups, conducted one-on-one interviews, made presentations, and had casual conversations over lunch or while munching on a snow cone bought from a set of entrepreneurial children. We chatted on the porch swings of residents' houses, talked about college football with local shop owners and hospital administrators, and had conversations with elementary-aged children about their favorite subjects in school or their new puppy. We sought to understand the five communities in our study as much as is possible as an outsider so that we could expose the social elements that allow NTDs—diseases considered by many physicians, scientists, and policy-makers to only be present in low-income countries—to thrive in the United States.

In this chapter, we detail the beliefs and attitudes of community residents. We use their voices to describe the challenges they face, the cycle of poverty that exists in their communities, and the components that put them at risk of NTDs. Although all five communities are classified as communities of extreme poverty, they are not all the same. They have different histories, different challenges, and different visions of the future. In this chapter, we have tried to capture their stories to give voice to the struggles of many rural Americans, and many people of color, living in the Southern United States. We have chosen to use pseudonyms for each community and the residents we spoke to in order to provide anonymity for the residents that participated in this study. The information contained in this chapter seeks to detail the NTD infection risk factors that we witnessed firsthand and expose the social, political, and economic structures (both formal and informal) that create these risk factors.

STUDY METHODS

Community Selection

In the United States, NTDs are concentrated almost exclusively in areas of extreme poverty. Therefore, to examine the likely prevalence of NTDs in the United States, we focused on the most high-risk communities throughout the American South. Our reasoning for selecting only communities located in the South was twofold. The Southern United States has a unique combination of high poverty rates and a suitable climate for NTDs, making many Southern communities at elevated risk for infection. Additionally, although there are pockets of extreme poverty in urban areas, we chose to focus on rural areas because there is higher prevalence of NTDs among rural populations globally and the unique challenges for health access, adequate infrastructure, and knowledge development faced by low-income rural communities.[4] In a small, isolated town with no industry, there are very few jobs to be had. This means that members of the community have to choose between unemployment and leaving their home, where generations of their family have lived. Additionally, there is a real, physical barrier to health-care access. Individuals in rural communities may have to travel hours to get medical care. For those without a car or money for travel, this makes accessing basic healthcare nearly impossible. And finally, isolation means that most Americans have never heard of these communities. They are not confronted with images of poverty in rural communities throughout the South. These conditions create the greatest risk for prevalence of NTDs and, therefore, we choose to focus on them for our study.

To select the appropriate communities for inclusion in this study, we identified rural counties that had a poverty rate of 50 percent or greater. We began by looking at county level data, because accurate information at the town-level was difficult to obtain. After identifying counties with a poverty rate of 50 percent or greater, we looked for communities with median family incomes of under $25,000 and a high percentage of people of color. We looked for communities with a high percentage of people of color because previous research indicates that people of color are disproportionately affected by NTD infections.[5] Lastly, we targeted rural areas of the county.

The U.S. Census Bureau defines rural as everything that is left after individual urban areas have been defined.[6] In order to define urban, the U.S. Census Bureau looks at population thresholds, density, land use, and distance. Other departments have different definitions regarding what qualifies as rural, but for this study, we chose to use a measure of total population and proximity to urban centers. With one exception, the average population in the communities that participated in this study was around 2,500 and a minimum of an hour's drive from the nearest urban center or city. The one exception to this was the community Marigold, Texas which has a population of over 100,000 people and would be defined by the U.S. Census Bureau as an urban area. The reason Marigold was included in the study is because of its identity as a border community, the high population of refugees and immigrants—who are at high risk for NTD infection and can be isolated from the surrounding health system—and the rural isolation of the surrounding colonias.

Upon identifying communities that fit the study parameters, we began contacting local churches, nonprofits, health departments, schools, and local government officials to solicit interest in the project. Many people we contacted did not respond or were suspicious of our intentions. Eventually, one community agreed to participate and had connections with other nonprofits in some of our target communities. Through this snowball effect, we were able to recruit the remainder of communities for the project.

Data Gathering

Data for this project was gathered through focus groups and one-on-one interviews conducted by multiple members of the research team. Local community leaders, whether they were directors of a local nonprofit, leaders in the faith community, elected government officials, or city employees, played a central role in recruiting individuals to participate in focus groups and interviews. These local leaders served as a go-between for our research team, talking to community members, distributing information, setting up interviews and attendance at various community meetings, and getting residents to the focus group location.

One focus group was held in each community, for a total of five focus groups. For each focus group we aimed to have four to eight individuals participate, with the average focus group hosting six individuals. The average age of focus group participants varied by community, but ranged from individuals in their mid-twenties to individuals in their early seventies. Eighty-three percent of focus group participants were female and 17 percent were male. Fifty-nine percent of participants were African American, 31 percent were white, and 10 percent were Latino. All conversations within the focus group discussion were captured via audio recording. The purpose of audio recording focus group conversations was to ensure accuracy in the information we obtained from residents.

A total of forty-three one-on-one interviews were conducted over the course of this project. Approximately ten to fifteen one-on-one interviews were collected per community, with the exception of Poppy, Mississippi, where only two one-on-one interviews were conducted. Information gained through one-on-one interviews was recorded only through the use of hand-written notes. We determined that interview subjects felt more comfortable and were willing to speak more openly in a one-on-one setting when they were not being recorded. Members of the research team worked to catch as much detail as possible, including exact quotes, with hand-written notations.

Data Analysis

Once all data was obtained from residents throughout the community, the audio recordings and hand-written notes were transcribed by members of the research team. Data was separated by community and by topic. This allowed the research team to conduct a comparative case study on low-income rural communities in the American South. There were numerous areas of overlap, but each community had different opinions of the primary issue or concern. Using the comparative case study method to identify similarities, differences, and patterns across the five cases, we built a picture of the components that put these communities at risk for NTD infection and discussed the broad challenges they face in issues that result from and are related to NTDs, such as poverty, health care access, and social dynamics.

The following chapter provides descriptions for each community, along with historical context. Each community that participated in the study was unique, despite overlapping in a number of issues. For this reason, it is important to understand the specific context for each community and our research team's experience working with them. Following the individual community descriptions, we have combined all information gained from the communities into relevant topic areas. As a reminder, the names of communities and residents have been changed in order to provide the communities with confidentiality.

COMMUNITY OVERVIEW

Peony, Louisiana

Meandering down the two-lane highway, one cannot help but be struck by the sense of calm here. Rain has come through recently as both the potholes in the road and the fields are inundated with water. Everything is still and quiet. The sun shines down through the car windows and the fields are a brilliant shade of green. Large farm houses can be seen on both sides of the highway, with combines and sprayers tucked away in a shop or near a grain elevator. Slowly, the peace of the fields gives way to the outskirts of a small town and the mood changes. Both sides of the streets are lined with small, dilapidated houses and trailers. Some have tarps where a roof should be; some look altogether abandoned. But block after block of deteriorating buildings show signs of life: Kids toys strewn across the front yard, recently vacated chairs on the front porch, the occasional decoration on the door.

Peony is situated along the banks of the Mississippi River and offers beautiful views along with an abundance of wildlife. The natural beauty of the area even compelled a visit from an American president. Running parallel with the town's scenic history, however, is a long and violent history of racial discrimination. The area once held massive cotton plantations and thousands upon thousands of slaves. White plantation owners became wealthy as a result of the work of enslaved Africans and the social structure of white supremacy was firmly established. The Civil War brought upheaval to the region and the presence of Union troops became a regular occurrence, with many of Peony's slaves fleeing behind Union lines for safety. While the Emancipation Proclamation provided hope for enslaved people, and Peony experienced a growth in African American land ownership that was rare in the post–Civil War South, white residents worked quickly to reestablish the previous social and economic structure. Like most former plantation communities in the South, sharecropping became the new way of life for former slaves. The post-Reconstruction Era brought with it the continuation of white supremacist policies, especially the use of Jim Crow laws. As a majority

African American community, there were clashes during the Civil Rights Movement of the 1960s as African American residents fought against the white supremacy that engulfed Peony.

Today, Peony is, in many ways, typical of Southern former plantation communities; still trying to sweep an ugly history of discrimination under the rug. Life moves slower here and the friendly exterior barely hides the suspicion they feel at our presence. While some residents welcome us openly, the community still fights a daily battle against white supremist ideals and the inescapable current of racial discrimination.

As we wind our way through town, we note tires stacked in yards, standing water, a lack of screens on the windows. All things that we, as disease researchers, are trained to identify as risk factors for infection. The observation regarding the lack of window screens stings with irony as we realize that many of the homes have holes in them. During our first visit to Peony we are greeted warmly by Matthew, the community organizer that helped orchestrate the focus group, and he is happy to tell us all he can about the town. As other residents file in they all wear a smile and engage in friendly, spirited conversation. Their manner immediately makes you feel like you have known them for years rather than thirty seconds. Their charm and joyousness stands in stark contrast to the jarring poverty of the town. The reasons are hard to put your finger on, but something about these residents makes you fall in love with Peony; makes you see its beauty through all the hardship.

Peony is highly segregated with the white neighborhood on one side of town and the African American neighborhoods on the other. The difference in income between the African American neighborhoods and the white neighborhood is clear. In Peony, the white neighborhood is composed of well-kept brick houses with well-maintained yards. Many of the African American neighborhoods contained decaying homes. Matthew drove us to the "white" school and explained that this private school had been established after the federal government declared separate but equal unconstitutional as an attempt by the white community to maintain the segregated education system. Even today, the town's private school is almost exclusively white with the public school made up of almost exclusively African American students. As Duncan and Coles (1999) noted in their work on poverty in rural America, this practice of privatization took place all over the South following desegregation and was not just limited to schools.[7] Almost anything that could be privatized as a measure to avoid integration, was privatized.

The downtown of Peony is now mostly empty, with the majority of its buildings both vacant and uninhabitable. The crumbling store fronts tell a story of a different time. A time when shops lined the streets and people bustled around doing their shopping and visiting neighbors. A time when Peony had been prosperous. Many African American community members speak fondly of this economic prosperity even while acknowledging the overt Jim Crow discrimination of those years. This time had long since passed, however, and now dozens of young people move away every year in search of jobs.

As the American economy transitioned and technological innovation reached every corner of the United States, agrarian communities like Peony experienced the swift elimination of employment opportunities. What used to require ten workers could now be accomplished by one driving a machine. As jobs were eliminated, the lack of economic diversity in towns like Peony became inescapable. Aside from farming, there were no other opportunities and as a middle-aged African American resident named Rosyln explained, "Ain't everybody want to be a farmer. It's not the easiest job in the world. You've got to have your roots down there. I mean, you can't just all of a sudden decide you want to farm."

The lack of job opportunities that presented in the wake of mechanization drove residents further into poverty and deeply eroded their ability to escape the quickly deteriorating social and economic circumstances of their lives. Though, not all residents suffered. Most African Americans in the community had been sharecroppers. The mechanization of farming relieved their servitude but the white farmers had spent decades preventing other businesses from entering the community for fear they would lose their farm labor. Thus, when farming mechanized, the white farming community remained prosperous, while the African American community continued to suffer.

The majority of the residents we spoke with in Peony were African American. The only white residents that spoke with us were individuals who worked with the African American community and all of them were transplants to the town. It is important to note that there was disagreement among the residents with regards to the role racism played in daily life and the perpetuation of poverty. Some residents felt that it was not a problem in their community anymore, while others disagreed. The white residents who we spoke to stated very clearly that racism was still a significant problem and that the town remained highly segregated. We were surprised by the disagreement regarding the role of race in the community, but it is probable that the residents did not feel comfortable speaking freely on the topic with outsiders. The white residents who moved from outside the community noted that the idea of racial progress is relative. They stated that while things may be better in Peony compared to thirty or forty years ago, the racial norms were still far behind the curve of progress made in other places. On numerous other topics, however, all residents spoke more openly.

Residents of Peony are realistic about the obstacles they face in relieving the extreme poverty of the town, but there are several areas that they consider most pressing. These areas are: health care, unemployment, and housing.

Racial tensions and political oppression play important roles in perpetuating the health, employment, and housing challenges in Peony and, as such, residents discussed those social issues at length also and that is the reason that the topics have been included in this book. Residents believe that the political, social, and economic issue areas result from and contribute to the extreme poverty of the community, causing them to play a central role in the threat of NTDs within the community.

Poppy, Mississippi

The first time we visited Poppy a severe thunderstorm blanketed the town. Rain clanged loudly on the tin roof of the after-school center as we hurried inside. The downtown consists of a few buildings along one side of the street. Most are abandoned, some are caved in, but two or three have recently become occupied. Across from the short row of buildings sits what is typically a small creek. That day, due to excessive amounts of rain, the muddy brown water threatened to climb over the sides and into the streets. Houses sit perched on either side of the creek. Many of which are in need of repair. The condition of the housing is always one of the most startling elements of the communities we worked with in this study, but the day of our first visit to Poppy it was particularly notable as we wondered how many are cold and wet inside. Some may have even been filling with water as rain came unobstructed through holes in the roofs or broken windows.

Poppy is small and isolated. Large-scale farms radiate out in every direction but agriculture appears to be completely separate from the town. Unlike some of the other communities in this study, the farms are largely commercially run rather than farmed by members of the community and the African American residents of the town are completely separate from the surrounding agriculture. This is not a significant change from the agricultural history of the area, however, as even in the 1850s and 1860s many of the plantations were owned by absentee landlords and controlled by overseers. We are told that Poppy used to be approximately 50 percent white and 50 percent African American (though the historical data shows that African Americans always greatly outnumbered whites) but the white population began an exodus in the 1970s. The town is now almost 100 percent African American. Despite its current racial homogeneity, remnants of its Jim Crow past remain. The "white school" is boarded up, having been condemned years ago. The "black school" now hosts all the elementary and middle school-aged children in town. Even this school looks in need of repair, however.

The streets of Poppy are narrow and not well maintained. Some look like an alley way rather than a regular street and there is no industry to speak of in the entire region. This town, and many others like it, exists because of slavery. Large plantations used to dot the landscape and white supremacy reigned as the principal cultural doctrine in both the pre– and post–Civil War era. A young African American man named Josiah, who considered himself to be involved in the politics of Poppy, said that slavery never ended in this area. "It's transformed," he said while eating one of the cookies we had dropped off at the center, "the state of Mississippi spends more money on people in jail that haven't been to trial yet, than they do on child protective services . . . When you're keepin' poor people in jail . . . they don't have access to basic rights; they're bein' arrested but not bein' tried."

Following the Civil War, Poppy continued its previous social and economic structure through the implementation of sharecropping and Jim Crow laws. The community remained separate and extremely unequal. Economic prosperity was virtually impossible for the majority of African American residents. The Civil Rights Movement of the 1960s saw political protest in Poppy, like it did in many other places throughout the South, but the movement did not fully reach this community until the mid-1970s into the early 1980s. Residents speak proudly about the fight of the older generation of African Americans to win equal treatment, political representation, and voting rights.

Social change was not something that many white residents were willing to accept and as the federal government became more involved in undoing the structure of the Jim Crow era in the 1970s, most of the white residents decided to go elsewhere. This began the decline of the town's population, which has decreased by almost 30 percent over the last several decades. Despite its difficult history, residents speak fondly of their town. "My favorite thing about the community is the closeness of the people" an African American woman in her late seventies named Sherry said with a smile. This is a sentiment repeated over and over again in all the communities we worked with. There is extreme poverty and frustration over social and economic injustices, but there is also a true and obvious love for the town and the people. An African American resident in his late twenties, named Samuel, explained, "I love my family and I love my people, but at the same time we have some major issues here. And these issues are not just coincidental, it's deliberate."

All the residents we spoke to in Poppy were African American, with the exception of two community organizers who were white women in their mid to late twenties. Like the community of Peony, the white residents we spoke with were transplants to the community and were not representative of the few remaining lifelong white residents. We spoke with residents of all ages, who included retired teachers, politicians, church leaders, and the unemployed. The goal of our conversations with the residents of Poppy was to examine the social and political factors contributing to the extreme poverty of the town. As with all the other communities, we sought to demonstrate how the social and political structures allow for NTDs to persist. Residents spoke a great deal about education, as will be discussed later in the chapter, but they also touched on topics such as water quality, food insecurity, and lack of adequate housing and sanitation, all red flags for infection from NTDs.

"Nobody cares about us outside this area," Josiah told us when we started inquiring about some of the challenges the community faced. The community is in an extremely isolated area of the rural South and has never had much political power, even in the time of cotton plantations. Arguably, the majority of Americans likely do not even know this region of the South exists. Despite this invisibility, the region played an indispensable part in American history both during the antebellum era, Reconstruction, both world wars, and on through the Civil Rights movement. The residents we spoke to are proud of their town and its history but, more than any other community we worked with, they convey frustration with both the state and federal government. They even expressed feelings that the state and country are purposefully looking the other way. "We are never going to get that kind of attention," Sherry told us, referring to the news coverage of Flint, Michigan's water crisis, "because we don't have the numbers and because the systems don't want us to get the attention. They want to keep the people here oppressed."

Examining the history of the community, it is easy to see why the residents feel this frustration. From slavery to Jim Crow and sharecropping they have spent the better part of 150 years struggling under political, economic, and social oppression. Today, African Americans here and throughout the United States suffer significant differences in net wealth, owed largely to the "head start" whites were given in accumulating wealth and passing it on to the next generation.[8] This well-documented explanation for wealth differences between whites and African Americans—even when income is controlled for—known as the historical legacy thesis, is further compounded when one takes into account that wealth plays an enormous role in academic achievement.[9] Additionally, the structural racism within the housing and credit markets allows for the wealth gap to be sustained.[10]

Poppy, like many other communities, experiences this firsthand and is continuously fighting against poverty, poor education, food insecurity, poor water quality, and a lack of proper sanitation. There is little focus on health among the residents of Poppy, though this is changing with a new health initiative undertaken by the town's alderman, Stephen. While there might be little focus on health, residents are acutely aware that they lack access and resources. For some, the state is, in part, responsible for their lack of adequate health care. They tell us about how the state's governor refused to accept the Medicaid extension offered under the Affordable Care Act. "The state and federal [governments] don't care," the residents told us repeatedly.

For African Americans in Poppy, poverty has always been a central component of life. Attempting to express the extent of the problem, Stephen explained, "The systemic poverty and generational poverty is unlike anything else in the country." For Poppy, the lack of jobs, lack of quality education, and lack of opportunities for the younger generation has helped to continue a cycle of poverty and the majority of younger residents have a difficult time seeing a way out. Many of the things that most Americans take for granted are not accessible, available, or feasible in the extreme poverty of Poppy. The residents who are employed are employed by the school and, outside of these jobs, residents tell us that there are not many other options for employment.

The extreme poverty of the community creates a number of serious issues, particularly for health. "The quality of housing is bad," one of the community organizers, Samantha, explained, "so you have mold inside and leaky roofs." This confirms our worry that many residents are not just at risk for NTDs, but also for respiratory diseases. When residents do get sick, making a trip to the doctor is not easy. "If a kid is sick in these smaller towns, parents don't always have a car or money for gas to get these kids to the doctor or pharmacy," another community organizer named Jacqueline, who is familiar with several communities in the region, tells us. Similar to the situation in Peony, those who are employed cannot take time off of work to take their child to the doctor. Even the movement toward telemedicine is not a solution for Poppy. "When you're looking at hospitals, they use more of the online," Sherry told us, "but how do you do that without basic internet?" In Poppy, which has limited to no internet access, often loses power, and has low levels of computer literacy, tele-medicine does not offer a solution.

Basic services that many Americans take for granted, are either not an option or are not reliable in Poppy. The town does not have a grocery store. There is no bus system or other form of public transportation, so for the low-income residents of Poppy, they are at the mercy of the few chain businesses that exist in close proximity. "The same loaf of bread that is 88 cents at Walmart is $1.25 at Dollar General," a young African American man named Alex, who leads a gardening program at the elementary school tells us, demonstrating how a bad situation is made worse as the only place to buy food is the Dollar General. Many of the residents explain how the systemic poverty that exists in the community is made worse by the community's isolation. Samantha summed up their troubles eloquently stating, "It is expensive to be poor. Everything costs more."

Marigold, Texas

After hours of driving in darkness the first light of morning begins to appear around us. The road we have been traveling is already busy and the landscape on each side combined with the birds flying overhead signal that we are near the beach. Long sand dunes and patchy grasses inspire a short conversation about taking a driving break and visiting the beach, but these aspirations are quickly derailed when we look at the time. Instead, we continue down the two-lane road toward our first meeting in the bustling border community of Marigold. After several more miles, the road begins to carry us away from the water and we continue traveling through small town after small town, each one becoming bigger as we go along. Soon, the highway expands into several lanes each direction, tall, thin palm trees decorate the roadside, and our destination looms before us. Marigold is different from all the other communities that we worked with in this study for a number of reasons. It is a large multicultural, international, urban metropolis, whereas all the other communities are small, isolated rural locations. The population of this city is easily dozens of times larger than the next largest community participating in this project and, admittedly, we are initially concerned that it will not appropriately fit our study.

Despite the differences between this urban community and other rural communities in this study, we determine that the city does, in fact, have more in common with our other communities than meets the eye. Importantly, there are large disparities between rich and poor, with the poor residents residing far below the poverty line. Marigold is one of the poorest communities in the state of Texas with official statistics showing that approximately 25 percent of the population lives in poverty. There is no shortage of housing with inadequate infrastructure, as the housing landscape alternates between large mansions, smaller middle-class homes, and decaying trailers. Low-income residents, especially those living in the surrounding rural communities known as colonias, have the same complaints about raw sewage in their homes as do residents of other communities in this study. And despite numerous, state-of-the-art hospitals, health access is difficult, if not impossible, for much of the population. The rate of uninsured residents still hovers around 30 percent, despite improvements over the last few years. Close to 80 percent of Marigold's population is Latino, many of them immigrants and refugees—whether documented or undocumented. The community has a strong connection to its sister city on the other side of the border—though the U.S. State Department has used a Level 4: Do Not Travel warning for that area of Mexico. Those of undocumented status have especially limited access to care and none live without the daily fear of deportation. Recent changes in immigration laws have created a palpable level of discomfort throughout the community, both for immigrants and for Border Patrol. For these reasons, combined with the evidence that at least one NTD already exists throughout this region of Texas, we decide it is not only appropriate, but important that Marigold be included in the study.

We travel down the freeway, passing hotels, HEBs, and Walmarts, searching for our exit. Once we find it and exit, we look for the office of the community organizer named Ellen who is helping us set up discussions with residents. We spot the building just off the feeder road surrounded by houses with sagging roofs and chipping paint. The driveway leading into the building's parking lot is steep and the bottom of the car scrapes along it as we drive in. The building is small and unassuming with bars covering the windows. We walk hurriedly inside, trying to get out of the cold winter weather. The front door is locked with signs in both English and Spanish instructing visitors to ring the doorbell. We do so and are greeted by the organization's assistant director, Maria. She is a middle-aged Latina woman, friendly and eager to help, but her English is difficult to understand. She directs us to a community room and offers us coffee. As we wait, we learn that she travels regularly between the United States and Mexico, offering assistance to those in need on both sides of the border. Because of her frequent crossings and her work in Mexico, she is witnessing first hand many of the changes and new challenges faced by people on both sides. In some ways, the economic disparities here are more striking than the other communities and in some ways less so. Here in Marigold, they are pockets hidden within a thriving metropolis. While this is common in cities throughout the United States, the location of this city, along the U.S. border with Mexico, makes many of these low-income neighborhoods as isolated as if they were located hundreds of miles away from the urban community. This is especially true as anti-immigration rhetoric builds throughout the country. Notably, most residents of the city, including the white, U.S.-born residents, are against the Trump Administration's stance on immigration and speak openly of their opposition to a wall along the border. While the U.S.-Mexican border and immigration policy is one of the central issues in national politics, the people we spoke to in Marigold say that they are largely ignored by both the state and federal government. Though this might sound like a surprising statement given the border's prominence in national politics, it became increasingly clear to us over the fourteen months we worked with the community, that their complaints were valid.

Marigold, and other border communities throughout the United States are in a challenging situation. They are left out of policy conversations by both parties, but they are right in the middle of policy implementation. No one is asking what their challenges are or what the community needs, rather they are directing them to adapt to national political priorities. We were told by many residents that the local government is "very active" in the humanitarian crisis. Ellen talked about the community-level programs that have been established in spite of the national level arguments and policies. She stated, almost with exasperation, "We can't let people flounder without water and shelter." With the federal government focused on what residents believe are the wrong issues, the community has taken things into their own hands. During our time in Marigold, we spoke mostly to white residents, as fear of deportation or the general hostility toward immigrants, made it difficult to speak with members of the Latino community. We were, however, able to speak with three individuals who had immigrated to the United States many years earlier. Most of the white residents we spoke to were nonprofit leaders, physicians, and community health care professionals. Through these conversations we learned about the extent of the healthcare challenges in Marigold.

Marigold is unique in that it faces multiple serious disease challenges and has a well-documented history of inadequate housing and infrastructure. As mentioned previously, colonias are very common along the U.S.-Mexico border. These colonias are occupied mostly by immigrants, though many U.S.-born individuals also live in the communities. Most importantly, colonias are notorious for lacking water and sanitation infrastructure, through no fault of their own. Thus, the community concerns for Marigold, even ones that might seem the same on the face of the issue, vary greatly from the other communities in the study. Marigold has water and sanitation issues, but these issues do not only result from extreme poverty. They are also a result of predatory. (formerly) state supported reality practices. Marigold also has significant issues with health access, not because the nearest hospital is two hours away, but because some residents must decide whether to risk deportation or suffer with their illness. The city has numerous, multifaceted concerns, but we chose to only address the ones directly related to the threat of NTDs.

Primrose, South Carolina

Depending on which direction you come into Primrose you will either wind down a two-lane road with beautiful live oak trees draped in Spanish moss, which form a tunnel as their limbs arch over the roadway from each side, or you will pass a government facility protected by a huge gate resembling something you would see at the entrance of a military base and quiet fields surrounded by decaying fences and a few cows here and there. Regardless of whether you take the picturesque way into town or not, once you arrive on the outskirts of Primrose you would never guess that it is only about an hour away from one of the nation's most popular tourist cities. The community is tucked away in a region of the state that few tourists pass through; an area condemned to high levels of poverty and violence. Primrose is a medium-sized small town, complete with a number of fast food restaurants and a Walmart. It even has a small hospital with an emergency room capable of handling low-level emergencies. This hospital serves the town of Primrose and the surrounding region. Having a hospital located right in the community is a great advantage for Primrose, but, as we found out during our time there, it cannot solve all the challenges of health inequality and access. One of the most notable things about Primrose is that it has a university branch campus located in a neighboring town, though residents give no indication that the university is part of either community in more than physical presence.

The county in which Primrose resides survives primarily on agriculture and serves as one of the state's leading producers of watermelon. As one drives through the town, the view along the roadway is an even mix of trees and sprawling fields. Despite the on-paper demographic similarities, all the communities that took place in this study are unique, with a strongly defined identity and Primrose is no different. The area in which Primrose resides was a thriving home for Native American communities prior to the arrival of Europeans. Years later, it played a role in the Revolutionary War. Following the Revolutionary War, Primrose, like so many other communities in the South at the time, adopted the plantation system and began producing large amounts of cotton. Soon, the slave population in Primrose and the surrounding county outnumbered the white population.

In the early years of the twentieth century, the highway brought in a large tourist industry and the nearby government facility offered steady employment. This boom would not last, however. A new interstate, which allowed traffic to bypass Primrose entirely, meant travelers no longer came through the county and the government facility was eventually downsized. Today the outlook is much bleaker. More than a third of the population lives in poverty and one-fourth of all children in the county are born to teenage mothers; this is a rate 2.5 times higher than the state average. Additionally, statistics show that 41 percent of mothers receive inadequate prenatal care, likely contributing to the county's infant mortality rate, which is double the state average. Even this rate hides health disparities, however, as infant mortality among African American infants is almost twice as high as that among white infants. In almost every conceivable health measure, the county in which Primrose resides ranks last. These health rankings are something that members of the hospital board along with the town's long-time physician are highly aware of and working diligently to improve.

The first time we visited Primrose, we drove around town and took note of the large, beautiful homes coexisting only blocks away from the trailers and small, decaying homes of the town's poorest residents. Traveling through town we were made uncomfortably aware that we were outsiders. Cars slow to watch us, suspicion written all over the faces of the occupants. Individuals walking the sidewalks glanced our way with unhappy, almost hostile glares. They looked over the Texas A&M logos on our shirts and quickly decided that we are up to no good. Out of all the communities we visited, Primrose was the most outwardly hostile. The general feelings of the community, however, stand in stark contrast to the warm, friendly nature of the community organizers and hospital personnel that helped us coordinate focus groups and interviews with residents. All of these individuals are happy to see us and happy to help. They listened intently as we talked about the project and openly shared their goals and vision for the town. They expressed hope that collaborating with us on this study could help improve some areas of health in Primrose.

We began our conversations with residents of Primrose the way we always do, asking them what they love about their community. Residents told us that they love the small town, that there is family close by and someone is always willing to help you out if you need it. When we asked them what the biggest problems were in their community, the answers we received were not at all what we expected. "Too much gun violence," an African American woman in her mid-thirties named Latoya responded immediately when asked this question. Another, older African American woman named Sharon added, "It was better when we were in school. We could go out and not have to worry about anybody shooting. We could play outside and not have to worry about a drive by." All of the residents confirmed that this was a significant problem in their community. We were told that there was a gang problem and many mothers in Primrose worried about their children being shot if they were outside playing.

Admittedly, we were caught off-guard by these comments. It seemed unusual to us that a small, rural community would have such high levels of gang violence. We were told that the gang violence was even worse in two of the neighboring counties.

In addition to concerns about gun violence, most of the residents we spoke to expressed concern about the number of people with AIDS in Primrose. Many of them said they knew at least one individual personally who was HIV positive and they blamed the increase in the disease on "the younger generation's" sexual promiscuity. This was an interesting perspective since some of the residents who expressed this opinion were in their mid-twenties. The concern about what residents viewed as an AIDS epidemic is palpable. One resident even asked us if it was possible to get AIDS from mosquitoes. Most residents, both young and old, felt that it was not a lack of education that was allowing HIV to spread in the community, rather that people no longer cared about spreading disease to other people, whether it be the common cold or HIV. There was a clear lack of trust among members of the community and many seemed to view other residents as a threat rather than as their neighbor.

Magnolia, Alabama

A two-lane road weaves its way through the hilly countryside. Tall, brilliantly green trees so thick that it is impossible to see more than a few feet into them, line both sides of the road. The humidity hangs in the air, creating a haze which drapes over the endless green canopy. Every now-and-then a red dirt road cuts off to one side or the other and the trees part to reveal a pasture, with cows chomping lazily and looking for pockets of shade to escape the heat. It is some of the most breathtakingly beautiful landscape in the country, but the vast majority of Americans will never see it. We are over an hour from the nearest city in a Deep South state that easily falls into the category of a "flyover" state.

Finally, the outskirts of a town begin to appear. Near the town's grocery store, the road splits; one route taking traffic around the downtown and the other road heading straight for the heart of the little community. We follow the latter. Less than a mile later a tiny downtown appears with well-maintained, but obviously old brick buildings and a large, imposing courthouse. The entire downtown is encompassed in two square blocks but is alive with people. Magnolia appears to be thriving, which is unusual for the communities we worked with throughout this study. Despite the nicely kept buildings and the residents bustling about, however, it is the county seat of the poorest county in one of the poorest states in the country. The median annual income for the county hovers around $13,000 and, like many communities, this median income hides the large economic disparity that exists. Some members of Magnolia are making good, steady incomes that are much higher than this median. While others, in fact a large percentage of the population, are living below the poverty line and bringing in an annual income far below this meager median.

On our first visit, we drive around the town before heading to the courthouse, where we are scheduled to meet the community organizer and talk with some of the residents. Magnolia only has about 2,000 residents but enough churches to accommodate a population twenty times that size. They dot the landscape every 50 yards or so as we travel along, ranging from small, one room structures to picturesque, 200-hundred-year-old buildings that served the community's very first residents.

As we move further from downtown, the buildings and homes become more sparse. We come across a park in poor condition and two elderly African American gentlemen sitting in the shade of the pavilion. Upon striking up a conversation with the men we learn that they "watch over the park." It is unclear whether this is an official designation or something they voluntarily do out of concern for the park's propensity to support illegal activities. Both men are lifetime residents of the town and look to be in their eighties. They tell us that the park does not get much use anymore aside from the softball games and warn us that if we decide to take the walking trail, we need to keep an eye out for snakes. Both are friendly and seem interested in the strange outsiders that have descended on their park. They ask us why we have come to Magnolia and we provide a brief summary of the project. They nod and shrug, not breaking from their slow, slightly distracted demeanor. We ask them if they have ever heard of hookworm. "Oh yes," one of them says with clear recognition, "my grandmama start tellin' me about that when I was six years old." The other man looked at us with concern and asked, "That still a problem here?" We explained that we believed it was and that's why we were here. The conversation started to wind down and we headed back to our car. As we climbed in and got ready to drive away, one of them yelled after us, "Y'all try to stay out of the heat!"

We drove away from the park and headed further down the road toward the river. We noticed signs directing traffic toward a state park and decided to take a look. When we arrived, we were the only car in the parking lot. Down a short path we could see a portion of a playground and a hint of the river. As we walked slowly down the heavily wooded path, we had no idea what to expect once we reached the water. Suddenly the path opened up to reveal two playgrounds, a number of picnic tables and the wide, slow-moving river. A long, sandy beach with a designated swimming area stood just ahead and the river was lined with thick, beautifully green trees. "Wow!" one of the members of our research team commented, "This is amazing." We stood and took in the scene for a few minutes but it was only 9:30 a.m. and already in the mid-nineties. It was not long before a desire to get out of the heat drove us back to the car.

From the state park we headed back downtown to meet the community organizer, a loud and joyful African American woman in her late thirties named Tamera. She had gathered some residents for us to talk with at the courthouse. The courthouse is easily the largest building in town; at least double the size of the next largest building. Giant, white columns frame the front and there was a steady stream of people going in and out. We chatted briefly with the security officer as we stepped one-by-one through the metal detector and then headed to the room that had been designated for our focus group that day. We chose this community as part of our project because it exhibits a number of risk factors for the presence of NTDs. Magnolia and surrounding counties were part of the vast cotton empire that served as the major economy for much of the South. The entire county where Magnolia resides relied heavily on slave labor on the large cotton plantations and the tradition of harsh and absolute discrimination carried well into the twentieth century.

Although the county historically has been, and remains, majority African American, this majority had very little political or economic power. For more than 100 years, almost no African Americans voted anywhere in the county. In the 1964 election, the white voters of the county did not even allow Lyndon Johnson to appear on the ballot because of their strong opposition to Civil Rights. By 2016, however, Hillary Clinton won the county with more than 70 percent of the vote, demonstrating a dramatic shift in the county's political power.

During our time in Magnolia, we talked to individuals from all across town and the surrounding countryside. They were the kindest, friendliest individuals we have ever come across—which is saying something for people who spend a lot of time in the rural South. Each and every one of them went out of their way to ask how they could help with the project and to talk with us about their community. Everything moves slower here and each person indicated that they had all the time in the world to work with us or help us in any way that they could. They showed no suspicion of outsiders; though this was probably helped by our partnership with one of the big state universities, of which even residents who never went to college show strong allegiance.

Another notable difference between this community and the others that partook in this study is that we were able to speak with members of both the white and black community. Both races willingly gave up their time, drove us—ultimately complete strangers—around town, and invited us to make ourselves comfortable around their homes. We spoke with many of the poor residents, but also middle- and upper-class individuals. This gave us a fuller picture of the issues facing the community as a whole and not just the largest segment of it.

Like all of the communities we work with, residents in Magnolia express a love for the close-knit community. "What I like is that everybody knows everybody," an African American man in his early twenties named Christopher told us, adding with a smile, "That's a good thing and could be a bad thing." All the residents we spoke with talked about how much they enjoyed living near family and how anyone in town would help you out if you needed it. But like many other rural Southern communities, they expressed frustration with the many challenges they faced. "The county is so poor and close to bankruptcy," a middle-aged white woman named Leanne told us, trying to give us an idea of how dire the economic situation had become. "They would rather build prisons than homes," a younger African American woman named Jasmine said off-handedly, going on to talk about how there are more registered voters in the county than there are people of voting age. There seemed to be a feeling that crooked local politicians scammed their way into office and then spent money in ways that did not benefit the residents.

Magnolia is a small town with a big history. It, and the towns surrounding it, played a central role in the slave economy, as the region has fertile soil for growing cotton. Decades later, the region around Magnolia became a main player in the Civil Rights Movement. Some of the most well-known moments in Civil Rights history happened just right down the road, so to speak. Magnolia is a town shaped by this history as a notable economic divide still exists between white residents and African American residents. Unlike some of the other communities in this study, however, racial tension is not bubbling over the surface. Residents of all races and ethnicities appeared to genuinely enjoy each other's company and there was more of a feeling here than in any other community that the fates of everyone, regardless of race, were intertwined. Residents lamented their lack of access to healthcare and openly discussed the issues they had with water and sanitation infrastructure. On the whole, they seem to have discussed, or at least considered, all of these problems before and were motivated to find solutions.

COMMUNITY CONCERNS AND NTD RISK FACTORS

Health Access

All five of the communities that participated in this project discussed the challenges they faced with health access. A high-spirited Catholic nun named Margaret, who had lived in Peony for almost two decades explained, "geographically, we are an hour and twenty minutes—hour and thirty minutes—to get to [town name retracted]. For a lot of people that's a burden to try to go that far. It takes a lot of planning." The isolation of each community is indeed a problem when it comes to gaining access to medical care. In Peony, for those who own a car it might only take half a day, but many of Peony's residents do not own cars. For those individuals, there are two options: pay someone to drive you to your appointment or take the Medicaid van. "If you have a Medicaid card you can go in the van, but if they're picking people up along the way that would be an all day thing," Rosyln explained to us earnestly, trying to convey the obstacles people face to simply see a doctor, "And if you go there with a child, you have to have enough money to feed yourself and the child. There is some—a lot of deterrence there—a lot of obstacles."

This problem was echoed by the community of Primrose. The residents, physicians, and hospital administrators alike in Primrose expressed numerous concerns and frustrations about healthcare access. John, the hospital administrator, is a middle-age white man with a friendly disposition and a genuine concern for the health of residents in the community. He explained that the closest trauma center is an hour and a half away. He said one of the benefits is that there is county insurance for life flights—meaning that even uninsured residents are airlifted to better equipped hospitals at no cost to them—but that many residents have trouble with primary care access. "Compared to the rest of the state," he said, "we have three times the number of nonessential ER visits because people are seeking primary care in the emergency department." When we pressed him on why people used the ER for primary care, he said it was a combination of lack of health insurance and lack of transportation. He told us that Primrose used to have free public transportation, which allowed residents to easily get to the doctor when they needed to, but the grant they had received for the project ended and it was not renewed. "Now," he explained, "people have to pay their relatives to drive them." This is a common theme that we heard in all five communities we worked with: in order to get to a doctor, residents must pay someone else to drive them, even if that someone is their mom or sibling or cousin.

When asked what the number one challenge was for the community of Magnolia, Christopher told us, "Without a doubt, resources. Resources when it comes to everything just about." Specifically, residents of Magnolia felt that there was a lack of health resources. The community does not have a hospital and "people don't have [access] to the care they need" even for the simplest things. If a resident needs to see a specialist they have to travel over an hour to get to the appropriate doctor. As a middle-aged African American resident named Connie explained, "You don't know or can't get the care that you need right here, so I pray to the Lord God that you don't have a heart attack or stroke." Many of Magnolia's residents said that the lack of access to care makes it extremely important that people take care of themselves, but that most residents neglect their health.

In many of the communities that participated in this study, physical access to healthcare is not the only health access problem that they face. For most, financial barriers provide a secondary obstacle that must be overcome. "If you have to go to the doctor and you don't have no insurance, that would come out of your pocket," Sharon from Primrose said, "and sometimes you don't have it so you don't go to the doctor to get it treated." To the residents of Primrose, the cost of seeing a doctor must always be weighed against how serious they felt their illness was. For many residents, particularly those living in poverty, the cost of healthcare was too high unless they thought they were dying.

The cost of seeing a doctor was not the only prohibitive cost within the healthcare system that residents of Primrose shared with us. Many of them discussed how the cost of medication was typically so high that they could not afford it, even for those that had insurance. "Medicine is expensive" we were told many times. Latoya was happy to tell us as much as we wanted to hear about the challenges of health in Primrose. She said, "Yeah, because your co-pay could be like $10, but your medicine could be like $100." The statement she was making was that if you had insurance, you could possibly afford to go to the doctor, but you still might not be able to afford the medicine you need to get better. In these cases, the question for residents becomes: should you waste your time going to the doctor at all?

The question of whether it was worth going to the doctor at all came up in other areas. Mary, an older African American woman, who served as a member of Primrose's hospital board, said that a lot of people decided not to get treatment because they didn't believe they would be able to survive the treatment. In the majority of cases she was talking about individuals diagnosed with cancer, but had numerous examples of residents who had chosen to forgo treatment because they had so many comorbidities that they deemed treatment worthless. This was a disheartening thing to hear: residents were not or could not maintain their health on a regular basis and, thus, chose not to seek treatment for deadly diseases.

Lack of access to affordable healthcare was a widespread problem in Primrose and a reality for many of the residents we talked to. Tara, an African American woman in her mid-thirties, who did have access to healthcare, told us, "Sometimes, it's best to put the people first. I work at a law firm. We come across these clients that want to go to the doctor and get treatment but they can't. Or they can take some doctors but the doctors want the money upfront. Sometimes it's just a sad situation. Sometimes just don't make it about the money because . . . really they took an oath to help people." There was some sense among Primrose's poor residents that those in the healthcare profession were more interested in financial gain, though this was not the impression we received with talking to any of the people working at the hospital. Dr. Rodriguez, a middle-aged Latino man, who had served as the town's primary physician for over two decades, told us that he believes medical schools have a significant deficiency in their training. "There are no courses in understanding populations and cultures," he explained, "we need to start training medical students to work in rural areas and to understand their patients." He went on to say that he had overseen many residents on rotations from the nearby city and, universally, they had all failed to comprehend the challenges of serving a rural, low-income population. One of the other members of the hospital's board, an older African American man named Joseph, talked about how Primrose was located in a poor and underrepresented county. "We recognize health challenges," he said, "and we are doing the best we can with what we got."

With regard to financial resources, a young African American resident from Magnolia told us, "healthcare is just another bill," to which the man standing next to him added, "they say I don't have insurance and I don't want to go. I have a car, a kid, and rent. If I go to the doctor I'm going to have a bill and if the bill doesn't get paid it's going to go to collections to your credit. You're trying to get ahead in life." This was a sentiment we heard expressed over and over: taking care of one's health was too expensive. Most residents were just trying to make it from one day to the next. They were trying to put food on the table, gas in their car, clothes on their kids. Adding one more bill would be the straw that broke the camel's back and, therefore, health is viewed as a luxury.

In Magnolia, what was clear was that most residents could not afford healthcare even if they wanted to. Additionally, everyone in the county was aware that if they ever had a significant medical issue, they likely would not make it to a hospital in time. The only way to get there was to be airlifted and there was only one helicopter available for the region. We were told of a boy who had been bitten by a poisonous snake and had died because he wasn't able to get to a hospital in time.

The burden of obtaining medical care, while the largest obstacle, is not the only problem that residents in all these communities are concerned about in relation to health. They acknowledge that the stress of daily life, trying to pay their bills, coping with unemployment, caring for children, often distracts residents from getting the care they need. "The most important thing that our younger peoples here [is] being aware of the disease that are going on and for them to understand how important it is," Mary, a middle-aged African American woman who worked in Peony's social services department, explains, "They workin' trying to pay a bill. They just don't take the time to go get it examined to find out." In many of the communities, residents we talked to about the community's attitudes toward health seemed to describe a combination of ignorance is bliss and survival mode. Describing this balance, Mary, clearly frustrated by the situation, stated, "It has nothing to do with can't pay for it, because just like I said, most everybody just about has a Medicaid card. It's just, I don't know." She trails off, partly exasperated and partly exhausted by a problem that has persisted in the community for years. Her friend steps in and finishes her sentence, "Won't have to deal with it."

What the two women described gives voice to the challenges and choices many in Peony and other communities of poverty face. They are just trying to survive day-to-day, trying to provide a better life for the next generation and, as such, adding an illness or unexpected medical diagnosis to the multiplicity of their problems, is simply too much. For many, it is better to not know they are sick than to direct resources to addressing it.

For many people we spoke with, there was the belief that some level of purposeful neglect played a role in the health outcomes of the community. "They just livin' like they livin' and they not payin' attention to their children or themselves," Mary explains, "because if they take better care of themselves, they would take better care of their children." This lack of attention to health throughout all the generations has led to higher rates of infant mortality, low rates of vaccination, and low adherence to the well-child check-up schedule.

In Magnolia, the other reason we were told people do not go to the doctor was pride. This was unique among all the communities we worked with in this study. Nowhere else had residents told us that it was customary to deal with your health challenges on your own. The phenomenon was best explained by Christopher who stated, "It's like a custom thing. It's like we don't want to go to the doctor because we don't want to find out. I ain't going because if something is wrong I'm just going to pray to God. We are very religious people down in the South South [*sic*], so we believe God can fix anything—which he can, but some things we have to fix ourselves like get up and go to the doctor." It was true that all the Magnolia residents we spoke to were highly religious people who turned to God both out of faith and out of necessity, as there were no other resources. What was difficult to decipher from our conversations was whether or not they would seek healthcare if they could afford it and they had the resources available in town, or if the pride and the custom of individualism prevent them from utilizing them regardless of physical and financial access.

Every community we worked with as a part of this study had significant issues with health access, but the health access issues within Marigold were more nuanced than lack of access to a doctor. They involved fear, shame, and one's health literally residing in the hands of Border Patrol. Many individuals we spoke with discussed the shame placed on patients who come to the doctor with advanced illnesses. They described this as one of the reasons some people do not seek medical attention at all. One medical professional named Dr. Johnson said, "We see here a lot of doctors and nurses who blame or shame patients in the ICU for their conditions." This is to say that when individuals finally do seek medical help, doctors and nurses say things to them like, "You let your diabetes get out of control." Some residents told us that many people punish or blame themselves for their illnesses. They believe the illness is their fault because they are poor and could not go to the doctor. Others blame themselves for not being able to figure out the "rules of the healthcare game," which made them unable to access treatment. Whatever the source of shame, it was evident during our time in Marigold that it played a central, important role in why people choose not to seek medical treatment even when they are very ill.

For those that are able to figure out the healthcare system and can access a doctor, they run into another set of issues ranging from legal status to health insurance. We are told by residents and local medical professionals alike that health access used to be much easier in Marigold. Dr. Johnson, who has worked in Marigold for decades explained to us, "Now Border Patrol checks for papers routinely on the roads so individuals won't venture out . . . [it's not] that individuals aren't interested or don't care about their health. These individuals have to be pretty clever. They have to adjust their schedules around the Border Patrol." Residents that have a hard time accessing care include children born in the colonias. Some of these children do not have documentation, even though they were born in the United States. "You're not going to be able to go across the border and get care" Dr. Smith told us, explaining that many undocumented immigrants used to go into Mexico for medical care, adding that the Trump Administration "has cut individuals off from that safety valve." He went on to explain the ways that health access has changed since he first started practicing in Marigold, detailing how it used to be possible to write a letter to Border Patrol explaining the health situation and sending the individual, even if undocumented, to a better hospital to get cancer treatment. The inability to treat patients as a result of their immigration status is one of the largest, most significant changes he has noticed in the last few years. It is important to acknowledge that despite the negative portrayal of Border Patrol in the popular media every community activist and/or organizer that we spoke to during this project spoke highly of the Border Patrol personnel in their community. They often viewed them as team members, helping community groups provide safety and services to people crossing the border. There were not, however, the same positive feelings about Immigration and Customs Enforcement (ICE).

Unlike the other communities, we worked with in this study, the health of Marigold was controlled largely by federal politics and a larger percentage of the population is uninsured. The reason for high levels of uninsured individuals appears to be the inability of many to qualify for Medicaid, partly a result of the state's choice not to expand the program. Maria told us, "To buy medical insurance is very expensive. Neither my husband nor I can afford insurance. We don't qualify for free insurance or discounted because we are considered middle class, but we can't afford to pay $300 a month either." Other residents who were able to travel back and forth across the border told us that their only option was to get medical care and pharmaceuticals in Mexico because they could not afford the American health system. This is true of white, U.S.-born Americans as well, who travel from all parts of the state to seek care in Mexico because they cannot afford healthcare in the United States. A female resident named Jessica, who had numerous negative experiences with the Medicaid system, expressed her frustration with Medicaid access by saying, "If you are diabetic, supposedly you get Medicaid. Not true. You have to lose your leg to be eligible and there are no advocacy groups to help you." Unlike many of the other communities in the study, federal programs were no help to many residents of Marigold and they remained stuck; unable to access health care in Mexico or the United States.

To overcome this lack of access in the past, Marigold has turned to the use of mobile health units. Mobile health units, as the name implies, are clinics on wheels that can travel to some of the most disadvantaged neighborhoods to provide medical care. In Marigold, mobile units travel to the colonias and other communities in need, offering basic medical services without the requirement of documentation. While these have been very successful in the past, national rhetoric surrounding immigration has dampened its impact. Residents and health care providers alike tell us that now when mobile units go into marginalized communities, people are afraid to show up because they lack documentation or they are afraid it might actually be ICE trying to trick people. Additionally, one of the largest mobile clinics is run by the Texas National Guard. The idea of the National Guard offering free healthcare without the need to show immigration status seems to many who need the care, as a rouse to draw out undocumented immigrants. Fear of using mobile units combined with high uninsured rates and an inability to access health care in Mexico means that most of the neediest members of Marigold have no options for healthcare. Compounding all of these issues is an underlying anger from local leaders directed at the federal government. A feeling that things are worse with the new policies rather than better. "We can't just sit back," Tony, a middle-aged white man, told us, "The local police and local government does their best to work and resolve the problems we have. We aren't Washington, DC."

With this level of lack of access, the parasitic diseases we study are not even on residents' radar in any of the communities we worked with. Aside from hookworm, none of the residents we spoke to had heard of NTDs and, even if they had, there was nowhere for them to be tested for infection. Like so many low-income, rural communities, the residents in this study were at a disadvantage. Not only because they were at high risk for NTD infections, but also because they did not have the physical or financial access to care even if they had been aware of their risk status.

Water and Sanitation

NTDs thrive in areas with unclean water and inadequate sanitation. These components are two of the main predictors for the presence of diseases such as hookworm. For Poppy, the struggle for clean water and proper sanitation is an ongoing issue. Samantha told us, "When I first moved here the water wasn't drinkable." She went on to explain that there was a boil water notice in effect for the first ten months that she lived in the community. In our conversations with residents it seemed that boil water notices were a regular occurrence in Poppy. "We have leaky pipes so contaminants get into the water," a middle-aged African American named Constance told us. "If we lose power for more than 10 seconds, our whole filtration system shuts down and it takes days to fix," Jacqueline added, "Power cuts down several times a day because it is a rural area."

While the boil water notices provide information to the residents, many of them admit that boiling water every time you have to cook, clean, or brush your teeth is simply too difficult. Many shared that they do not have the time and instead end up using the contaminated water as is rather than boiling it. They also do not see their current situation changing anytime in the near future. "The towns do not have the resources to fix things," Stephen explained to us while inspecting a flooded area of his yard, "so you have all these small towns going after the same grants to try and fix the same problems everywhere here."

Not having regular access to clean water is not the only infrastructure challenge faced by Poppy. Many, if not all, parts of the town also do not have proper sanitation systems. Proper waste disposal was one of the most important developments in modern disease control and countries throughout the world that lack proper sanitation experience high levels of illness and death. The same is true for Poppy. Infant mortality rates in this region are almost twice as high as the national average. There have been no studies conducted on the impact of inadequate sanitation on the health of residents in Poppy, but the people we spoke to expressed concern and outrage. "There's a street where they are not connected to the sewer," Jacqueline said animatedly, trying to convey how unacceptable it was, "When it rains like this, you don't drive by. The water overflows in the ditch and runs out into the road." What she was describing was the regular overflow of human waste into the street.

It is not just sewage overflowing into the streets, however. Sherry explained, "When it floods, which happens quite a bit because we are not far above sea level, all the stuff backs up and it's gross." The lack of proper sanitation infrastructure in Poppy means that many residents suffer with their sewage backing up into their homes during times of heavy rain. Not only does this expose residents to a number of NTDs, but to several other diseases that are not the focus of this study.

Of all the challenges we discussed with Poppy's residents, it was issues with water and sanitation that seemed the most challenging to solve. Improving infrastructure requires a large financial investment, something that is beyond the reach of this particular community. Some residents are aware that there are grants that would provide funding for these improvements and are focused on completing applications for this funding.

The residents of Marigold experience similar water and sanitation infrastructure issues to those experienced by the residents of Poppy. They worried about the lack of adequate water and sanitation in many areas. Over the course of this project, which as previously mentioned lasted approximately fourteen months, Marigold experienced three floods. Ellen told us, "We had an ugly flood six months ago. Ugly. Ugly. Water was right up there on that road," pointing out to the road in front of her. A middle-aged gentleman named Miguel expanded on why the flooding is such a significant problem, "This past flood we had," he said, "the sewer system broke down. So it was very hard for people . . . some people could not go back to live in their houses."

The flood and sanitation challenges exist in what could be considered the city's suburbs, but they are an even larger problem in the colonias. Ellen told us, "There were some terrible conditions out here in the colonias that just got ignored." She went on to explain that when there is flooding or sewer issues, the city might come out and condemn the areas, giving the residents no other options of where to live. In other cases, the city completely ignores the issues and leaves people to deal with the standing water and raw sewage entirely on their own. "There's always those issues in the poor colonia areas," several residents told us.

In all of our conversations about water and sewer issues in Marigold, it was apparent that the modernized, economically prosperous areas of the city had no issues, but the rural colonias rarely, if ever, had clean drinking water or proper waste disposal. Many parts of the colonias might not even have electricity. Part of the water and sewer issues in the colonias was the result of predatory housing practices, as previously mentioned, but the state has recently passed laws making it illegal to build colonia subdivisions without water and sewer.[11] Many living in the colonias worked hard to accumulate enough money to build a home, but many colonias have no paved roads, no running water, and no sanitation system. The new ordinances are aimed to prevent this underdevelopment. Unfortunately, there is no retroactive prohibition for the colonias already in existence. Put simply, there are many colonias that still do not have access to basic necessities.

Magnolia was another community with significant water-related challenges. One portion of the county did not even have water access. In a matter-of-fact way, Connie explained, "they showed on the tv—showed on the national news—where they were putting up the jugs to the thing to get water and also the dogs were going there drinking and licking the water from the same fountain!" She was talking about the area of the county that had no water access so residents had to walk with jugs to a water spicket on the side of the road, fill the jugs, and carry the water back to their homes. "If you're anything of a Christian it's going to bother you," Tamera added, referencing the individuals who had to walk to get their water.

Even in areas of the county that have access to water, many people do not drink it. "Someone here warned me about the tap water from a certain faucet in the building," a white, middle-aged man named Michael told us, "So I stopped drinking it from that source, but I get my tap water from the kitchen here now and I wonder if it's any better. I mean, aren't they all from the same source?" Leanne told us that she does not drink the water at all. She said there is no water specialist in town to tell them if the water is contaminated or not, but they believe that it is. We were told that many residents believe they have gotten sick from drinking the water in the county because it is so heavily contaminated. Those that can afford it, drink bottled water. Those who cannot boil it, if they have the time, but many have to drink the water as is.

In addition to the contaminated drinking water, many Magnolia residents talk about the river that runs just outside of town. Giving us a glimpse of the folklore surrounding the river, a lifelong resident named Elizabeth stated, "There are people that say, you live on a certain side of the river, you're more likely to get cancer, but I don't know if any study has been done." Many residents spoke about the mill outside of town and how they believed it contaminated the water and the air. Most residents believed that this contamination caused cancer, but few felt that they could do anything about it. They seemed resigned to live with contaminated water and the increased health risks that came along with it.

When we spoke with residents of Magnolia, they all spoke openly about the lack of septic tanks and the raw sewage throughout the county. One resident told us that there are a lot of people living in trailers that are piping their raw sewage out onto the ground. Another resident told us that the building they worked in had to be closed twice because of raw sewage. Everyone in the county is supposed to get a permit and is required by law to have adequate septic systems, but Tamera explained, "Once again you're talking about money. Most of the time they're just thinking about how they barely got the living situation, so now I got somewhere to live so I cannot afford trying to get the septic done." The lack of financial resources leads many individuals to construct their own waste disposal systems, most commonly running the sewage into their backyards.

Even for those trying to install proper sanitation, the soil in Magnolia does not percolate and the county gets a lot of rain every year. Some residents told us that they do not believe the sewage treatment even works and that when there is a lot of rain, sewage flows everywhere. In the park we visited when we first arrived, there was a septic mound right next to the play set. The old men in the pavilion told us that the ground does not percolate so they run the sewage into that mound. It struck us that putting a septic mound right in the middle of a park where children play would make it much more likely for diseases like hookworm to persist. It appeared that everyone understood sanitation was an issue, they simply did not have the resources to solve it.

Housing

As has been discussed in the previous chapters, adequate housing, or the lack thereof, is a significant risk factor for infection with NTDs. A lack of window screens leaves residents vulnerable to mosquito bites and some houses have even larger problems. An African American resident from Peony who was in her early forties explained that there are houses in town that have a "big hole in the middle of the floor and the ceiling and the wall." These types of conditions make it easy for water to get into a house, which causes health issues beyond NTDs. Mold grows in some homes and it is impossible to create a healthy living environment for children.

When speaking to Matthew in Peony he said, "I'm worried about the condition of the housing also. From mold to bugs to just the elements being able to get in from outside." This concern was echoed by everyone that we talked to. They mentioned the fact that many houses have mold and lead paint. "The condition of the housing be [*sic*] causing some of the sickness," a middle-aged woman, Martha, explained to us, "especially in the children."

Lack of adequate housing is a problem that Peony's residents are all very aware of, but there seems to be some hopelessness in what to do about it. The white side of town does not have the same housing issues. All the houses on that side of town are brick, nicely maintained, and do not suffer from the same holes, mold, and lead paint problems as the house on the African American side. The divide between the quality of housing is immediately striking. It is indicative of the large financial divide between the farmers and the majority of the town's residents. Outside of the white residents, or the "farmers" as they are referred to, unemployment and economic hardship make day-to-day life a challenge and makes dealing with the housing problem all but impossible. "They don't have enough finances to help themselves," Mary said, and it is true. The problem of adequate housing in Peony is staggering but residents are left with limited options on how to improve the situation.

Many of the poor residents of Primrose live in trailers that are in varying stages of decay. Even those that live in traditionally built homes, however, express frustration with the conditions. "We have these landlords that have the old houses," Sharon said, "and they're just renting and they're not concerned with mold or asbestos or stuff that's there." There was a feeling among many of the poorest residents that the landlords they rented houses from were unconcerned with the health of tenants. Candace, a young African American woman even implied that a landlord lied to her grandmother just so that they would not have to fix the problem. She stated, "My grandmother, I told her, 'that's mold'. She called her landlord. He went up in the attic and said, 'that's not mold. That's just some weather that got in the roof'. She paid for the house, had somebody inspect it. Mold." She made the last part of the statement matter-of-factly, as if to say, "we all knew it was mold."

The hot, humid climate of Primrose means that if weather gets inside the trailers and homes, mold can become a significant problem and it was the main problem that residents were concerned about. They worried about thevhealth implications of mold, which include allergic reactions and asthma attacks in individuals with asthma. The presence of mold could also mean that people in these homes are at risk of certain NTDs. If a home is exposed to the elements in any way it means that mosquitoes and other vectors could also enter the home. These are dangerous, though more invisible, threats of inadequate housing.

Unemployment

Peony is plagued with high rates of unemployment. In fact, upward of 50 percent of the population is currently without work. It is not for a lack of trying, however. The challenge in Peony, as mentioned previously, is that it was and still is a farming community. Thus, the tragic irony of the unemployment problem is that it was largely created by residents right there in the community. Martha, remembering the days when sharecropping was the primary economic driver of Peony, described the actions of the white farm owners in the 1940s, 1950s, and 1960s, as companies tried to establish themselves in the town, "The thing is they didn't realize that they needed to keep jobs. When they blocked the jobs back then when factories wanted to come and they wouldn't let them come. The commerce got together and voted it out. They wouldn't let them come in because they were risking their chance of people working on their farm." White farmers in Peony were fearful of losing their sharecroppers and to ensure that they would always have people to work the land, they actively excluded competing forms of employment.

At the time that farmers in Peony were blocking factories and other types of industry from coming into town, they continued employing a large number of people. Some residents recalled, "The farmers used to have a lot of employees and nowadays they have three people working with all this technology." Even for those farmers working to maintain as many positions as possible, the extra numbers do not come close to making a dent in the unemployment rate. "That's what they didn't realize," Martha said, eyes cast downward, "they was [*sic*] killing their own town by not letting factories come here."

Food Insecurity

Close to 100 percent of students in Poppy are part of the free and reduced lunch program. One of the biggest concerns expressed by residents, particularly those working in the schools, was the widespread food insecurity faced by Poppy's children. "My kids don't know that they're poor or food insecure because they have Ramen and Rotel at home," a young woman named Natalie told us, "If everyone is the same, you don't see it." Her statement captured the extent of the food security problem in Poppy. Everyone in the community is poor and food insecure, so kids do not know that this is not how everyone in America lives.

Some residents felt that federal policies and lack of attention to isolated areas like the region where Poppy is located only make the problem worse. "They stick a Dollar General there because technically Dollar General provides you with enough things to say there's not a food desert," Alex, who runs a local gardening program, explained in frustration, "that lets the government say that there's no longer a food desert because you can get access to a Dollar General." He went on to discuss how this not only does not solve the problem of food insecurity, but it only gives residents access to poor quality foods. In a community that does not have access to healthcare, unhealthy diets compound the many health issues.

Like they are in addressing all the challenges they face, Poppy is working on innovative solutions to help alleviate food insecurity. Members of the community said that they need local farmers and a farmers market that feeds the community, but that when they tried to do that it failed. "All of the farmers are growing cash crops like soybeans and corn," Josiah said, "not food to eat." The failure of the farmer's market did not dissuade residents, however. They continued to search for creative solutions to their problems, focusing on programs they could develop without the need for outside assistance. Recently, they have begun a gardening program. They have developed a class within the school district that teaches the children in the community how to grow their own fruits and vegetables. Residents believe that if the younger generation can learn to grow and maintain some of their own food supply then they will have more and healthier food options in the future.

The gardening program implemented at the elementary school has had some success, but it is not without obstacles. The history of slavery and oppression is so entrenched in the community that Alex admits that getting children to garden has been extremely challenging. "Their parents and grandparents were tenant farmers," he explained. For the younger generation this has come to mean that they should never again have to work the land. Though community organizers have not yet found a way to overcome this challenge, they continue to work on improving and expanding the gardening program. For many residents, it offers a realistic way to alleviate food security and provide healthier food options for everyone.

Education

Throughout our conversations with residents in Poppy, they continuously returned to the issue of education. For members of the community, the best way for them to reduce poverty in their community was to produce better, more highly educated students. Residents we spoke with were passionate about making sure that the younger generation had the ability to succeed, but acknowledged that the lowest income families often have a hard time making education a priority in their households.

Due to the inability to prioritize education, they are struggling to make improved education a reality. A retired teacher pointed out how the lack of resources in the community made it difficult for them to improve the education system. "The problem is we don't have highly qualified lower level teachers because once we get them here, there is nothing here to attract these families to keep them here," Sherry said. She was not only talking about a lack of services when she discussed the challenges of keeping qualified teachers in the area. When discussing the difficulty of retaining qualified teachers, she explained, "you're the lowest paid teachers in an incredibly isolated area" and what about those conditions would make qualified teachers want to stay in Poppy?

While holding a teaching position in Poppy sounds like a difficult job—high poverty students, low pay, isolation, and little government support—residents spoke fondly and proudly about the teachers they had. Sherry told us, "It's about the passion, because the teachers are great. They come early. They stay late when they can. It's not that they don't want to help, but when they don't have backup or support it makes it like they have to give up." Although a seemingly straight-forward statement, the nuances of the lack of support warrant some discussion. Poppy suffers from a lack of support from both the state and federal government, but this is not the only issue for teachers. In a community where parents are struggling with extreme poverty, not able to work, or working several jobs to make ends meet, they cannot always be involved in their children's schooling. In some instances, parents do not have enough education themselves to help or support their children in their school work. This already difficult environment for quality education is made more complicated by placing all of the burden of education on the teachers and community residents speak indirectly about this burden's effect on teacher burnout.

The final concern several residents express is the state's apparent focus on punishment rather than education. "You would think they would take those funds that they're using for the prisons to build schools and educate the population," Josiah said matter-of-factly, "but instead they would rather take that money and build prisons. If you want to see the school to prison pipeline in action, our schools are probably the best place to see it." Several residents were in agreement with this statement, suggesting to us that their state does not have the proper priorities. The lack of funding for education at the state level is particularly impactful in communities of extreme poverty like Poppy. Regardless of the passion residents feel for developing quality education and all the work they are doing on their own, without support from the state or federal government, many of Poppy's children face insurmountable obstacles.

Threat of Disease

Unlike many of the other communities we work with, infectious diseases are on everyone's radar in Marigold. "The Zika virus," Maria told us when asked what diseases she was concerned about, "That's a scary one and we saw several people having it. My daughter-in-law was pregnant last year and I was very worried about it." Many residents we talked to expressed concern about Zika, though it is hard to go anywhere in the state without hearing radio ads or seeing posters talking about the threat of infection and how residents can protect themselves. The state has become active in Zika education and awareness throughout all the at-risk areas and it shows in this community. Some residents mentioned that there needed to be more targeted education about Zika in poor areas because the people were more susceptible to the virus, but Ellen said she is not sure of what efforts were already underway in those neighborhoods.

Aside from specific concerns about Zika, residents also expressed concerns about vaccine-preventable diseases. This was again unique, as no other community had mentioned this concern. It is possible the focus on vaccine-preventable diseases can be explained by the high-profile battle between the anti-vaccine movement and health professionals across the state. This battle has been raging in schools, neighborhoods, and even the halls of the state capitol for the past few years. We were still caught by surprise, however, as that county that Marigold resides in has some of the highest vaccination coverage rates in the state. To express his concern about vaccine-preventable diseases Miguel, who came over from Mexico in his younger years, explained to us, "I get concerned. I don't know much about it, but the vaccine war [is a concern]." He continued by saying, "People arguing about vaccinating their children and what not. I grew up in an era where you don't get your vaccination and you might have your hand fall off!"

The majority of residents we spoke to were highly aware of most of the disease threats in their community, particularly threats from mosquito-borne diseases. This knowledge came both through experience and extensive education and outreach done by state health officials and university extension offices. Understanding the threats posed by vector-borne diseases gives members of Marigold an advantage in prevention. They are aware that vectors carry disease and have some base knowledge on how to prevent infection, even if they cannot fully implement the prevention recommendations. Additionally, there are existing mechanisms in place to increase disease awareness, which could help increase residents' awareness of NTDs.

Race

As with any town in the South, one cannot understand the history of a place without understanding the role that slavery, Jim Crow laws, and the Civil Rights Movement played in shaping the modern-day community and the extreme poverty it suffers from. As mentioned previously, Peony has a long and violent history of racism and oppression, but, on a whole, many residents felt that there had been improvement since the 1960s. Some African American residents said that when it was important, the whole community, black and white, were able to come together. Residents from every area of the community pointed out ways that race and social relations had improved over the last generation. "Everything is different and we need to know how to come together and also you have to think it's not all about race and looks and about who is this or who is this. It's just the way you carry yourself to make an impact on people" a younger African American resident, Jennifer, explained to us. She continued by saying, "I work in both areas and I seen that I can just draw everybody together, but if I have an issue going on you best believe they all come. Both races."

There were many other residents who felt a similar way when discussing race issues and the impact they had on the community, "I've been here all my life," Jennifer said, "I love the people. You have some good areas. You have some bad areas, but the people show love." For the African American residents of Peony, the relationship between whites and blacks has increased tremendously. Most white members of the town express the same feelings, though there are a handful of both white and African American residents that are a little more cautious to praise the progress too heavily, "People are good, but it is a small community," Roslyn said matter-of-factly, "It is very difficult for people to speak out. There's fear of retaliation." "It is a very divided community," she continued when we asked her for more explanation, "economically and race wise."

While residents of Peony are right in saying that racial tensions are not as bad as they were prior to the 1970s, it is clear to us, as outsiders, that there is still a stark division between them. An older white male resident declined to even speak with us because he said we (meaning researchers and other outsiders) are "in the business of misquoting us." Many of the white residents in town felt that they had been made to look like villains in the past because of the town's racial divide.

There is a divide, however, and it is both economic and in physical location. The vast majority of those unemployed are African American. The vast majority of those living in inadequate housing are African American and African American and white residents literally live on two different sides of town. Some African American residents do not blame all the economic division on the town's history, however. Roslyn told us, "in some areas, some do get held back because of the community where they over here like the farmers—they got big money coming and we over here—we ain't got nothing coming because we made nothing." In Roslyn's mind, the economic divide has less to do with race and more to do with the failure of community members to create a prosperous life for themselves.

As we listened to a group of African American residents talk about how they believed race was no longer a problem in the community, Matthew, who later told us of his own experience watching the racial dynamics of the community, interjected, "I do have to wonder if some of the peaceableness and the good feelings between the communities and between the class levels . . . depends on maintaining the status quo—be happy with what's there and don't go pushing too much or saying too much." This comment brought up a real question in everyone's minds: would everything be so congenial if the status quo was tested? It is an impossible question to answer without testing the status quo, but it appeared that the residents in the group saw some truth in the statement.

The reality for Peony, as it relates to residents' risk of infection from NTDS, is that racism is the primary catalyst for the poverty around them. The historical and modern-day structural and overt racism puts African American residents at risk of infection from diseases such as *Toxocara canis*, hookworm, and West Nile Virus. The historical economic structure that prohibited African American residents from building wealth are integral to Peony's story today; to the social and economic factors that support NTD prevalence.

On the other hand, one can see the beginnings of efforts by some in the white and African American community to create one whole community rather than one divided by race. The next challenge will be to determine whether these bridges reduce the extreme poverty of African American residents and, in turn, reduce their risk of NTDs.

Politics

Politics in the South is vested in tradition and, in many ways, elitism. And like any town in the Deep South, Peony has had its share of political contests. Its experiences range from complete political control by white residents and violent disenfranchisement of African American residents, to the struggle for African American voting rights and the eventual ability for African Americans to have a political voice. But as central as the struggle for voting rights was to Peony, many residents implied that active political involvement from African American residents was a thing of the past. "I hear it all the time, 'Well my vote doesn't count'," Roslyn told us, "And it kills me. Regardless, do you know what people went through so that we could vote?! All you have to do now is take a piece of paper up in the voter register's office and register. Do you know how many people died behind this!?" She expressed frustration for what many older residents viewed as the younger generation's disrespect for the pain and sacrifice of previous generations. For an African American in Peony in the 1960s and 1970s one was taking their life, or at least their livelihood, in their hands if they wanted to have a political voice.

While it is easier for African Americans to vote in Peony today, much of what is discussed is a discomfort about being too political. Jennifer explained, "It is a small community so if you did say things . . . by the time you get home everybody know that so and so talked and said this and said that . . . It's just like, most of us younger people are quiet." Emphasizing the point, Roslyn adds, "And if you show up and the rumor mill is going to go around again. *Who do they think they are showing up to this meeting or how dare they speak up?*" In Peony there is clearly a feeling that organizing for political purposes is an unwise thing to do. It might not be dangerous like it was in decades past, but it will not go unnoticed. Older African American residents express strong pride and respect for the political activism of previous decades, "they used to have meetings," Martha explains proudly, "and they were very political and they would get out and say these are the people that are trying to help us and this and that. And somebody told me, they're up in the church talking politics and I say, that was the only place blacks had to talk politics was up in the church."

African American residents are not the only ones that have a strained relationship with the political system however. Matthew described the division between upper-class and working-class whites by saying, "This is the Bible Belt. Deep South. Evangelical. Conservative evangelical faith traditionally has said, you don't get involved in politics. That's not something that good Christians ought to deal with or be involved with. There are exceptions to that rule, of course. I grew up in that world so I know it very well." He explained that, coming from a blue-collar home, political involvement was not something you spent time on. That was something that the wealthier families, people who had attended college, concerned themselves with and there was a general, even if misguided, trust that they were doing what was best for everyone.

In the realm of politics, it seemed that most members of the community were relatively uninvolved aside from the few individuals who ran for city council or the mayor's office. That does not mean that they did not have opinions, or that there was no controversy in some elections, but the status quo seemed to be for "the farmers" to drive the political direction of the town. In our discussions, we are reminded of a quote from Melissa Fay Greene's book, *Praying for Sheetrock,* "People's lives do not consist, on the whole, of politics and large ideals, but of children and groceries and laundry and paychecks."[12] Residents of Peony have their opinions, but the deep poverty that consumes them leaves them little time to participate.

When discussing their representatives at the state level, many African American residents of Peony waved their hands in dismissal. "They only care about the interests of the farmers" they told us. None of them felt that these representatives were at all concerned with the broader issues facing their community. This lack of political voice at the local, state, and federal level is vital to understanding how extreme poverty persists in Peony and the other communities in this study and, in turn, why NTDs are ignored or overlooked. In a speech delivered at the Annual World Bank Conference on Development Economics in 2001, Morten Rostrup said, "The focus on poverty alleviation tends to focus attention on economic inequity—it does not expose the political role in creating and sustaining inequity and the political solutions above and beyond good policy that are required to generate real progress in health and society."[13] Poverty and the NTDs associated with it, is not strictly a problem of economics. Rather, it is a political and social problem, rooted in issues like racism, disenfranchisement, and other forms of social and political marginalization. For this reason, it is vital that we discuss issues of racism and political marginalization when confronting NTDs in the United States.

Low-income and marginalized residents of Primrose had a number of concerns about the health of their community, but another major theme that they discussed was their lack of power to do anything about it. The county is roughly 75 percent African American and 25 percent white, with a poverty rate hovering around 40 percent. Of individuals living in poverty, 90 percent are African American. More importantly, employment data in the county shows wage disparities between whites and African Americans working the same jobs, with African Americans making 35 percent less in some occupations. The income inequality also translates into social and political inequality.

"I guess if you don't have a title it don't mean nothin' really," Latoya told us when asked about how much power there was in the community to make change. Overall, residents' feelings regarding political power ranged from apathy to charges of overt oppression. "I think it's based on mostly the rich ones that are in this community trying to keep it the same instead of bringing change," Sharon explained. There was a feeling among several Primrose residents that individuals with money in the community did not want the low-income individuals to improve their economic, social, and political situation.

This mild sense of helplessness sometimes even expressed itself in conversations with Primrose's healthcare professionals. They were continuously searching for greater resources and were proud of the times they had been able to secure funding or push a piece of legislation through, such as county insurance for life flights. The helplessness came out, however, when they mentioned that grants had ended so programs could not be continued or in talking about how severe the diabetes epidemic was. In these cases, even some of the more powerful members of Primrose felt the crushing weight of the poverty that surrounded them and a lack of power to change it.

WHAT'S NEXT?

Peony, Louisiana

The challenges faced by Peony are massive—for white and African American residents alike. They are a small, rural, isolated town that seems to have been all but forgotten about by the rest of the country. This is a story common to rural communities throughout the United States. The residents talk about ways that they can work to improve the lives of fellow community members. When talking about how to overcome the obstacles, particularly in the realm of health, Roslyn states, "It's about how we going to get our younger ones to start doing these things for themselves so their children will be able to do these things for themselves." Many residents echoed this sentiment. There is a strong feeling in Peony that people need to be more aware of health threats and how they can minimize their risks. To make the biggest improvements, though, Martha told us, "It's how we prioritize our life." That is to say that this resident recognizes that in attempting to survive people have to prioritize putting the food on the table above going to see a doctor. Putting food on the table is always going to be the most important, but they expressed that people have to increase health on their list of priorities and begin taking actions to protect their health.

All the residents of Peony are pondering the enormous questions of: how do we get more medical care right here in our community? How do we educate people on how to take care of themselves? How do we make health a priority when there are so many other competing factors? These are not easy questions to answer. The town struggles with terrible living conditions, high unemployment, teenage pregnancy, and a lack of access to medical care. All of the risk factors for the presence of NTDs exist in the community, but so do all the risk factors for dozens of other major public health issues. The community is swimming upstream but they want a better future and are committed to improving conditions and helping people live fuller, healthier lives. All they need now are the tools.

Poppy, Mississippi

Poppy faces significant challenges and great risk for infection by NTDs. A lack of clean water and proper sanitation threatens the health of residents and suggests that hookworm infection is likely. Additionally, the stray dogs throughout the community raise concerns about the presence of *Toxocara canis*. The challenges faced by the community, not just in the area of health, are substantial. For more than a century, the community has been isolated, mostly ignored or forgotten by the rest of the country and even the state and federal governments. Despite the hardships, people in the community have faith that there are better days ahead. "I believe a revitalization is coming," Sherry told us enthusiastically. "We may not see it. We may not be here, but it's going to happen. There's enough good people that see the potential that will work to make it better."

Residents desire to improve their community and the obstacles they face to doing so was summed up perfectly by Josiah who said, "I think if we had more resources, that there are a lot of people that would make a huge difference here."

Marigold, Texas

Marigold faces a number of challenges similar to all the other communities in this study, but these challenges are, in many ways, compounded by the spotlight Washington, DC is shining on the region. There was unanimous agreement among all the residents we spoke with, whether foreign-born or U.S.-born, that they were frustrated with the inability of residents to access medical care. Lack of insurance combined with all-consuming fear of deportation means that many residents do not go to the hospital until they are dying or that they never seek care at all. The number of infectious diseases in the region also means that healthcare is necessary to protect the lives and health of the entire community, which includes immigrants and refugees. People infected with mosquito-borne diseases, or other NTDs such as Chagas—which disproportionately impacts immigrant communities—need to be able to report their infections and get treated. Otherwise, the infection can spread undetected by authorities until it is endemic within a population (regardless of nationality or citizenship).

To solve some of these issues, people need to feel safe in accepting care from mobile units. Health education and outreach needs to be provided in languages other than English and Spanish so that the marginalized populations of refugees from tribal areas of Central America can get the information they need. The national rhetoric and policies are only making health and health access worse in Marigold. Acknowledging that providing medical care to immigrants and refugees will help preserve the health of all Americans is the first step to addressing some of Marigold's issues.

Primrose, South Carolina

Residents of Primrose would love to see health improve in their community. As we have mentioned numerous times, NTDs are diseases of poverty. They exist, in large part, because of the economic and social circumstances that exist within society. Without these circumstances, there would be little ability for NTDs to infect people. Primrose has all the risk factors—biologically, ecologically, and socially—for NTDs. Some older residents even recalled receiving mandatory deworming medicine before they were allowed to begin the school year back in the 1950s. Free treatment for parasites has ended, but the environment has not changed. Without access to care, NTD infections become long-term or chronic conditions pushing individuals further into poverty.

Magnolia, Alabama

Magnolia had a number of challenges that could not easily be solved. They needed more resources, better access to healthcare, more education, greater awareness, clean water, and proper sanitation. Making it more difficult is the increasing divide many residents are starting to feel within the community. Jasmine explained, "We are so divided. The county is a little bit more divided now than it's ever been . . . I think it has a lot to do with politics, even now with the race. White and black. We're back there again and it sucks." With regards to the racial divide in the community, Christopher told us, "It's an issue no one wants to talk about. No one wants to bring it up, but in order to fix it, we have to talk about it." In a community that we viewed as being less divided than any of the other communities in the study, it was disheartening to hear that the felt modern politics was beginning to pull the community apart.

For this community, addressing the division head on is one of the first steps to fixing the more tangible issues. Until the divide is addressed, many poorer members of the community do not feel like they can change their circumstances. "I just never feel like I have power with anything," a cashier at the local grocery store named Elaine told us. Like this cashier, the poorest members of the county feel that they are crushed by the culture and politics of the region. They feel that their thoughts and opinions do not matter, and even if they speak up, these opinions are not heard. Overcoming these social and political obstacles and increased resources would go a long way toward helping the community tackle the issues related to NTDs.

Conclusion

Every community that we worked with in this study was chosen because, on paper, they are similar and display all the major risk factors for the presence of NTDs. What we discovered from working with the communities and talking with residents about the challenges they face is that, while there is overlap on issues like water and sanitation, each community is starkly different. Some communities have more extreme social challenges, such as overt racism or active political oppression. Others have more severe logistical challenges, such as physical or financial barriers to healthcare. What we hope to show with this chapter is that rural America is not a monolith. These mostly forgotten communities struggle everyday with challenges that many Americans do not even consider. What do you do when you cannot reach a hospital in an emergency? How do you keep your family from getting sick when raw sewage floods your home every time there's a heavy rain? How do you seek healthcare when you are afraid to leave your home? The social, political, and economic challenges of the five communities that participated in this study are not isolated incidents. There are thousands of communities across the United States struggling with the same or similar issues. The people in these communities face many daily struggles, including the risk of NTD infection. With this knowledge, it is no longer acceptable for our response to developing policies or providing health services for such diseases to be, "those don't exist in the United States."

NOTES

1. Peter Hotez, personal communication, September 14, 2018.
2. Catriona Davies, "Poverty, like Apartheid, is Man-Made, Says Mandela," *The Telegraph*, last modified February 4, 2005, https://www.telegraph.co.uk/news/uk news/1482735/Poverty-like-apartheid-is-man-made-says-Mandela.html.
3. Morten Rostrup, "The Role of Nongovernmental Organizations in Providing Health Care," Text delivered at the Annual *World Bank Conference on Development Economics*, p. 6. 2001.
4. Peter Hotez, "Hookworm and Poverty," *Annals of the New York Academy of Sciences* 1136, no. 1 (2008): 38–44.
5. Hotez, *Blue Marble Health.*
6. Ratcliffe et al., "Defining rural at the US Census Bureau," *American Community Survey and Geography Brief* 1, no. 8 (2016).
7. Cynthia Duncan and Robert Coles, *Worlds Apart: Why Poverty Persists in Rural America* (New Haven: Yale University Press, 1999).
8. Dalton Conley, "Decomposing the Black-White Wealth Gap: The Role of Parental Resources, Inheritance, and Investment Dynamics," *Sociological Inquiry* 71, no. 1 (2001): 39–66.
9. Conley, "Decomposing the Black-White Wealth Gap: The Role of Parental Resources, Inheritance, and Investment Dynamics"; Donald Easton-Brooks and Alan Davis, "Wealth, Traditional Socioeconomic Indicators, and the Achievement Debt," *The Journal of Negro Education* (2007): 530–541.
10. Conley, "Decomposing the Black-White Wealth Gap: The Role of Parental Resources, Inheritance, and Investment Dynamics."
11. Barton et al., "Las colonias in the 21st Century: Progress along the Texas-Mexico Border," *Federal Reserve Bank of Dallas*, 2015.
12. Melissa Fay Greene, *Praying for Sheetrock* (Boston: Da Capo Press, 2006), 253.
13. Rostrup, "The Role of Nongovernmental Organizations in Providing Health Care."

Conclusion

What's Next?

THE OVERALL PICTURE

Over the past decade, the conversation about NTDs in the United States—a conversation spearheaded by Dr. Peter Hotez at Baylor College of Medicine in Houston, Texas—has appeared to make the majority of Americans uncomfortable. As Dr. Hotez wrote in his 2016 book titled *Blue Marble Health: An Innovative Plan to Fight Diseases of the Poor amid Wealth*, "It has become apparent to me that NTDs in the United States represent an inconvenient truth."[1] This inconvenient truth is that we have the level of poverty in the United States that allows NTDs to not only exist, but thrive. In his 1962 landmark book about poverty in America, Michael Harrington wrote, "There is a familiar America. It is celebrated in speeches and advertised on television and in magazines. It has the highest mass standard of living the world has ever known. While this discussion is carried on, there existed another America."[2]

The "Other" America that Harrington wrote about in 1962 is not a thing of the past. As discussed in chapter 2, there are more Americans living in \$2/day poverty today than there were fifteen years ago, due largely to changes in the cash welfare system. There are millions of Americans living without enough food, clean drinking water, and adequate shelter. Hotez (2016) described the images he has witnessed in the poorest areas of Houston, saying "I saw abandoned buildings, dilapidated housing with no window screens, uncollected garbage, clogged drainage ditches that smelled like sewage, discarded tires filled with water, and packs of stray and roaming dogs. I thought to myself, these images look just like the standard global disease movie typically shown to first-year public health or medical students. A little bit of Lagos (Nigeria's largest city) right here in Texas."[3]

In February of 2019, a story published in BBC News named Escobares, Texas, the poorest city in the United States.[4] The city, situated on the Rio Grande, is a border community with 62 percent of residents living below the poverty line. It has very little in the way of employment opportunities and it has seen an increase in crime over the past several years as a result of cartels active on the Mexican side of the border. Unfortunately, the story of Escobares is not an outlier nationally, or along the U.S.-Texas border. A 2013 article in Texas Monthly named McAllen and Brownsville, two border cities in Texas, numbers 1 and 2 of America's poorest cities. The article states that 10.6 percent of households in Brownsville make less than $10,000 per year and 37 percent of the McAllen population does not have health insurance.[5]

All up and down the Texas border, but particularly in the Rio Grande Valley, poverty rates double the state poverty rate.[6] Additionally, the child poverty rate in McAllen, Texas is the highest in the state at 42.4 percent. Brownsville, Texas, however, is not far behind with a child poverty rate of 39.2 percent.[7] The Texas border's poverty challenges deepen in the colonias. As we have discussed previously in this book, almost half the colonias in the United States are located along the Texas-Mexico border in Hidalgo County.[8] "According to estimates, roughly half a million people live in colonias along the Texas piece of the U.S.-Mexico border alone. While nearly exclusively of Latino origin, almost three-quarters of the people living in Texas colonias hold U.S. citizenship and two-thirds are U.S. born."[9] The poverty rates in these communities are six times the state average.[10] Additionally, Medicaid and the Affordable Care Act are only available to U.S. citizens, meaning that undocumented immigrants who become ill often end up dying from a lack of access to healthcare.[11] On this front, however, the promotora network has had much success bringing healthcare to underserved communities.[12] In many ways, the poverty and social disadvantages of the colonias become a lifelong problem. As Guilamo-Ramos and Thimm-Kaiser (2018) observe, "Disadvantage among Latino adolescents in colonia communities does not exclusively manifest itself as poverty or poor health. Disadvantage among colonia youth includes being shut out of opportunities to acquire skills and preparation for success and good health later in life."[13]

As with the case of Escobares, the extreme poverty along the Texas-Mexico border is also not an outlier. Similar poverty statistics can be observed in the Mississippi Delta, the Alabama Black Belt, and the Appalachian region. "The Mississippi Delta is known as the poorest corner of the poorest state in America."[14] Roughly 22 percent of the population of Mississippi is food insecure and that number only increases when looking at food insecurity in the Delta.[15] Many Delta communities do not have grocery stores or a means of public transportation to get them to one.[16] Overall poverty has declined from the time of Robert Kennedy's poverty tour from over 50 percent to around 34 percent, but there is still a general feeling that the region is regressing.[17] In summing up the situation in the Delta, Cummins (2017) states, "Overall access to health is still abysmal, keeping the Delta's high rates of diabetes, heart disease, hypertension, and obesity among the worst in the nation. Employment prospects remain dismal. Schools are dilapidated and receive rock-bottom ratings from the Mississippi Department of Education. Economic development remains a constant struggle."[18]

In Appalachia, the region Johnson made famous for its high levels of rural poverty, self-blame and the opioid epidemic ravage many communities. Beattyville, Kentucky was featured by *The Guardian* in 2015 as the "poorest white town in America."[19] In Beattyville, life expectancy is well below the national average, more than one-third of teenagers dropout of high school, and there remain virtually no economic prospects.[20] Many in the community report that they feel the rest of the country looks down at them and even laughs at them, rather than viewing them as a community struggling.[21] Those who do not feel this sense of ridicule, mostly feel invisible. "Half a century later, while poverty levels have fallen dramatically in some parts of the country in good part thanks to Johnson, the economic gap between the region and much of the rest of America is as wide. And its deprivation is once again largely invisible to most of the country."[22]

Like the Texas-Mexico border, the Mississippi Delta, and Appalachia, the Alabama Black Belt is known for its extreme poverty, but also for its prominent role in the Civil Rights Movement. "The pervasiveness of high poverty in the Black Belt is an example of a faulty social structure. From slavery to sharecropping, to displaced agricultural workers, economic opportunities have been systematically curtailed for blacks in the area."[23] Many places in Alabama's Black Belt lack basic water and sanitation infrastructure, something that has been heavily reported on in the last few years.[24] Interestingly, many within the Black Belt do not believe that it is the role of the government to fix these issues, believing strongly in the local community.[25] Thus, communities throughout the Black Belt battle systemic poverty, a lack of adequate resources, and the feeling of invisibility within the American system. Like the communities on the border or in the Delta or in Appalachia, poverty, and the issues that come with it, are not a political talking point; they are a lived reality. Businesses closing or moving elsewhere (taking the few remaining jobs with them), inability to get to a grocery store, hungry children, and homes full of mold are the day-to-day challenges faced by the poorest in America.

While it might be unbelievable to some Americans that these conditions exist, the project that produced this book took us all over the Southern United States. It took us to small towns and large cities. We witnessed firsthand raw sewage pooling in backyards surrounded by children's toys and houses leaning so dramatically that they looked like they might collapse at any moment.

We would argue, however, that the descriptions produced by Harrington and Hotez are not the "Other" America. Instead, they are America. This is what America is: a country where wealth and extreme poverty persist side-by-side. Prosperity and despair; record low unemployment rates and communities where 70 percent of the population is unemployed; housing over-construction and a lack of adequate housing. In America, persistent inequality—whether between races or socioeconomic levels or rural-urban residents—is the reason that NTDs infect millions of Americans in the year 2019. But it does not have to be this way.

ECONOMIC IMPACT

While the social and structural components that contribute to poverty and allow for the existence of NTDs in the United States are critical, understanding the economic impacts of these diseases is equally so. Many NTDs have symptoms that can be overlooked or that can be mistaken for something else. However, their existence in communities of extreme poverty further dilutes the economic prospects of the city or town.

Given that the existence of NTDs in the United States has scarcely been studied since the 1950s, estimates of their economic impact are limited. The most extensive investigation of the issue, as discussed in chapter 1, was conducted by Bleakley (2009) and it looked at the economic impact at the turn of the nineteenth century; drawing a comparison in the before and after of the Rockefeller Campaign. His findings, however, showed large economic impacts as hookworm was eliminated and demonstrated a dramatic increase in school attendance.[26] Outside of this specific examination of the economic impacts of NTDs in the United States, knowledge is limited. For this reason, we draw on international data to demonstrate the devastating economic impacts of these diseases.

Soil-transmitted helminths, which include hookworm, are some NTDs that have been proven to currently infect people in low-income communities in Alabama.[27] Globally, the World Health Organization estimates that the elimination of such infections would result in an economic benefit of $95.7 billion USD from 2012 to 2030.[28] Norris et al. (2012) found that for every $1 spent on deworming for soil-transmitted helminths, society gains $30. Additionally, the study found that deworming programs increased school attendance in Kenya by 25 percent.[29] These are substantial benefits from the control and/or elimination of just one set of NTDs and there are several types that affect Americas.

Another disease that is known to exist in pockets of the United States is Chagas Disease. As we described in previous chapters, infection is most common in Texas, Louisiana, and California. Lenk et al. (2018) estimate that controlling or eliminating Chagas globally, would result in a savings of $7.5 billion USD from 2021 to 2030.[30] In the United States, the total annual costs (healthcare costs plus productivity losses) per Chagas-infected person is $15,762.[31] In total productivity, it is estimated that the United States losses $861 million USD annually to Chagas Disease. How might the economic prospects of some of America's poorest communities be different with the elimination of these infections?

The economic benefits that result from the control of other types of NTDs are just as significant. Trachoma, a disease caused by *Chlamydia trachomatis* which can lead to blindness, results in an estimated $2.9 million USD in productivity losses annually.[32] In China, schistosomiasis control resulted in a gain of $6.20 USD for every $1 spent.[33] Another study of schistosomiasis in China found that 29.8 percent of all enrolled participants had a complete loss of work capacity due to infection.[34] In Africa, where schistosomiasis is more prominent, the economic benefits of its elimination could be even greater.

The countrywide and global figures that illustrate the economic impacts of NTDs serve as a warning of the economic losses likely occurring in the United States. Millions, if not billions, of dollars lost in productivity. Children unable to attend school and, thus, reducing their workforce contribution. Because there is limited study of NTDs in the United States, we do not know the extent of the productivity losses that accompany these infections. These losses do not only affect the individuals that can no longer work, they also affect the economic prosperity of the community and the country as a whole. Therefore, the problem of NTDs in the United States is a two-part problem: the social and moral questions surrounding poverty in America and the microeconomic and macroeconomic impacts.

WHAT IS NEEDED?

The hardship that can be caused by NTD infection can be seen through graphic images from low-income countries as organizations like the Gates Foundation dedicate millions of dollars to ridding these places of NTDs. In many ways, NTD prevention is a great investment. As stated earlier in the book, "Fifty cents per person per treatment, on average, is the cost to treat and prevent the most common NTDs."[35] What's more, "every dollar spent on NTD prevention is estimated to turn into more than $50 in productivity."[36] The reality is that the United States government *does* spend money to fight NTDs. In the 2019 fiscal year, the U.S. government allocated $103 million for NTDs.[37] Unfortunately, all of this money was allocated to fight NTDs in other countries. Fighting NTDs in the countries most affected is critical and we are not arguing that this money should not be allocated to USAID to run NTD control and elimination programs. It should. The work being done by USAID, nonprofits, and other organizations focused on controlling NTDs is vital to people around the world. Our argument, instead, is that in addition to funding NTD control abroad, we must also fund it right here in the United States.

Scientists and public health officials understand what NTDs are, how to prevent them, how to diagnose them, and how to treat them. These are diseases that are entirely preventable but that cause significant physical and economic burden to those infected. Thus, preventing such diseases makes great humanitarian and economic sense. The curse of NTDs in America, however, is that addressing them demands that we acknowledge that there are Americans living in extreme poverty and that these diseases do, in fact, exist in a place like the United States. Awareness must be raised and the political will must be mustered to allocate resources to address this problem domestically.

EDUCATION AND OUTREACH

One of the most important and necessary responses that must occur with regards to NTDs in the United States is community-level education and outreach. These programs should be aimed at raising NTD awareness among doctors, nurses, health departments, and health care professionals, as well as among residents in at-risk communities. The types of activities should vary depending on the needs of the community, but a combination of flyers (or other informational material) available in extension centers, doctor's offices, community centers, etc. and workshops or training programs for local leaders and healthcare professionals could be effective in raising awareness. In order to create a program with the greatest chance of success, it is important to include multiple types of interventions. As Philips et al. (2018) found in their study of community-based health interventions, "intervention programs that engage the population through multiple activities or activities that are spaced over the entire duration of the program are more successful than the ones based on a single activity."[38] Other studies have found that delivering health information face-to-face (when feasible) is often a welcome and effective method of raising awareness among a population.[39]

Selecting the appropriate methods for an education and outreach campaign is very important because many studies in the health promotion literature have demonstrated that increased awareness reduces infection rates.[40] Additionally, in their 2017 study, Shariatpanahi et al. found that "as public knowledge of various diseases, increases, people are more likely to seek early care if needed."[41] There does seem to be some discrepancy in how effective awareness campaigns are based on the type of health issue for which awareness is being raised. Awareness campaigns appear to be more effective for communicable diseases than for noncommunicable diseases.[42] Finally, media campaigns and education programs in universities are effective in increasing disease awareness.[43] A 2015 study that utilized a type of mathematical modeling called an SIS model, found that media campaigns designed to raise awareness were able to effectively lower infection rates.[44] With regards to school-based programs, there is evidence to suggest that college students that receive health information are more likely to act on that information than other subpopulations.[45] In this way, they serve as effective information promoters because they not only change their own behavior, but they take the information they have learned back to their family and friends who are not part of the college community.[46]

In primary and secondary schools, health education can also have a positive impact on health outcomes. A study by Collins et al. (2009) found that when health programs deploy a diffusion process that provides teachers curriculum based on scientific evidence, that there are positive health outcomes.[47] Thus, school-based education programs appear to have a positive impact at all grade levels.

For the education and outreach component of this project, we have developed one-page informational materials and, as of this writing, have begun to coordinate training workshops for various groups within the communities that participated in this study. By and large, all the communities that participated in this study have been highly interested in programs that can raise community awareness of NTDs and lessen the risk of infection. There has been a strong commitment from both community leaders and local residents to see a tangible, effective outcome from this project and there is hope that overall awareness levels will eventually be increased.

What is vital to creating effective education and outreach programs, however, is to create programs that work within the culture of each individual community and provide community involvement and ownership over the program. Each community has strengths that they can bring to a project and their involvement in program development and implementation is vital to creating an effective program. In communities that have a university extension presence, the extension office can be the perfect place to house such programs, as they have the expertise and experience for program management, but are also a part of the local community.

Diverse, well-structured education and outreach programs, designed with the help of the community and driven by local community members, rather than members of a research team is the most effective way to increase awareness regarding NTDs and the first small step that can be taken to reduce the number of Americans suffering from these infections.

FEDERAL AND STATE-LEVEL INVOLVEMENT

Education and outreach programs are vitally important to increasing understanding of NTDs at the local level—both among residents and healthcare providers—but that alone will not end the problem of NTDs in the United States. In order to fully address, not only the diseases, but the social and economic factors that contribute to their existence, there must be federal and state-level involvement. Throughout the course of this project we had numerous conversations with state health organizations and Congressional offices about the problem of NTDs in the United States. Understanding of the problem ranged from a complete lack of awareness about NTDs to a somewhat patronizing disinterest in them to a desire to address them directly. And while we did run into barriers with individuals who did not want to hear about the problem, overall, we found that Congressional offices on both sides of the aisle were concerned about NTDs and were in agreement that something needed to be done. We had numerous phone calls, one-on-one meetings, and other communications where both Republican and Democratic staffers gave up their time—most talking with us on several occasions—and showed a genuine interest in the problem. This has made us optimistic about the future, but there is still much that needs to be done.

As of this writing, there are only five official pieces of legislation that have been introduced to address NTDs, whether globally or in the United States. Three of them, H.R. 826, which was introduced in January 2019 by Rep. Christopher Smith (R-NJ), S.2481, introduced September 2019 by Senator Sherrod Brown (D-OH), and S.2675 introduced in October 2019 by Senator Cory Booker (D-NJ) address NTDs in the United States. H.R. 826 and S.2481, which contain almost exactly the same language, both call for the Department of Health and Human Services to submit a report to Congress on NTDs in the United States. Additionally, the bills propose that the Centers for Disease Control and Prevention enter into cooperative agreements that would allow them to address NTDs in the United States. Aside from these two pieces of legislation, H.R. 3400, which was also introduced by Rep. Christopher Smith, calls for funding and work for NTDs, but only in the international context.

The most recent, and comprehensive, piece of federal legislation to address NTDs in the United States is Senate Bill 2675, which was introduced by Senator Cory Booker (D-NJ) on October 23, 2019. This bill, known as the STOP (Study, Treat, Observe, and Prevent) Neglected Diseases of Poverty Act, does four main things. First, the Act would create an Interagency Task Force to prevent, diagnose, and treat NTDs in the United States.[48] Second, the Act provides resources for an NTD surveillance system.[49] Third, it requires the Department of Health and Human Services, specifically the secretary, to "implement educational programs to raise awareness" of these diseases.[50]

Lastly, the legislation is aimed at helping to facilitate research for new diagnostic tools and treatments.[51] Of the legislation Dr. Peter Hotez stated, "This legislation fills an important void in terms of health disparities in America. It is among the first comprehensive pieces of legislation to address the previously hidden poverty-related neglected diseases in the United States. These illnesses are not rare, in fact, they are common, but seldom diagnosed, treated, or prevented because they occur almost exclusively in Americans living in extreme poverty."[52] In all, the bill is the most direct attempt made to address the issue of NTDs in the United States, but it remains in committee discussions with no guarantee of making it to the floor for a vote.

The Federal government is not the only place where NTDs are being overlooked, however. There is also very little being done at the state level. As of this writing, the state of Texas is the only state with a program addressing NTDs. This program, which is a few years old, is part of the Infectious Disease Control Unit and provides information on seventeen NTDs that either have a history in Texas or could be transmitted in Texas. The diseases included in this program are Ascariasis, Chagas, Dengue, Echinococcosis, Fascioliasis, Hookworm, Leishmaniasis, Leprosy, Paragonimiasis, Rabies, Taeniasis, and Trichuriasis, and, under the program, all of them are reportable diseases. In addition, the Texas Chagas Taskforce is an active organization made up of Chagas experts from across the state. Over the past five years, the Texas Chagas Taskforce has focused on raising awareness of Chagas among physicians and other healthcare professionals. Prior to the work of the Taskforce, many physicians in Texas knew little to nothing about Chagas, and those that knew about the diseases did not believe it occurred in the United States. The Taskforce has had great success in changing these perceptions and developing greater Chagas awareness.

Another important program in the state of Texas is the Texas A&M University Colonias Program. The program was founded by the Texas State Legislature in 1991 and serves colonias in the Western, Central, and Lower Rio Grande Region.[53] The program conducts extensive outreach and training along the Texas-Mexico border, including training programs for community health advisers and community health workers; two groups that are vitally important in border communities. Though the Colonias Program is providing valuable outreach and training, it has little to no focus on NTDs.

Following a 2017 study, which identified hookworm infection in Lowndes County, the Alabama Department of Public Health launched the Lowndes County Unincorporated Waste Water Project with the goal of providing low-income residents with septic tanks.[54] The program was launched in January 2019 and costs recipients $20/month as well as a one-time fee of $500 for conventional systems or $1,000 for engineered systems. This program is taking important steps toward addressing some of the infrastructure factors that contribute to hookworm infection, but there is concern that it is still cost-prohibitive for most low-income residents in the areas of greatest infection risk.

In addition to Texas and Alabama, there is some limited NTD information available on the websites for the South Carolina Department of Health and Environmental Control and the Louisiana Department of Health. To the best of our knowledge, there are no formal programs within these departments. The South Carolina Department of Health and Environmental Control provides information on Rabies and West Nile Virus, while the Louisiana Department of Health provides extensive information about Chagas, including disease information and testing guidelines. The Louisiana Health Department also provides some more limited information on Leishmaniasis.

Lastly, there is work being conducted as universities across the country that is directed at NTDs. Both Mississippi State University and the Task Force for Global Health—which has a collaboration with Emory University—focus on NTDs in the international context. The School of Public Health and Tropical Medicine at Tulane University, the National School of Tropical Medicine at Baylor College of Medicine, and several departments at Texas A&M University, including the Bush School of Government and Public Service, where we reside, are examining NTDs in the United States. All of these programs are extremely important to developing a greater understanding of the extent of the problem in the United States and what can be done to reduce infection rates. Ultimately, however, much greater effort must be made at both the state and federal level to address the prevalence of NTDs in the United States.

CONCLUSION

Kofi Annan, former secretary general of the United Nations and Nobel Prize laureate, famously said, "It is my aspiration that health will finally be seen not as a blessing to be wished for but as a human right to be fought for."[55] This is the same mentality that should be used to address NTDs, not just throughout the world, but right here in the United States. Americans and global citizens alike have the right to be protected from easily preventable diseases. In a country with as vast of resources as the United States, it is unacceptable to allow these diseases to persist.

State and local health departments, members of Congress, researchers, and activists have begun to question the mentality that NTDs do not exist in the United States, as evidenced by the progress in legislation and programs described in this chapter. Unfortunately, this acknowledgement is coming slowly and there is still a larger contingent that tunes out when the topic of NTDs in the United States comes up. The reality is, however, that the presence of NTDs in the United States has important implications, eloquently summed up by Berlinguer (2004), "Health has a dual moral value: it is essential for the quality of life and life itself, and is instrumental as a precondition of freedom."[56] Communities throughout the United States are suffering from NTD infection and we, as a society, are obligated to pay attention. As Philip Alston explained, "denial does not eliminate responsibility, nor does it negate obligations."[57] We can deny the existence of these diseases in our poorest communities, but that does not remove them from existence and it does not eliminate our responsibility to address them. The time to address NTDs in the United States is now.

NOTES

1. Hotez, *Blue Marble Health*, 135.

2. Michael Harrington, *The Other America: Poverty in the United States* (New York: Penguin Books, 1962), 1.

3. Hotez, *Blue Marble Health*, 3.

4. Celia Barria and Mohamed Madi, "Escobares, Texas: Life in the Poorest City in the US," published February 1, 2019, https://www.bbc.com/news/av/world-us-canada-47171130/escobares-texas-life-in-the-poorest-city-in-the-us.

5. Jason Cohen, "Rio Grande Valley Tops List of 'America's Poorest Cities,'" *Texas Monthly*, published January 21, 2013, https://www.texasmonthly.com/articles/rio-grande-valley-tops-list-of-americas-poorest-cities/.

6. Alexa Ura and Elbert Wang, "Poverty in Texas Drops to Lowest Levels in More Than a Decade," *Texas Tribune*, published September 13, 2018, https://www.texastribune.org/2018/09/13/texas-poverty-census-2017-lowest-levels-decade/#targetText=And%20families%20living%20in%20the,that's%20double%20the%20state%20figure.&targetText=The%20latest%20estimates%20released%20Thursday,of%2018.5%20percent%20in%202011.

7. Ura and Wang, "Poverty in Texas Drops to Lowest Levels in More Than a Decade."

8. Gaby Galvin, "On the Border, Out of the Shadows," *US News & World Report*, published May 16, 2018, https://www.usnews.com/news/healthiest-communities/articles/2018-05-16/americas-third-world-border-colonias-in-texas-struggle-to-attain-services.

9. Vincent Guilamo-Ramos and Marco Thimm-Kaiser, "Youth Living in Settlements at US Border Suffer Poverty and Lack of Health Care," *The Conversation*, published October 10, 2018, http://theconversation.com/youth-living-in-settlements-at-us-border-suffer-poverty-and-lack-of-health-care-103416.

10. Chris McGreal, "America's Poorest Border Town: No Immigration Papers, No American Dream," *The Guardian*, published November 19, 2015, https://www.theguardian.com/us-news/2015/nov/19/americas-poorest-border-town-no-immigration-papers-no-american-dream.

11. McGreal, "America's Poorest Border Town: No Immigration Papers, No American Dream."

12. Galvin, "On the Border, Out of the Shadows."

13. Guilamo-Ramos and Thimm-Kaiser, "Youth Living in Settlements at US Border Suffer Poverty and Lack of Health Care."

14. Paul Adams, "Poverty and Progress in the Mississippi Delta," *BBC News*, published January 4, 2012, https://www.bbc.com/news/magazine-16385337.

15. Ruth Cummins, "Decades Go By, Yet Child Hunger and Poverty Endure in the Delta," *University of Mississippi Medical Center*, published July 17, 2017, https://www.umc.edu/news/News_Articles/2017/July/-decades-go-by,-yet-child-hunger-and-poverty-endures-in-the-delta.html.

16. Cummins, "Decades Go By, Yet Child Hunger and Poverty Endure in the Delta"; Emily Pettus, "Entrenched Poverty Tough to Shake in the Mississippi Delta," *Clarion Ledger*, last modified August 8, 2017, https://www.clarionledger.com/story/news/2017/08/07/mississippi-delta-poverty/544601001/#:~:targetText=Although%20opportunities%20have%20improved%20in,it's%2030%20to%2040%20percent.

17. Cummins, "Decades Go By, Yet Child Hunger and Poverty Endure in the Delta"; Adams, "Poverty and Progress in the Mississippi Delta."

18. Cummins, "Decades Go By, Yet Child Hunger and Poverty Endure in the Delta."

19. Chris McGreal, "America's Poorest White Town: Abandoned by Coal, Swallowed by Drugs," *The Guardian*, published November 12, 2015, https://www.theguardian.com/us-news/2015/nov/12/beattyville-kentucky-and-americas-poorest-towns.

20. McGreal, "America's Poorest White Town: Abandoned by Coal, Swallowed by Drugs."

21. McGreal, "America's Poorest White Town: Abandoned by Coal, Swallowed by Drugs."

22. McGreal, "America's Poorest White Town: Abandoned by Coal, Swallowed by Drugs."

23. Andrew A. Zekeri, "The Causes of Enduring Poverty in Alabama's Black Belt," *In the Shadows of Poverty: Strengthening the Rural Poverty Research Capacity of the South* (Mississippi State, MS: Mississippi State University, Rural Policy Research Institute's Rural Poverty Research Center, 2004).

24. Lyndsey Gilpin, "The Rural South's Invisible Public Health Crisis," *Montgomery Advertiser*, published July 6, 2018, https://www.montgomeryadvertiser.com/story/news/local/alabama/2018/07/06/story-first-series-ways-communities-addressing-rise-poverty-related-tropical-diseases-poor-sewage/754311002/.

25. Carlos Ballesteros, "Alabama has the Worst Poverty in the Developed World, U.N. Official Says," *Newsweek*, published December 10, 2017, https://www.newsweek.com/alabama-un-poverty-environmental-racism-743601.

26. Hoyt Bleakley, "Economic Effects of Childhood Exposure to Tropical Disease," *American Economic Review* 99, no. 2 (2009): 218–223.

27. McKenna et al., "Human Intestinal Parasite Burden and Poor Sanitation in Rural Alabama," 1623–1628.

28. William K. Redekop et al., "The Socioeconomic Benefit to Individuals of Achieving the 2020 Targets for Five Preventive Chemotherapy Neglected Tropical Diseases," *PLoS Neglected Tropical Diseases* 11, no. 1 (2017): e0005289.

29. Norris et al., "Social and Economic Impact Review on Neglected Tropical Diseases," *Economic Policy/Briefing Paper* (Washington, DC: Hudson Institute, 2012).

30. Edeltraud J. Lenk et al., "Socioeconomic Benefit to Individuals of Achieving 2020 Targets for Four Neglected Tropical Diseases Controlled/Eliminated by Innovative and Intensified Disease Management: Human African Trypanosomiasis, Leprosy, Visceral Leishmaniasis, Chagas Disease," *PLoS Neglected Tropical Diseases* 12, no. 3 (2018): e0006250.

31. Lee et al., "Global Economic Burden of Chagas Disease," 342–348.

32. Norris et al., "Social and Economic Impact Review on Neglected Tropical Diseases."

33. Xiao-Nong Zhou et al., "An Economic Evaluation of the National Schistosomiasis Control Programme in China from 1992 to 2000," *Acta tropica* 96, nos. 2–3 (2005): 255–265.

34. Tie-Wu Jia et al., "Quantifying Quality of Life and Disability of Patients with Advanced Schistosomiasis Japonica," *PLoS Neglected Tropical Diseases* 5, no. 2 (2011): e966.

35. Ellen Agler and Mojie Crigler, *Under the Big Tree: Extraordinary Stories from the Movement to End Neglected Tropical Diseases* (John Hopkins University Press, 2019), 4.

36. Agler and Crigler, *Under the Big Tree: Extraordinary Stories from the Movement to End Neglected Tropical Diseases*, 13.

37. *KFF*, "The U.S. Government and Global Neglected Tropical Disease Efforts," published January 28, 2020, https://www.kff.org/global-health-policy/fact-sheet/the-u-s-government-and-global-neglected-tropical-diseases/.

38. Mappalakayil Phinse Philip, Srinivasan Kannan, and Neetu Ambali Parambil, "Community-based Interventions for Health Promotion and Disease Prevention in Noncommunicable Diseases: A Narrative Review," *Journal of Education and Health Promotion* 7 (2018): 149.

39. Chris Bullen, "Taking Public Health to the Streets: The 1998 Auckland Meningococcal Disease Awareness Program," *Health Education & Behavior* 27, no. 3 (2000): 363–370.

40. Bullen, "Taking Public Health to the Streets: The 1998 Auckland Meningococcal Disease Awareness Program"; Shariatpanahi et al., "Assessing the Effectiveness of Disease Awareness Programs: Evidence from Google Trends Data for the World Awareness Dates," *Telematics and Informatics* 34, no. 7 (2017): 904–913; Priti Kumar Roy, Shubhankar Saha, and Fahad Al Basir, "Effect of Awareness Programs in Controlling the Disease HIV/AIDS: An Optimal Control Theoretic Approach," *Advances in Difference Equations* 217, no. 1 (2015): 1–18.

41. Shariatpanahi et al., "Assessing the Effectiveness of Disease Awareness Programs," 904.

42. Shariatpanahi et al., "Assessing the Effectiveness of Disease Awareness Programs."

43. Roy, Saha, and Al Basir, "Effect of Awareness Programs in Controlling the Disease HIV/AIDS: An Optimal Control Theoretic Approach"; Ashley N. Plaster et al., "University Students' Knowledge, Attitudes, and Sources of Information about Zika Virus," *Journal of Community Health* 43, no. 4 (2018): 647–655.

44. Roy, Saha, and Al Basir, "Effect of Awareness Programs in Controlling the Disease HIV/AIDS: An Optimal Control Theoretic Approach."

45. Plaster et al., "University Students' Knowledge, Attitudes, and Sources of Information about Zika Virus."

46. Plaster et al., "University Students' Knowledge, Attitudes, and Sources of Information about Zika Virus."

47. Janet Collins et al., "Programs-that-Work: CDC's Guide to Effective Programs that Reduce Health-Risk Behavior of Youth," *Journal of School Health* 72, no. 3 (2002): 93–99.

48. Cory Booker, "Booker Introduces Legislation to Help Eliminate Neglected Diseases of Poverty in the United States," published October 23, 2019, https://www.booker.senate.gov/?p=press_release&id=999.

49. Booker, "Booker Introduces Legislation to Help Eliminate Neglected Diseases of Poverty in the United States."

50. Booker, "Booker Introduces Legislation to Help Eliminate Neglected Diseases of Poverty in the United States."

51. Booker, "Booker Introduces Legislation to Help Eliminate Neglected Diseases of Poverty in the United States."

52. Booker, "Booker Introduces Legislation to Help Eliminate Neglected Diseases of Poverty in the United States."

53. "Who We Are," Texas A&M University Colonias Program, accessed 2019, https://colonias.arch.tamu.edu/about/who-we-are/index.html.

54. McKenna et al., "Human Intestinal Parasite Burden and Poor Sanitation in Rural Alabama."

55. Ruth Dreifuss, "What We Owe to Kofi Annan's Legacy in Global Health," *Kofi Annan Foundation*, published May 22, 2019, https://www.kofiannanfoundation.org/changing-drug-policy/what-we-owe-to-kofi-annans-legacy-in-global-health-by-h-e-ruth-dreifuss/.

56. Giovanni Berlinguer, "Bioethics, Health, and Inequality," *The Lancet* 364, no. 9439 (2004): 1088.

57. Philip Alston, "Statement on Visit to the USA," *United Nations Human Rights, Office of the High Commissioner*, published December 15, 2017, https://www.ohchr.org/EN/NewsEvents/Pages/DisplayNews.aspx?NewsID=22533&LangID=E.

Bibliography

AAP Council on Community Pediatrics. "Poverty and child health in the United States." *Pediatrics* 137, no. 4 (2016): e20160339.

Adams, Paul. "Poverty and progress in the Mississippi Delta." *BBC News*. Published January 4, 2012. https://www.bbc.com/news/magazine-16385337.

Agler, Ellen, and Mojie Crigler. *Under the Big Tree: Extraordinary Stories from the Movement to End Neglected Tropical Diseases*. Baltimore: John Hopkins University Press, 2019.

Alaimo, Katherine, Christine M. Olson, and Edward A. Frongillo. "Family food insufficiency, but not low family income, is positively associated with dysthymia and suicide symptoms in adolescents." *The Journal of Nutrition* 132, no. 4 (2002): 719–725.

———. "Food insufficiency and American school-aged children's cognitive, academic, and psychosocial development." *Pediatrics* 108, no. 1 (2001): 44–53.

Albuquerque, Catarina de. *Promotion and Protection of All Human Rights, Civil, Political, Economic, Social and Cultural Rights, Including the Right to Development*. New York: United Nations General Assembly Human Rights Council, 2011. https://doi.org/10.1163/2210-7975_HRD-9970-2016149.

Alewu, B., and C. Nosiri. "Pesticides and human health." In *Pesticides in the Modern World—Effects of Pesticides Exposure*, pp. 231–250. InTech, 2011.

Alexander, Karl L., Doris R. Entwisle, and Linda S. Olson. "Schools, achievement, and inequality: A seasonal perspective." *Educational Evaluation and Policy Analysis* 23, no. 2 (2001): 171–191.

Allsworth, Jenifer E., Jane Alyce Ratner, and Jeffrey F. Peipert. "Trichomoniasis and other sexually transmitted infections: Results from the 2001–2004 NHANES surveys." *Sexually Transmitted Diseases* 36, no. 12 (2009): 738–744.

Alston, Philip. "Report of the Special Rapporteur on extreme poverty and human rights on his mission to the United States of America." *United Nations*. Published May 4, 2018. http://digitallibrary.un.org/record/162953.

———. "Statement on visit to the USA, by Professor Philip Alston, United Nations Special Rapporteur on extreme poverty and human rights." *New York: United Nations Office of the High Commissioner for Human Rights*. Published December 15, 2017. www. ohchr. og/EN/NewsEvents/Pages/DisplayNews. aspx.

Alto, Barry W., and Steven A. Juliano. "Temperature effects on the dynamics of *Aedes albopictus* (Diptera: Culicidae) populations in the laboratory." *Journal of Medical Entomology* 38, no. 4 (2001): 548–556.

American Society for the Prevention of Cruelty to Animals. "Pet statistics." Accessed August 19, 2019. https://www.aspca.org/animal-homelessness/shelter-intake-and-surrender/pet-statistics.

Americans with Disabilities Act (ADA). "Americans with Disabilities Act of 1990, Pub. L. No. 101–336, 104 Stat. 328." (1990).

Anderson, Alice L., and Thomas Allen. "Mapping historic Hookworm disease prevalence in the southern US, comparing percent prevalence with percent soil drainage type using GIs." *Infectious Diseases: Research and Treatment* 4 (2011): IDRT-S6762.

Anglin, Mary K. "Lessons from Appalachia in the 20th century: Poverty, power, and the "grassroots"." *American Anthropologist* 104, no. 2 (2002): 565–582.

Arcaya, Mariana C., Alyssa L. Arcaya, and S. V. Subramanian. "Inequalities in health: Definitions, concepts, and theories." *Global Health Action* 8, no. 1 (2015): 27106.

Arcipowski, Erin, John Schwartz, Lisa Davenport, Meghan Hayes, and Tracy Nolan. "Clean water, clean life: Promoting healthier, accessible water in rural Appalachia." *Journal of Contemporary Water Research & Education* 161, no. 1 (2017): 1–18.

Arnold, Carrie. "Can America cope with a resurgence of tropical disease?" *Wellcome Trust*. Published August 10, 2015. https://mosaicscience.com/story/america-tropical-disease/.

Attanasio, Orazio P., and Luigi Pistaferri. "Consumption inequality." *Journal of Economic Perspectives* 30, no. 2 (2016): 3–28.

AVMA. "Mandatory spay/neuter laws." Accessed August 20, 2019. https://www.avma.org/Advocacy/StateAndLocal/Pages/sr-spay-neuter-laws.aspx?mode=full.

Bailey, Martha J., and Nicolas J. Duquette. "How Johnson fought the war on poverty: The economics and politics of funding at the office of economic opportunity." *The Journal of Economic History* 74, no. 2 (2014): 351–387.

Balestra, Carlotta, and Richard Tonkin. "Inequalities in household wealth across OECD countries: Evidence from the OECD wealth distribution database." *OECD Working Paper No. 88* (2018). http://www.oecd.org/officialdocuments/publicdisplaydocumentpdf/?cote=SDD/DOC(2018)1&docLanguage=En.

Ballesteros, Carlos. "Alabama has the worst poverty in the developed world, U.N. official says." *Newsweek*. Published December 10, 2017. https://www.newsweek.com/alabama-un-poverty-environmental-racism-743601.

Baptiste, Nathalie. "This black community has filed a civil rights complaint over unsanitary sewage conditions." *Mother Jones*. Published October 4, 2018. https://www.motherjones.com/environment/2018/10/this-black-community-has-filed-a-civil-rights-complaint-over-unsanitary-sewage-conditions/.

Barnwell, Paul. "Why teachers quit: It's not about money (or low-pay)." *The Atlantic*. Published May 27, 2015. https://www.theatlantic.com/education/archive/2015/05/the-ongoing-struggle-of-teacher-retention/394211/.

Barria, Celia, and Mohamed Madi. "Escobares, Texas: Life in the poorest city in the US." Published February 1, 2019. https://www.bbc.com/news/av/world-us-canada-47171130/escobares-texas-life-in-the-poorest-city-in-the-us.

Bartfeld, Judith, Craig Gundersen, Timothy Smeeding, and James P. Ziliak, eds. *SNAP Matters: How Food Stamps Affect Health and Well-Being*. Palo Alto: Stanford University Press, 2015.

Barton, Jordana, Emily Ryder Perlmeter, Elizabeth Sobel-Blum, and Raquel Marquez. "Las colonias in the 21st century: Progress along the Texas-Mexico border." *Federal Reserve Bank of Dallas* (2015).

Bartram, Jamie, and Sandy Cairncross. "Hygiene, sanitation, and water: Forgotten foundations of health." *PLoS Medicine* 7, no. 11 (2010): e1000367.

Bassil, Kate L., Catherine Vakil, M. Sanborn, D. C. Cole, Judith S. Kaur, and K. J. Kerr. "Cancer health effects of pesticides: Systematic review." *Canadian Family Physician* 53, no. 10 (2007): 1704–1711.

Bean, Frank D., Cynthia Feliciano, Jennifer Lee, and Jennifer Van Hook. "The new US immigrants: How do they affect our understanding of the African American experience?" *The Annals of the American Academy of Political and Social Science* 621, no. 1 (2009): 202–220.

Beaumier, Coreen, Melissa N. Garcia, and Kristy O. Murray. "The history of dengue in the United States and its recent emergence." *Current Tropical Medicine Reports* 1, no. 1 (2014): 32–35.

Beil, Laura. "The parasite on the playground." *The New York Times*. Published January 16, 2018. https://www.nytimes.com/2018/01/16/health/toxocara-children-new-york-playgrounds.html.

Berlinguer, Giovanni. "Bioethics, health, and inequality." *The Lancet* 364, no. 9439 (2004): 1086–1091.

Bern, Caryn, Sonia Kjos, Michael J. Yabsley, and Susan P. Montgomery. "Trypanosoma cruzi and Chagas' disease in the United States." *Clinical Microbiology Reviews* 24, no. 4 (2011): 655–681.

Bershadker, Matt. "Acting on the critical link between pets, people, and poverty." *American Society for the Prevention of Cruelty to Animals*. Published February 26, 2019. https://www.aspca.org/blog/acting-critical-link-between-pets-people-and-poverty.

Bhattacharya, Jay, and Janet Currie. "Youths at nutrition risk: Malnourished or misnourished?" In *Risky Behavior Among Youths: An Economic Analysis*, pp. 483–522. University of Chicago Press, 2001.

Bickel, Gary, Mark Nord, Cristofer Price, William Hamilton, and John Cook. "Guide to measuring household food security." (2000).

Bjerede, Marie. "Rural districts face challenges and opportunities with technology access." *Technology Solutions That Drive Education*. Published January 2, 2018. https://edtechmagazine.com/k12/article/2018/01/rural-districts-face-challenges-and-opportunities-technology-access.

Bjørling-Poulsen, Marina, Helle Raun Andersen, and Philippe Grandjean. "Potential developmental neurotoxicity of pesticides used in Europe." *Environmental Health* 7, no. 1 (2008): 50.

Bleakley, Hoyt. "Disease and development: Evidence from hookworm eradication in the American South." *The Quarterly Journal of Economics* 122, no. 1 (2007): 73–117.

———. "Economic effects of childhood exposure to tropical disease." *American Economic Review* 99, no. 2 (2009): 218–223.

Blumenthal, Sidney. "Katrina comes home to roost." *The Guardian*. Published September 2, 2005. https://www.theguardian.com/world/2005/sep/02/hurricane katrina.usa10.

Boccaccio, Mary. "Ground itch and dew poison the Rockefeller Sanitary Commission 1909–14." *Journal of the History of Medicine and Allied Sciences* 27, no. 1 (1972): 30–53.

Bockarie, Moses J., Louise A. Kelly-Hope, Maria Rebollo, and David H. Molyneux. "Preventive chemotherapy as a strategy for elimination of neglected tropical parasitic diseases: Endgame challenges." *Philosophical Transactions of the Royal Society B: Biological Sciences* 368, no. 1623 (2013): 20120144.

Bolin, Robert C. "Disaster impact and recovery: A comparison of black and white victims." *International Journal of Mass Emergencies and Disasters* 4, no. 1 (1986): 35–50.

Booker, Cory. "Booker introduces legislation to help eliminate neglected diseases of poverty in the United States." Published October 23, 2019. https://www.booker.s enate.gov/?p=press_release&id=999.

Bor, Jacob, Gregory H. Cohen, and Sandro Galea. "Population health in an era of rising income inequality: USA, 1980–2015." *The Lancet* 389, no. 10077 (2017): 1475–1490.

Bouri, Nidhi, Tara Kirk Sell, Crystal Franco, Amesh A. Adalja, D. A. Henderson, and Noreen A. Hynes. "Return of epidemic dengue in the United States: Implications for the public health practitioner." *Public Health Reports* 127, no. 3 (2012): 259–266.

Boustan, Leah Platt, Fernando Ferreira, Hernan Winkler, and Eric Zolt. "Income inequality and local government in the United States, 1970–2000." *No. w16299*. National Bureau of Economic Research, 2010.

Bradberry, Sally M., Alex T. Proudfoot, and J. Allister Vale. "Glyphosate poisoning." *Toxicological Reviews* 23, no. 3 (2004): 159–167.

Brady, David, Andrew S. Fullerton, and Jennifer Moren Cross. "More than just nickels and dimes: A cross-national analysis of working poverty in affluent democracies." *Social Problems* 57, no. 4 (2010): 559–585.

Bretveld, Reini W., Chris M. G. Thomas, Paul T. J. Scheepers, Gerhard A. Zielhuis, and Nel Roeleveld. "Pesticide exposure: The hormonal function of the female reproductive system disrupted?" *Reproductive Biology and Endocrinology* 4, no. 1 (2006): 30.

Brouqui, Philippe, and Raoult, Didier. "Arthropod-borne diseases in homeless." *Annals of the New York Academy of Sciences* 1078, no. 1 (2006): 223–235.

Brown, Karl. "Managing sexually transmitted diseases in jails." *TheBodyPro*. Published September 1, 2003. https://www.thebodypro.com/article/managing-sexually-transmitted-diseases-jails.

Bullard, R. D. *Dumping in Dixie: Race, Class, and Environmental Quality*. Boulder, CO: Westview, 1990. http://www.ciesin.org/docs/010-278/010-278chpt1.html.

Bullen, Chris. "Taking public health to the streets: The 1998 Auckland meningococcal disease awareness program." *Health Education & Behavior* 27, no. 3 (2000): 363–370.

Burkholder, J. E., T. C. Allison, and V. P. Kelly. "Trypanosoma cruzi (Chagas) (Protozoa: Kinetoplastida) in invertebrate, reservoir, and human hosts of the lower Rio Grande valley of Texas." *The Journal of Parasitology* 66, no. 2 (1980): 305–311.

Byard, Jim. "Workforce information Lowndes County AL unemployment underemployment." *Lowndes County*. Accessed October 3, 2018. https://lowndescountyedc.com/doing-business/workforce-information.

Byrne, Brian. "A shocking number of Americans don't have a toilet." *The Week*. Published November 24, 2015. https://theweek.com/articles/590312/shocking-number-americans-dont-have-toilet.

Caldwell, Leigh Ann, and Dan Merica. "America's longest war." Last modified January 8, 2014. https://www.cnn.com/2014/01/08/politics/war-on-poverty-50-years/index.html.

Camarota, Steven. "Immigrants in the United States: A profile of America's foreign-born population." *Center for Immigration Studies*. Published August 8, 2012. https://cis.org/Immigrants-United-States-Profile-Americas-ForeignBorn-Population.

Cantor, Jacob, Leigh-Anne Krometis, Emily Sarver, Nicholas Cook, and Brian Badgley. "Tracking the downstream impacts of inadequate sanitation in central Appalachia." *Journal of Water and Health* 15, no. 4 (2017): 580–590.

Cao, Junji, Hongmei Xu, Qun Xu, Bingheng Chen, and Haidong Kan. "Fine particulate matter constituents and cardiopulmonary mortality in a heavily polluted Chinese city." *Environmental Health Perspectives* 120, no. 3 (2012): 373–378.

Carcavallo, Rodolfo U., and Susana Curto de Casas. "Some health impacts of global warming in South America: Vector-borne diseases." *Journal of Epidemiology* 6, no. 4sup (1996): 153–157.

Carey, J. Christopher, Mark A. Klebanoff, John C. Hauth, Sharon L. Hillier, Elizabeth A. Thom, J. M. Ernest, R. Phillip Heine, et al. "Metronidazole to prevent preterm delivery in pregnant women with asymptomatic bacterial vaginosis." *New England Journal of Medicine* 342, no. 8 (2000): 534–540.

Carrera, Jennifer. "Sanitation and social power in the United States." PhD dissertation, University of Illinois at Urbana-Champaign, 2014.

Carrera, Jennifer S., and Catherine Coleman Flowers. "Sanitation inequity and the cumulative effects of racism in colorblind public health policies." *American Journal of Economics and Sociology* 77, no. 3–4 (2018): 941–966.

Casey, Patrick H., Kitty Szeto, Shelly Lensing, Margaret Bogle, and Judy Weber. "Children in food-insufficient, low-income families: Prevalence, health, and nutrition status." *Archives of Pediatrics & Adolescent Medicine* 155, no. 4 (2001): 508–514.

Castro, Gilbert A. "Helminths: Structure, classification, growth, and development." In *Medical Microbiology*. 4th edition. University of Texas Medical Branch at Galveston, 1996.

Cauthen, Nancy K., and Sarah Fass. "Measuring poverty in the United States." *National Center for Children in Poverty*. Published June 2008. http://www.nccp.org/publications/pub_825.html.

Cavaca, Aline Guio, Tatiana Breder Emerich, Paulo Roberto Vasconcellos-Silva, Edson Theodoro dos Santos-Neto, and Adauto Emmerich Oliveira. "Diseases neglected by the media in Espírito Santo, Brazil in 2011–2012." *PLoS Neglected Tropical Diseases* 10, no. 4 (2016): e0004662.

Ceccarelli, Soledad, Agustín Balsalobre, Paula Medone, María Eugenia Cano, Rodrigo Gurgel Gonçalves, Dora Feliciangeli, Darío Vezzani, et al. "DataTri, a database of American triatomine species occurrence." *Scientific Data* 5 (2018): 180071.

Center for Poverty Research. "How is poverty measured in the United States?" *University of California at Davis*. Last modified December 18, 2017. https://poverty.ucdavis.edu/faq/how-poverty-measured-united-states.

———. "What is the current poverty rate in the United States?" *University of California at Davis*. Last modified October 15, 2018. https://poverty.ucdavis.edu/faq/what-current-poverty-rate-united-states.

Center on Budget and Policy Priorities. "Policy basics: Top ten facts about social security." Last modified August 14, 2019. https://www.cbpp.org/research/social-security/policy-basics-top-ten-facts-about-social-security#:~:targetText=Over%2063%20million%20people%2C%20or,young%20survivors%20of%20deceased%20workers.

Centers for Disease Control and Prevention. "Assessment of sexually transmitted diseases services in city and county jails—United States, 1997." *MMWR: Morbidity and Mortality Weekly Report* 47, no. 21 (1998): 429.

———. "Blood donor screening for Chagas disease—United States, 2006–2007." *MMWR: Morbidity and Mortality Weekly Report* 56, no. 7 (2007): 141.

———. "CDC—Chagas disease—General information." Last modified July 17, 2019. https://www.cdc.gov/parasites/chagas/gen_info/vectors/index.html.

———. "Dengue." Last modified February 14, 2002. https://www.cdc.gov/dengue/index.html?CDC_AA_refVal=https%3A%2F%2Fwww.cdc.gov%2Fdengue%2Ffaqfacts%2Findex.html.

———. "Diseases characterized by urethritis and cervicitis—2015 STD treatment guidelines." Last modified June 4, 2015. https://www.cdc.gov/std/tg2015/urethritis-and-cervicitis.htm.

———. "Elimination of malaria in the United States (1947–1951)." Last modified July 23, 2018. www.cdc.gov/malaria/about/history/elimination_us.html.

———. "Hookworm FAQs." Last modified December 16, 2014. https://www.cdc.gov/parasites/hookworm/gen_info/faqs.html.

———. "Neglected tropical diseases (NTDs)." Last modified September 14, 2018. https://www.cdc.gov/globalhealth/newsroom/topics/ntds/index.html.

———. "Ocular toxocariasis—United States, 2009–2011." *MMWR: Morbidity and Mortality Weekly Report* 60, no. 22 (2011): 734.

———. "Parasites—Ascariasis." Last modified February 15, 2018. https://www.cdc.gov/parasites/ascariasis/index.html.

———. "Parasites—Hookworm." Last modified January 10, 2013. https://www.cdc.gov/parasites/hookworm/index.html.

———. "Statistics and maps: Dengue cases in the US." Last modified March 13, 2020. https://www.cdc.gov/dengue/statistics-maps/index.html.

———. "Understanding food deserts." Last modified July 1, 2020. https://www.cdc.gov/Features/FoodDeserts/.

Chambers, John R., Lawton K. Swan, and Martin Heesacker. "Perceptions of US social mobility are divided (and distorted) along ideological lines." *Psychological Science* 26, no. 4 (2015): 413–423.

Chandra, Ranjit Kumar. "Nutrition and the immune system: An introduction." *The American Journal of Clinical Nutrition* 66, no. 2 (1997): 460S–463S.

Chapman, Jeff, and Jared Bernstein. "Immigration and poverty: How are they linked." *Monthly Labor Review* 126 (2003): 10–15.

Chaudry, Ajay, and Christopher Wimer. "Poverty is not just an indicator: The relationship between income, poverty, and child well-being." *Academic Pediatrics* 16, no. 3 (2016): S23–S29.

Chen, Linda. "The old and mysterious practice of eating dirt, revealed." *NPR*. Published April 2, 2014. https://www.npr.org/sections/thesalt/2014/04/02/297881388/the-old-and-mysterious-practice-of-eating-dirt-revealed.

Chesson, Harrell W., John M. Blandford, and Steven D. Pinkerton. "Estimates of the annual number and cost of new HIV infections among women attributable to trichomoniasis in the United States." *Sexually Transmitted Diseases* 31, no. 9 (2004): 547–551.

Chetty, Raj, David Grusky, Maximilian Hell, Nathaniel Hendren, Robert Manduca, and Jimmy Narang. "The fading American dream: Trends in absolute income mobility since 1940." *Science* 356, no. 6336 (2017): 398–406.

Chetty, Raj, John N. Friedman, Nathaniel Hilger, Emmanuel Saez, Diane Whitmore Schanzenbach, and Danny Yagan. "How does your kindergarten classroom affect your earnings? Evidence from project STAR." *The Quarterly Journal of Economics* 126, no. 4 (2011): 1593–1660.

Chetty, Raj, Michael Stepner, Sarah Abraham, Shelby Lin, Benjamin Scuderi, Nicholas Turner, Augustin Bergeron, and David Cutler. "The association between income and life expectancy in the United States, 2001–2014." *JAMA* 315, no. 16 (2016): 1750–1766.

Chetty, Raj, and Nathaniel Hendren. "The impacts of neighborhoods on intergenerational mobility II: County-level estimates." *The Quarterly Journal of Economics* 133, no. 3 (2018): 1163–1228.

Chien, Y. L., and Paul Morris. "Many Americans still lack retirement savings." *The Regional Economist* 26, no. 1 (2018).

Children's Defense Fund. "Child poverty in America 2017: National analysis." Published September 12, 2018. https://www.childrensdefense.org/wp-content/uploads/2018/09/Child-Poverty-in-America-2017-National-Fact-Sheet.pdf.

Chilton, Mariana, Michelle Chyatte, and Jennifer Breaux. "The negative effects of poverty & food insecurity on child development." *Indian Journal of Medical Research* 126, no. 4 (2007): 262.

Chitkara, Rajinder K., and P. S. Sarinas. "Dirofilaria, visceral larva migrans, and tropical pulmonary eosinophilia." *Seminars in Respiratory Infections* 12, no. 2 (1997): 138–148.

Chowell, Gerardo, Kenji Mizumoto, Juan M. Banda, S. Poccia, and Charles Perrings. "Assessing the potential impact of vector-borne disease transmission following heavy rainfall events: A mathematical framework." *Philosophical Transactions of the Royal Society B* 374, no. 1775 (2019): 20180272.

Christoffel, Tom, and Susan Scavo Gallagher. *Injury Prevention and Public Health: Practical Knowledge, Skills, and Strategies*. Burlington, MA: Jones & Bartlett Learning, 2006.

City of College Station. "Mosquito abatement program." Accessed August 1, 2019. https://www.cstx.gov/departments___city_hall/neighborhood/mosquito.

Coelho, Philip R. P., and Robert A. McGuire. "Racial differences in disease susceptibilities: Intestinal worm infections in the early twentieth-century American South." *Social History of Medicine* 19, no. 3 (2006): 461–482.

Cohen, Jason. "Rio Grande valley tops list of "America's poorest cities"." *Texas Monthly*. Published January 21, 2013. https://www.texasmonthly.com/articles/rio-grande-valley-tops-list-of-americas-poorest-cities/.

Coleman-Jensen, Alicia, Christian A. Gregory, and Matthew P. Rabbitt. "Definitions of food security." *United States Department of Agriculture Economic Research Service*. Last modified September 4, 2019. https://www.ers.usda.gov/topics/food-nutrition-assistance/food-security-in-the-us/definitions-of-food-security.aspx.

Coleman-Jensen, Alisha, Matthew P. Rabbitt, Christian A. Gregory, and Anita Singh. "Statistical supplement to household food security in the United States in 2017." *No. 2238-2019-2890* (2018).

Collins, Janet, Leah Robin, Susan Wooley, Dean Fenley, Peter Hunt, Julie Taylor, Deborah Haber, and Lloyd Kolbe. "Programs-that-work: CDC's guide to effective programs that reduce health-risk behavior of youth." *Journal of School Health* 72, no. 3 (2002): 93–99.

Colón-González, Felipe J., Carlo Fezzi, Iain R. Lake, and Paul R. Hunter. "The effects of weather and climate change on dengue." *PLoS Neglected Tropical Diseases* 7, no. 11 (2013): e2503.

Conley, Dalton. "Decomposing the black-white wealth gap: The role of parental resources, inheritance, and investment dynamics." *Sociological Inquiry* 71, no. 1 (2001): 39–66.

Cook, Angus, Jill Watson, Paul Van Buynder, Andrew Robertson, and Phil Weinstein. "10th anniversary review: Natural disasters and their long-term impacts on the health of communities." *Journal of Environmental Monitoring* 10, no. 2 (2008): 167–175.

Cooley, Aaron. "War on poverty." *Encyclopedia Britannica*. Accessed June 23, 2019. https://www.britannica.com/topic/War-on-Poverty.

Cotch, Mary Frances, Joseph G. Pastorek, Robert P. Nugent, Sharon L. Hillier, Ronald S. Gibbs, David H. Martin, David A. Eschenbach, et al. "Trichomonas vaginalis associated with low birth weight and preterm delivery." *Sexually Transmitted Diseases* 24, no. 6 (1997): 353–360.

Coumou, Dim, and Stefan Rahmstorf. "A decade of weather extremes." *Nature Climate Change* 2, no. 7 (2012): 491–496.

Coutinho, Eridan M., Frederico G. C. Abath, Constança S. Barbosa, Ana Lúcia C. Domingues, Marcelo C. V. Melo, Silvia M. L. Montenegro, Maria Anunciada F. Lucena, Sylvia A. M. Romani, Wayner V. Souza, and Amaury D. Coutinho. "Factors involved in Schistosoma mansoni infection, in rural areas of Northeast Brazil." *Memórias do Instituto Oswaldo Cruz* 92 (1997): 707–715.

Crosby, Molly C. *The American Plague: The Untold Story of Yellow Fever, the Epidemic That Shaped Our History*. New York, NY: Berkley Publishing Group, 2006.

Cross, John H. "Enteric nematodes of humans." In Baron, S. (editor). *Medical Microbiology* 4th Edition. Galveston, TX: University of Texas Medical Branch, 1996.

Crowley, Martha, Daniel T. Lichter, and Zhenchao Qian. "Beyond gateway cities: Economic restructuring and poverty among Mexican immigrant families and children." *Family Relations* 55, no. 3 (2006): 345–360.

Cubanski, Juliette, Wyatt Koma, Anthony Damico, and Tricia Neuman. "How many seniors live in poverty?" *Henry J Kaiser Family Foundation*. Published November 19, 2018. https://www.kff.org/medicare/issue-brief/how-many-seniors-live-in-poverty/.

Cudmore, Sarah L., Kiera L. Delgaty, Shannon F. Hayward-McClelland, Dino P. Petrin, and Gary E. Garber. "Treatment of infections caused by metronidazole-resistant Trichomonas vaginalis." *Clinical Microbiology Reviews* 17, no. 4 (2004): 783–793.

Cummins, Ruth. "Decades go by, yet child hunger and poverty endure in the Delta." *University of Mississippi Medical Center*. Published July 17, 2017. https://www.umc.edu/news/News_Articles/2017/July/-decades-go-by,-yet-child-hunger-and-poverty-endures-in-the-delta.html.

Cunha, Eleonora Lima Alves, Fernanda Karoline Vieira da Silva Torchelsen, Lucas Maciel Cunha, Maykon Tavares de Oliveira, Kátia da Silva Fonseca, Paula Melo Abreu Vieira, Cláudia Martins Carneiro, and Marta de Lana. "Benznidazole, itraconazole and their combination in the treatment of acute experimental Chagas disease in dogs." *Experimental Parasitology* 204 (2019): 107711.

Curtis, Rachel, Carolyn Hodo, Sarah Hamer, Karen Snowden, and Gabriel Hamer. "Chagas disease in Texas information for veterinary professionals with canine patients." *Texas A&M University School of Veterinary Medicine and Biomedical Sciences*. Accessed August 2019. https://kissingbug.tamu.edu/files/canine-chagas-disease-2.pdf.

Darling-Hammond, Linda. "Unequal opportunity: Race and education." *Brookings*. Published March 1, 1998. https://www.brookings.edu/articles/unequal-opportunity-race-and-education/.

Darmon, Nicole, Elaine Ferguson, and André Briend. "Do economic constraints encourage the selection of energy dense diets?" *Appetite* 41, no. 3 (2003): 315–322.

Data USA. "Lowndes County, Al." Accessed November 27, 2018. https://datausa.io/profile/geo/lowndes-county-al/.

Davies, Catriona. "Poverty, like apartheid, is man-made, says Mandela." *The Telegraph*. Published February 4, 2005. https://www.telegraph.co.uk/news/uknews/1482735/Poverty-like-apartheid-is-man-made-says-Mandela.html.

Davis, Dorland J., and T. D. Sullivan. "Complement-fixation tests for American trypanosomiasis in Texas." *Public Health Report* 61 (1946): 1083.

De Onis, Mercedes, Cutberto Garza, Cesar G. Victora, Adelheid W. Onyango, Edward A. Frongillo, and Jose Martines. "The WHO multicentre growth reference study: Planning, study design, and methodology." *Food and Nutrition Bulletin* 25, no. 1_suppl_1 (2004): S15–S26.

Deichstetter, Peggy. "The effect of climate change on mosquito-borne diseases." *The American Biology Teacher* 79, no. 3 (2017): 169–173.

Deitz, Shiloh, and Katie Meehan. "Plumbing poverty: Mapping hot spots of racial and geographic inequality in US household water insecurity." *Annals of the American Association of Geographers* 109, no. 4 (2019): 1092–1109.

Demers, Raymond Y., Robert Frank, Paul Demers, and Melvin Clay. "Leptospiral exposure in Detroit rodent control workers." *American Journal of Public Health* 75, no. 9 (1985): 1090–1091.

DeParle, Jason. "Harder for Americans to rise from lower rungs." *The New York Times*. Published January 4, 2012. https://www.nytimes.com/2012/01/05/us/harder-for-americans-to-rise-from-lower-rungs.html.

Desmond, Matthew. *Evicted: Poverty and Profit in the American City*. New York: Broadway Books, 2017.

Despommier, Dickson. "Toxocariasis: Clinical aspects, epidemiology, medical ecology, and molecular aspects." *Clinical Microbiology Reviews* 16, no. 2 (2003): 265–272.

Dick, Olivia Brathwaite, José L. San Martín, Romeo H. Montoya, Jorge del Diego, Betzana Zambrano, and Gustavo H. Dayan. "The history of dengue outbreaks in the Americas." *The American Journal of Tropical Medicine and Hygiene* 87, no. 4 (2012): 584–593.

Dickins, Dorothy, and Robert N. Ford. "Geophagy (dirt eating) among Mississippi Negro school children." *American Sociological Review* 7, no. 1 (1942): 59–65.

Dilulio, Jr., John J. "The future of compassion: President Bush's social program hasn't yet gotten a chance." *Brookings Institute* (2002).

Doar, Robert. "Consumption poverty and the official poverty measure." *AEIdeas*. Published September 18, 2017. https://www.aei.org/economics/consumption-poverty-and-the-official-poverty-measure/.

Doherty, Matthew. "Worst case housing needs have gotten … worse." *United States Interagency Council on Homelessness (USICH)*. Published September 28, 2017. https://www.usich.gov/news/worst-case-housing-needs-have-gotten-worse/.

Donné, Alfred. "Animacules observes dans les matieres purulentes et le produit des secretions des organes genitaux de l'homme et de la femme." *Comptes rendus de l'Académie des Sciences* 3 (1836): 385–386.

Douthit, N., Sakal Kiv, Tzvi Dwolatzky, and Seema Biswas. "Exposing some important barriers to health care access in the rural USA." *Public Health* 129, no. 6 (2015): 611–620.

Dreifuss, Ruth. "What we owe to Kofi Annan's legacy in global health." *Kofi Annan Foundation*. Published May 22, 2019. https://www.kofiannanfoundation.org/changing-drug-policy/what-we-owe-to-kofi-annans-legacy-in-global-health-by-h-e-ruth-dreifuss/.

Drewnowski, Adam, and Stephen E. Specter. "Poverty and obesity: The role of energy density and energy costs." *The American Journal of Clinical Nutrition* 79, no. 1 (2004): 6–16.

Dubini, Angelo. "New worm of the human intestine (Agchylostoma duodenale) constituting a sixth genus of nematodes found in man." In B. H. Kean, Kenneth E. Mott, and Adair J. Russell, eds. *Tropical Medicine and Parasitology: Classic Investigations*, vol. 2, pp. 287–291. Ithaca, NY: Cornell University Press, 1978.

Duhaime-Ross, Arielle. "Scientists think Alabama's sewage problem has caused a tropical parasite: The state has done little about it." *Vice News*. Published December 17, 2018. https://www.vice.com/en_us/article/pa5wdg/scientists-raised-the-alarm-about-hookworm-in-alabama-a-year-ago-the-state-has-done-little-about-it.

Dumonteil, Eric, Maria Elena Bottazzi, Bin Zhan, Michael J. Heffernan, Kathryn Jones, Jesus G. Valenzuela, Shaden Kamhawi, et al. "Accelerating the development of a therapeutic vaccine for human Chagas disease: Rationale and prospects." *Expert Review of Vaccines* 11, no. 9 (2012): 1043–1055.

Duncan, Cynthia, and Robert Coles. *Worlds Apart: Why Poverty Persists in Rural America*. New Haven: Yale University Press, 1999.

Duncombe, Chris. "Unequal opportunities: Fewer resources, worse outcomes for students in schools with concentrated poverty." *The Commonwealth Institute*. Published October 26, 2017. https://www.thecommonwealthinstitute.org/2017/10/26/unequal-opportunities-fewer-resources-worse-outcomes-for-students-in-schools-with-concentrated-poverty/.

Duong, Diane. "What do neglected tropical diseases have to do with nutrition?" *Global Citizen*. Published August 15, 2018. https://www.globalcitizen.org/en/content/neglected-tropical-diseases-ntds-nutrition/.

Dvorsky, George. "Why 'neglected diseases' are becoming a global danger." *Gizmodo*. Published November 20, 2014. https://io9.gizmodo.com/why-neglected-diseases-are-becoming-a-global-danger-1660705505.

Easton-Brooks, Donald, and Alan Davis. "Wealth, traditional socioeconomic indicators, and the achievement debt." *The Journal of Negro Education* 76, no. 4 (2007): 530–541.

Eaton, Danice K., Laura Kann, Steve Kinchen, Shari Shanklin, Katherine H. Flint, Joseph Hawkins, William A. Harris, et al. "Youth risk behavior surveillance—United States, 2011." *Morbidity and Mortality Weekly Report: Surveillance Summaries* 61, no. 4 (2012): 1–162.

Edin, Kathryn, and Laura Lein. *Making Ends Meet: How Single Mothers Survive Welfare and Low-Wage Work*. New York: Russell Sage Foundation, 1997.

Edin, Kathryn J., and Luke H. Shaefer. *$2.00 a Day: Living on Almost Nothing in America*. New York, NY: Houghton Mifflin Harcourt Trade & Reference Publishers, 2015.

Edsall, T. B. "Bush suspends pay act in areas hit by storm." *Washington Post*, 9, D3. Published September 9, 2005. https://www.washingtonpost.com/wp-dyn/content/article/2005/09/08/AR2005090802037.html.

Eggers, Frederick, and Fouad Moumen. "American housing survey: Housing adequacy and quality as measured by the AHS." *Available at SSRN 2284174* (2013).

Ehrenkranz, N. Joel, Arnoldo K. Ventura, Raul R. Cuadrado, William L. Pond, and John E. Porter. "Pandemic dengue in Caribbean countries and the southern United States—Past, present and potential problems." *New England Journal of Medicine* 285, no. 26 (1971): 1460–1469.

Elliot, Mark. "Prevalence and impacts of failing septic systems and straight pipes in rural Alabama." Presented at the *UNC Water and Health Conference*, Chapel Hill, NC. Last modified May 10, 2018. https://cfpub.epa.gov/ncer_abstracts/index.cfm/fuseaction/display.abstractDetail/abstract/10779/report/F.

Elliott, Mark, Parnab Das, Aaron Blackwell, Erdogan Aytekin, Yue Hu, Kevin White, Robert Jones, and Yuehan Lu. "Surface discharge of raw wastewater among unsewered homes in central Alabama." *AGUFM* 2017 (2017): PA24A-06.

Elman, Cheryl, Robert A. McGuire, and Barbara Wittman. "Extending public health: The Rockefeller Sanitary Commission and hookworm in the American South." *American Journal of Public Health* 104, no. 1 (2014): 47–58.

Elmayan, Ardem, Weihong Tu, Brandy Duhon, Preston Marx, Wendy Wolfson, Gary Balsamo, Claudia Herrera, and Eric Dumonteil. "High prevalence of Trypanosoma cruzi infection in shelter dogs from southern Louisiana, USA." *Parasites & Vectors* 12, no. 1 (2019): 322.

Environment Texas Research & Policy Center. "Raw sewage released by Hurricane Harvey." Published September 20, 2017. https://environmenttexascenter.org/reports/txe/raw-sewage-released-hurricane-harvey.

Ericsson, Charles D., Robert Steffen, Afzal A. Siddiqui, and Steven L. Berk. "Diagnosis of *Strongyloides stercoralis* infection." *Clinical Infectious Diseases* 33, no. 7 (2001): 1040–1047.

Eskenazi, Brenda, Asa Bradman, and Rosemary Castorina. "Exposures of children to organophosphate pesticides and their potential adverse health effects." *Environmental Health Perspectives* 107, no. suppl_3 (1999): 409–419.

Ettling, John. *The Germ of Laziness: Rockefeller Philanthropy and Public Health in the New South*. Cambridge, MA: Harvard University Press, 1981.

Evans, Desiree. "Doing time in the South." *Facing South*. Published March 5, 2009. https://www.facingsouth.org/2009/03/doing-time-in-the-south.html.

Evans, Mary Anna. "Flushing the toilet has never been riskier." *The Atlantic*. Published September 17, 2015. https://www.theatlantic.com/technology/archive/2015/09/americas-sewage-crisis-public-health/405541/.

Ewing, David Andrew, Christina A. Cobbold, B. V. Purse, M. A. Nunn, and Steven M. White. "Modelling the effect of temperature on the seasonal population dynamics of temperate mosquitoes." *Journal of Theoretical Biology* 400 (2016): 65–79.

Ewing, Reid, Shima Hamidi, James B. Grace, and Yehua Dennis Wei. "Does urban sprawl hold down upward mobility?" *Landscape and Urban Planning* 148 (2016): 80–88.

Farmer, Aaron, Thomas Beltran, and Young Sammy Choi. "Prevalence of Toxocara species infection in the US: Results from the National Health and Nutrition Examination Survey, 2011–2014." *PLoS Neglected Tropical Diseases* 11, no. 7 (2017): e0005818.

"Fast Facts About Food Insecurity." *Case Management Monthly* 16, no. 9 (2019): 2–3. http://search.ebscohost.com.srv-proxy2.library.tamu.edu/login.aspx?direct=true&db=ccm&AN=138447865&site=eds-live.

Faulkner, Charles T., Sharon Patton, and Sandra Strawbridge Johnson. "Prehistoric parasitism in Tennessee: Evidence from the analysis of desiccated fecal material collected from Big Bone Cave, Van Buren County, Tennessee." *The Journal of Parasitology* 75, no. 3 (1989): 461–463.

Federal Register. "Title 42 CFR Parts 1–60." (1988).

Ferguson, H. Bruce, Sarah Bovaird, and Michael P. Mueller. "The impact of poverty on educational outcomes for children." *Paediatrics & Child Health* 12, no. 8 (2007): 701–706.

Fillaux, J., and J. F. Magnaval. "Laboratory diagnosis of human toxocariasis." *Veterinary Parasitology* 193, no. 4 (2013): 327–336.

Finnigan, Ryan, and Kelsey D. Meagher. "Past due: Combinations of utility and housing hardship in the United States." *Sociological Perspectives* 62, no. 1 (2019): 96–119.

Fisher, Jonathan, David S. Johnson, and Timothy M. Smeeding. "Inequality of income and consumption in the US: Measuring the trends in inequality from 1984 to 2011 for the same individuals." *Review of Income and Wealth* 61, no. 4 (2015): 630–650.

Flowers, Catherine. "A county where the sewer is your lawn." *The New York Times*. Published May 22, 2018. https://www.nytimes.com/2018/05/22/opinion/alabama-poverty-sewers.html.

———. "Opinion: A county where the sewer is your lawn." *The New York Times*. Published May 22, 2018. https://www.nytimes.com/2018/05/22/opinion/alabama-poverty-sewers.htm.

Flowers, Catherine C., JoAnn K. Ward, and Inga Winkler. "Flushed and forgotten sanitation and wastewater in rural communities in the United States." *The Alabama Center for Rural Enterprise (ACRE), The Columbia Law School Human Rights Clinic, The Institute for the Study of Human Rights at Columbia University*. Published May 2019. https://www.humanrightscolumbia.org/sites/default/files/Flushed%20and%20Forgotten%20-%20FINAL%20%281%29.pdf.

Fogel, Catherine Ingram, and Michael Belyea. "The lives of incarcerated women: Violence, substance abuse, and at risk for HIV." *Journal of the Association of Nurses in AIDS Care* 10, no. 6 (1999): 66–74.

Forgan, Robert. "History of the treatment of trichomoniasis." *British Journal of Venereal Diseases* 48, no. 6 (1972): 522.

Forna, Fatu, and A. Metin Gülmezoglu. "Interventions for treating trichomoniasis in women." *Cochrane Database of Systematic Reviews* 2 (2003): CD000218.

Fothergill, Alice, and Lori A. Peek. "Poverty and disasters in the United States: A review of recent sociological findings." *Natural Hazards* 32, no. 1 (2004): 89–110.

Fox, Liana, Christopher Wimer, Irwin Garfinkel, Neeraj Kaushal, JaeHyun Nam, and Jane Waldfogel. "Trends in deep poverty from 1968 to 2011: The influence of family structure, employment patterns, and the safety net." *RSF: The Russell Sage Foundation Journal of the Social Sciences* 1, no. 1 (2015): 14–34.

Franco-Paredes, Carlos, Roberta Dismukes, Deborah Nicolls, Alicia Hidron, Kimberly Workowski, Alfonso Rodriguez-Morales, Marianna Wilson, Daniel Jones, Peter Manyang, and Phyllis Kozarsky. "Persistent and untreated tropical infectious diseases among Sudanese refugees in the United States." *The American Journal of Tropical Medicine and Hygiene* 77, no. 4 (2007): 633–635.

Freeman, Alexandra H., Kenneth A. Katz, Mark W. Pandori, Leah M. Rauch, Robert P. Kohn, Sally Liska, Kyle T. Bernstein, and Jeffrey D. Klausner. "Prevalence and correlates of Trichomonas vaginalis among incarcerated persons assessed using a highly sensitive molecular assay." *Sexually Transmitted Diseases* 37, no. 3 (2010): 165–168.

Freeman, Lance. "America's affordable housing crisis: A contract unfulfilled." *American Journal of Public Health* 92, no. 5 (2002): 709–712.

Friedman, Scott. "Identifying kissing bugs from similar bugs." *NBC 5 Dallas-Fort Worth*. Last modified January 7, 2016. https://www.nbcdfw.com/investigations/Hidden-Threat-Identifying-Kissing-Bugs-From-Similar-Bugs-353226731.html.

Galvin, Gaby. "An inside look into America's third world." *US News & World Report*. Published May 16, 2018. https://www.usnews.com/news/healthiest-communities/articles/2018-05-16/americas-third-world-border-colonias-in-texas-struggle-to-attain-services.

———. "On the border, out of the shadows." *US News & World Report*. Published May 16, 2018. https://www.usnews.com/news/healthiest-communities/articles/2018-05-16/americas-third-world-border-colonias-in-texas-struggle-to-attain-services.

Garber, Gary E. "The laboratory diagnosis of Trichomonas vaginalis." *Canadian Journal of Infectious Diseases and Medical Microbiology* 16 (2005): 35–38.

Garcia, Ana M. "Pesticide exposure and women's health." *American Journal of Industrial Medicine* 44, no. 6 (2003): 584–594.

Garcia, Melissa N., Laila Woc-Colburn, David Aguilar, Peter J. Hotez, and Kristy O. Murray. "Historical perspectives on the epidemiology of human Chagas disease in Texas and recommendations for enhanced understanding of clinical Chagas disease in the Southern United States." *PLoS Neglected Tropical Diseases* 9, no. 11 (2015): e0003981.

Garfield, Rachel, Anthony Damico, Jessica Stephens, and Saman Rouhani. *The Coverage Gap: Uninsured Poor Adults in States That Do Not Expand Medicaid—An Update*. Menlo Park, CA: Kaiser Family Foundation, 2016.

Garrett, Laurie. *Betrayal of Trust: The Collapse of Global Public Health*. New York: Hyperion, 2000.

Gasteyer, Stephen P., Jennifer Lai, Brittany Tucker, Jennifer Carrera, and Julius Moss. "Basics inequality: Race and access to complete plumbing facilities in the United States." *Du Bois Review: Social Science Research on Race* 13, no. 2 (2016): 305–325.

Gavrelis, Naida, Aylin Sertkaya, Liz Bertelsen, Becky Cuthbertson, Linda Phillips, and Jacqueline Moya. "An analysis of the proportion of the US population that ingests soil or other non-food substances." *Human and Ecological Risk Assessment: An International Journal* 17, no. 4 (2011): 996–1012.

Gee, Alastair. "America's homeless population rises for the first time since the great recession." *The Guardian*. Published December 6, 2017. https://www.theguardian.com/us-news/2017/dec/05/america-homeless-population-2017-official-count-crisis.

Genser, Bernd, Agostino Strina, Lenaldo A. dos Santos, Carlos A. Teles, Matildes S. Prado, Sandy Cairncross, and Mauricio L. Barreto. "Impact of a city-wide sanitation intervention in a large urban centre on social, environmental and behavicural determinants of childhood diarrhoea: Analysis of two cohort studies." *International Journal of Epidemiology* 37, no. 4 (2008): 831–840.

Gerba, Charles P., and James E. Smith. "Sources of pathogenic microorganisms and their fate during land application of wastes." *Journal of Environmental Quality* 34, no. 1 (2005): 42–48.

Gilen, Martin. *Why Americans Hate Welfare: Race, Media, and the Politics of Antipoverty Strategy*. Chicago: University of Chicago Press, 1999.

Gilpin, Lyndsey. "The rural South's invisible public health crisis." *Montgomery Advertiser*. Published July 6, 2018. https://www.montgomeryadvertiser.com/story/news/local/alabama/2018/07/06/story-first-series-ways-communities-addressing-rise-poverty-related-tropical-diseases-poor-sewage/754311002/.

Goins, R. Turner, Kimberly A. Williams, Mary W. Carter, S. Melinda Spencer, and Tatiana Solovieva. "Perceived barriers to health care access among rural older adults: A qualitative study." *The Journal of Rural Health* 21, no. 3 (2005): 206–213.

Gomberg-Muñoz, Ruth M. "Review essay: Law and migrant labor in the 20th century—Ghost workers and global capitalism." *Loyola University Chicago, Anthropology: Faculty Publications and Other Works*. Published 2018. https://ecommons.luc.edu/anthropology_facpubs/21/.

GoodRx. "Albendazole prices and Albendazole coupons." Accessed August 19, 2019. https://www.goodrx.com/albendazole.

Gottschalk, Peter, and Sheldon Danziger. "Inequality of wage rates, earnings and family income in the United States, 1975–2002." *Review of Income and Wealth* 51, no. 2 (2005): 231–254.

Gramling, Carolyn. "'Sunny day' high tide floods are on the rise along U.S. coasts." Published July 15, 2019. https://www.sciencenews.org/article/sunny-day-high-tide-floods-are-rise-along-us-coasts.

Gramm, Phil, and John F. Early. "The truth about income inequality." *The Wall Street Journal*. Published November 3, 2019. https://www.wsj.com/articles/the-truth-about-income-inequality-11572813786.

Greene, Melissa Fay. *Praying for Sheetrock*. Boston: Da Capo Press, 2006.

Greenough, P. Gregg, and Thomas D. Kirsch. "Hurricane Katrina. Public health response—Assessing needs." *New England Journal of Medicine* 353, no. 15 (2005): 1544–1546.

Greer, D. A. "Found: Two cases of Chagas disease." *Texas Health Bulletin* 9, no. 11 (1956): 11–13.

Gregg, II, Gary L. "George W. Bush: Domestic affairs." *University of Virginia, Miller Center*. Accessed December 1, 2019. https://millercenter.org/president/gwbush/domestic-affairs.

Griesinger, Wilhelm. "Klinische und anatomische Beobachtungen über die Krankheiten von Egypten." *Arch Physiol Heilkd* 13 (1854): 528–575.

Gross, Terry. "A 'forgotten history' of how the U.S. government segregated America." *NPR*. Published May 3, 2017. https://www.npr.org/2017/05/03/526655831/a-forgotten-history-of-how-the-u-s-government-segregated-america.

Gubler, Duane J. "Dengue and dengue hemorrhagic fever." *Clinical Microbiology Reviews* 11, no. 3 (1998): 480–496.

Guernier, Vanina, Michael E. Hochberg, and Jean-François Guégan. "Ecology drives the worldwide distribution of human diseases." *PLoS Biology* 2, no. 6 (2004): e141.

Guilamo-Ramos, Vincent, and Marco Thimm-Kaiser. "Youth living in settlements at US border suffer poverty and lack of health care." *The Conversation*. Published October 10, 2018. http://theconversation.com/youth-living-in-settlements-at-us-border-suffer-poverty-and-lack-of-health-care-103416.

Gundersen, Craig, Brent Kreider, and John Pepper. "Reconstructing the supplemental nutrition assistance program to more effectively alleviate food insecurity in the United States." *RSF: The Russell Sage Foundation Journal of the Social Sciences* 4, no. 2 (2018): 113–130.

———. "The economics of food insecurity in the United States." *Applied Economic Perspectives and Policy* 33, no. 3 (2011): 281–303.

Gundersen, Craig, and James P. Ziliak. "Food insecurity research in the United States: Where we have been and where we need to go." *Applied Economic Perspectives and Policy* 40, no. 1 (2018): 119–135.

Gurgel-Gonçalves, Rodrigo, Ed Komp, Lindsay P. Campbell, Ali Khalighifar, Jarrett Mellenbruch, Vagner José Mendonça, Hannah L. Owens, Keynes de la Cruz Felix, A. Townsend Peterson, and Janine M. Ramsey. "Automated identification of insect vectors of Chagas disease in Brazil and Mexico: The virtual vector lab." *PeerJ* 5 (2017): e3040.

Hahn, Robert A., and Benedict I. Truman. "Education improves public health and promotes health equity." *International Journal of Health Services* 45, no. 4 (2015): 657–678.

Halfon, Neal, and Paul W. Newacheck. "Childhood asthma and poverty: Differential impacts and utilization of health services." *Pediatrics* 91, no. 1 (1993): 56–61.

Hall, Andrew, Gillian Hewitt, Veronica Tuffrey, and Nilanthi De Silva. "A review and meta-analysis of the impact of intestinal worms on child growth and nutrition." *Maternal & Child Nutrition* 4 (2008): 118–236.

Hamer, Sarah. "Personal communication." December 5, 2018.

Hamer, Sarah A., Rachel Curtis-Robles, and Gabriel L. Hamer. "Contributions of citizen scientists to arthropod vector data in the age of digital epidemiology." *Current Opinion in Insect Science* 28 (2018): 98–104.

Han, Xinxin, Kathleen Thiede Call, Jessie Kemmick Pintor, Giovann Alarcon-Espinoza, and Alisha Baines Simon. "Reports of insurance-based discrimination in health care and its association with access to care." *American Journal of Public Health* 105, no. S3 (2015): S517–S525.

Hanford, Elaine Jennifer, F. Benjamin Zhan, Yongmei Lu, and Alberto Giordano. "Chagas disease in Texas: Recognizing the significance and implications of evidence in the literature." *Social Science & Medicine* 65, no. 1 (2007): 60–79.

Harrington, Michael. *The Other America: Poverty in the United States*. New York: Penguin Books, 1962.

Harriot, Michael. "Lowndes county, Ala: The place god forgot." *The Root*. Published April 27, 2018. https://www.theroot.com/lowndes-county-ala-the-place-god-forgot-1825483659.

Harris, John P., Miren Iturriza-Gomara, and Sarah J. O'Brien. "Estimating disability-adjusted life years (DALYs) in community cases of norovirus in England." *Viruses* 11, no. 2 (2019): 184. https://doi.org/10.3390/v11020184.

HealthyPeople.gov. "Sexually transmitted diseases." Last modified June 23, 2020. https://www.healthypeople.gov/2020/topics-objectives/topic/sexually-transmitted-diseases.

Heflin, David. "Chagas disease in dogs." *TexVetPets*. Published June 2014. https://www.texvetpets.org/article/chagas-disease-in-dogs/.

Henry J. Kaiser (KFF) Family Foundation. "Poverty rate by race/ethnicity." Last modified 2018. https://www.kff.org/other/state-indicator/poverty-rate-by-raceethnicity/?dataView=1&activeTab=map&currentTimeframe=0&selectedDistributions=total&sortModel=%7B%22colId%22:%22Location%22,%22sort%22:%22asc%22%7D.

Hernandez, Daisy. "Northern Virginia: 'Ground zero' for kissing bug disease." *The Atlantic*. Published July 24, 2014. https://www.theatlantic.com/health/archive/2014/07/northern-virginia-ground-zero-for-kissing-bug-disease/374383/.

Hero, Joachim O., Alan M. Zaslavsky, and Robert J. Blendon. "The United States leads other nations in differences by income in perceptions of health and health care." *Health Affairs* 36, no. 6 (2017): 1032–1040.

Herrmann, Nira, Lawrence T. Glickman, Peter M. Schantz, Marian G. Weston, and Linda M. Domanski. "Seroprevalence of zoonotic toxocariasis in the United States: 1971–1973." *American Journal of Epidemiology* 122, no. 5 (1985): 890–896.

Hicks, Lanis L. "Availability and accessibility of rural health care." *The Journal of Rural Health* 6, no. 4 (1990): 485–506.

Hirsch, Rebecca E. *Climate Migrants: On the Move in a Warming World*. Minneapolis: Twenty-First Century Books, 2016.

History.com. "Great society." Last modified August 28, 2018. https://www.history.com/topics/1960s/great-society.

Hlaing, Thein. "Ascariasis and childhood malnutrition." *Parasitology* 107, no. S1 (1993): S125–S136.

Hofstraat, Karlijn, and Wim H. van Brakel. "Social stigma towards neglected tropical diseases: A systematic review." *International Health* 8, no. suppl_1 (2016): i53–i70.

Hogben, Matthew, and Janet S. St. Lawrence. "HIV/STD risk reduction interventions in prison settings." *Journal of Women's Health & Gender-Based Medicine* 9, no. 6 (2000): 587–592.

Hoots, Brooke E., Thomas A. Peterman, Elizabeth A. Torrone, Hillard Weinstock, Elissa Meites, and Gail A. Bolan. "A Trich-y question: Should Trichomonas vaginalis infection be reportable?" *Sexually Transmitted Diseases* 40, no. 2 (2013): 113.

Hoppin, Jane A., David M. Umbach, Stephanie J. London, Paul K. Henneberger, Greg J. Kullman, Michael C. R. Alavanja, and Dale P. Sandler. "Pesticides and atopic and nonatopic asthma among farm women in the Agricultural Health Study." *American Journal of Respiratory and Critical Care Medicine* 177, no. 1 (2008): 11–18.

Hotez, P. J., D. H. Molyneux, A. Fenwick, E. Ottesen, S. E. Sachs, and J. D. Sachs. "Incorporating a rapid-impact package for neglected tropical diseases with programs for HIV/AIDS, tuberculosis, and malaria." *PLoS Medicine* 3, no. 5 (2006): e102.

Hotez, Peter J. *Blue Marble Health: An Innovative Plan to Fight Diseases of the Poor Amid Wealth*. Baltimore, MD: John Hopkins University Press, 2016.

———. *Forgotten People, Forgotten Diseases: The Neglected Tropical Diseases and Their Impact on Global Health and Development*. Sterling, VA: ASM Books, 2008. https://dukespace.lib.duke.edu/dspace/bitstream/handle/10161/16516/MP_2018_04_20_FinalDraft.pdf?sequence=1.

———. "Global urbanization and the neglected tropical diseases." *PLoS Neglected Tropical Diseases* 11, no. 2 (2017): e0005308.

———. "Hookworm and poverty." *Annals of the New York Academy of Sciences* 1136, no. 1 (2008): 38–44.

———. "Neglected diseases amid wealth in the United States and Europe." *Health Affairs* 28, no. 6 (2009): 1720–1725.

———. "Neglected infections of poverty in the United States of America." *PLoS Neglected Tropical Diseases* 2, no. 6 (2008): e256.

———. "Personal communication." Published September 14, 2018.

———. "Personal communication." Published September 18, 2018.

———. "Visceral and ocular larva migrans." *Seminars in Neurology* 13, no. 2 (1993): 175–179.

Hotez, Peter, Eileen Stillwaggon, Marian McDonald, Lynn Todman, and Lydia DiGrazia. "National summit on neglected infections of poverty in the United States." *Emerging Infectious Diseases* 16, no. 5 (2010): e1. https://wwwnc.cdc.gov/eid/article/16/5/09-1863_article.

Hotez, Peter J., Eric Dumonteil, Miguel Betancourt Cravioto, Maria Elena Bottazzi, Roberto Tapia-Conyer, Sheba Meymandi, Unni Karunakara, Isabela Ribeiro, Rachel M. Cohen, and Bernard Pecoul. "An unfolding tragedy of Chagas disease in North America." *PLoS Neglected Tropical Diseases* 7, no. 10 (2013): e2300.

Hotez, Peter J., Kristy O. Murray, and Pierre Buekens. "The Gulf Coast: A new American underbelly of tropical diseases and poverty." *PLoS Neglected Tropical Diseases* 8, no. 5 (2014): e2760.

Hotez, Peter J., Miriam Alvarado, María-Gloria Basáñez, Ian Bolliger, Rupert Bourne, Michel Boussinesq, Simon J. Brooker, et al. "The global burden of disease study 2010: Interpretation and implications for the neglected tropical diseases." *PLoS Neglected Tropical Diseases* 8, no. 7 (2014): e2865.

Hotez, Peter J., and Patricia P. Wilkins. "Toxocariasis: America's most common neglected infection of poverty and a helminthiasis of global importance?" *PLoS Neglected Tropical Diseases* 3, no. 3 (2009): e400.

Hotez, Peter J., and Sheila Jackson Lee. "US Gulf Coast states: The rise of neglected tropical diseases in "flyover nation"." *PLOS Neglected Tropical Diseases* 11, no. 11 (2017): e0005744.

Humphreys, Margaret. "How four once common diseases were eliminated from the American South." *Health Affairs* 28, no. 6. (2009): 1734–1744. https://www.ncbi.nlm.nih.gov/pubmed/19887414.

Hunt, Angie. "For food security, SNAP and WIC aren't redundant." *Futurity*. Published June 13, 2019. https://www.futurity.org/food-security-families-2082362-2/.

Hunt, Paul. "The human right to the highest attainable standard of health: New opportunities and challenges." *Transactions of the Royal Society of Tropical Medicine and Hygiene* 100, no. 7 (2006): 603–607.

Hunter, John M. "Geophagy in Africa and in the United States: A culture-nutrition hypothesis." *Geographical Review* 63, no. 2 (1973): 170–195.

Huppert, Jill S. "New detection methods for trichomoniasis may help curb more serious STIs." *Patient Care* 40, no. 5 (2006): 32–37.

Indiana State Department of Health. "Diseases involving sewage." Accessed August 15, 2019. https://www.in.gov/isdh/22963.htm.

Ingber, Sasha. "31 percent of U.S. households have trouble paying energy bills." *NPR*. Published September 19, 2018. https://www.npr.org/2018/09/19/649633468/31-percent-of-u-s-households-have-trouble-paying-energy-bills.

Institute for Policy Studies. "Inequality and health." Accessed December 1, 2019. https://inequality.org/facts/inequality-and-health/.

Isaacs, Julia B., Isabel V. Sawhill, and Ron Haskins. "Getting ahead or losing ground: Economic mobility in America." *The Brookings Institute*. Published 2008. https://www.brookings.edu/wp-content/uploads/2016/06/02_economic_mobility_sawhill.pdf.

Izenberg, Maxwell, Olivia Johns-Yost, Pauline D. Johnson, and Joe Brown. "Nocturnal convenience: The problem of securing universal sanitation access in Alabama's black belt." *Environmental Justice* 6, no. 6 (2013): 200–205.

Jackson, Lisa A., David H. Spaeh, Deborah A. Kippen, Naney K. Sugg, Russell L. Regnery, Merlyn H. Sayers, and Walter E. Stamm. "Seroprevalence to Bartonella quintana among patients at a community clinic in downtown Seattle." *Journal of Infectious Diseases* 173, no. 4 (1996): 1023–1026.

Jacobs, Ken, Zohar Perla, Ian Eve Perry, and Dave Graham-Squire. "Producing poverty: The public cost of low-wage production jobs in manufacturing." *UC Berkeley Center for Labor Research and Education*. Published May 10, 2016. http://laborcenter.berkeley.edu/producing-poverty-the-public-cost-of-low-wage-production-jobs-in-manufacturing/.

Jaeger, James W., Ian H. Carlson, and Warren P. Porter. "Endocrine, immune, and behavioral effects of aldicarb (carbamate), atrazine (triazine) and nitrate (fertilizer) mixtures at groundwater concentrations." *Toxicology and Industrial Health* 15, no. 1–2 (1999): 133–151.

James, Erwin. "Most offenders have low skills and prison is the place to put that right." *The Guardian*. Published February 3, 2012. https://www.theguardian.com/society/joepublic/2010/feb/03/prison-education-training-low-skills.

Jensen, Leif, Jill L. Findeis, and Qiuyan Wang. "Labor supply and underemployment in the Southern United States." *Journal of Rural Social Sciences* 16, no. 1 (2000): 5.

Jia, Tie-Wu, Jürg Utzinger, Yao Deng, Kun Yang, Yi-Yi Li, Jin-Huan Zhu, Charles H. King, and Xiao-Nong Zhou. "Quantifying quality of life and disability of patients with advanced schistosomiasis japonica." *PLoS Neglected Tropical Diseases* 5, no. 2 (2011): e966.

Johnson, Lyndon B. "The war on poverty." *First State of the Union Address.* Published January 8, 1964: 5.

Johnston, Matthew. "A brief history of income inequality in the United States." *Investopedia.* Last modified June 25, 2019. https://www.investopedia.com/articles/investing/110215/brief-history-income-inequality-united-states.asp.

Jyoti, Diana F., Edward A. Frongillo, and Sonya J. Jones. "Food insecurity affects school children's academic performance, weight gain, and social skills." *The Journal of Nutrition* 135, no. 12 (2005): 2831–2839.

Kanneganti, Kalyan, Jasbir S. Makker, and Prospere Remy. "Ascaris lumbricoides: To expect the unexpected during a routine colonoscopy." *Case Reports in Medicine* 2013 (2013).

Kapoor, Vikram, Indrani Gupta, A. B. M. Tanvir Pasha, and Duc Phan. "Real-time quantitative PCR measurements of fecal indicator bacteria and human-associated source tracking markers in a Texas river following Hurricane Harvey." *Environmental Science & Technology Letters* 5, no. 6 (2018): 322–328.

Katz, Cheryl. "People in poor neighborhoods breathe more hazardous particles." *Scientific American.* Published November 1, 2012. https://www.scientificamerican.com/article/people-poor-neighborhoods-breate-more-hazardous-particles/.

Keeley, Brian. "What's happening to income inequality?" In *Income Inequality: The Gap Between Rich and Poor.* Paris: OECD Publishing, 2015.

Keesing, Felicia, Lisa K. Belden, Peter Daszak, Andrew Dobson, C. Drew Harvell, Robert D. Holt, Peter Hudson, et al. "Impacts of biodiversity on the emergence and transmission of infectious diseases." *Nature* 468, no. 7324 (2010): 647–652.

Kehoe, Nicole. "How dangerous is pesticide drift?" *Scientific American.* Published September 17, 2012. https://www.scientificamerican.com/article/pesticide-drift/.

Kelman, Brett. "Tennessee suffered third-largest increase of uninsured people in the nation, census reports." *Tennessean.* Published September 11, 2019. https://www.tennessean.com/story/news/health/2019/09/11/tennessee-uninsured-residents-tenncare-census-report/2276127001/.

Ken Paxton, Office of the Attorney General of Texas. "Colonias prevention laws." Accessed September 15, 2019. https://www.texasattorneygeneral.gov/divisions/colonias-prevention/colonias-prevention-laws.

Kennedy, Bruce P., Ichiro Kawachi, Roberta Glass, and Deborah Prothrow-Stith. "Income distribution, socioeconomic status, and self rated health in the United States: Multilevel analysis." *BMJ* 317, no. 7163 (1998): 917–921.

KFF. "Health insurance coverage of the total population." Accessed November 15, 2019. https://www.kff.org/other/state-indicator/total-population/?currentTimeframe=0&selectedRows=%7B%22states%22:%7B%22kentucky%22:%7B%7D%7D%7D&sortModel=%7B%22colId%22:%22Location%22,%22sort%22:%22asc%22%7D.

———. "The U.S. government and global neglected tropical disease efforts." Published January 28, 2020. https://www.kff.org/global-health-policy/fact-sheet/the-u-s-government-and-global-neglected-tropical-diseases/.

Khalighifar, Ali, Ed Komp, Janine M. Ramsey, Rodrigo Gurgel-Gonçalves, and A. Townsend Peterson. "Deep learning algorithms improve automated identification of Chagas disease vectors." *Journal of Medical Entomology* 56, no. 5 (2019): 1404–1410.

Khuroo, Mohammed Sultan. "Ascariasis." *Gastroenterology Clinics of North America* 25, no. 3 (1996): 553–577.

Kim, Myoung, Jim Ohls, and Rhoda Cohen. "Hunger in America: 2001 National report prepared for America's second harvest." *No. d27650c180224c58bb7776dbb9283d15*. Mathematica Policy Research, 2001.

Kissinger, Patricia, and Alys Adamski. "Trichomoniasis and HIV interactions: A review." *Sexually Transmitted Infections* 89, no. 6 (2013): 426–433.

Kjos, S. A., K. F. Snowden, T. M. Craig, B. Lewis, N. Ronald, and J. K. Olson. "Distribution and characterization of canine Chagas disease in Texas." *Veterinary Parasitology* 152, no. 3–4 (2008): 249–256.

Klausner, Jeffrey D., Jefferson T. Baer, Katherine M. Contento, and Gail Bolan. "Investigation of a suspected outbreak of vaginal trichomoniasis among female inmates." *Sexually Transmitted Diseases* 26, no. 6 (1999): 335–338.

Klebanoff, Mark A., J. Christopher Carey, John C. Hauth, Sharon L. Hillier, Robert P. Nugent, Elizabeth A. Thom, J. M. Ernest, et al. "Failure of metronidazole to prevent preterm delivery among pregnant women with asymptomatic Trichomonas vaginalis infection." *New England Journal of Medicine* 345, no. 7 (2001): 487–493.

Kleinman, Ronald E., J. Michael Murphy, Michelle Little, Maria Pagano, Cheryl A. Wehler, Kenneth Regal, and Michael S. Jellinek. "Hunger in children in the United States: Potential behavioral and emotional correlates." *Pediatrics* 101, no. 1 (1998): e3.

Klemm, Rolf, Yaobi Zhang, Emily Toubali, Whitney Goldman, and Victoria Quinn. *Linking undernutrition and selected neglected tropical diseases*. New York: Helen Keller International, 2015.

Knab, Brian Russell. "Infectious disease and the South Texas colonias." PhD diss., *University of Texas Libraries*, 2016. https://repositories.lib.utexas.edu/handle/2152/44560.

Kochhar, Rakesh, and Anthony Cilluffo. "Income inequality in the US is rising most rapidly among Asians." *Pew Research Center*. Published 2018. https://www.pewsocialtrends.org/2018/07/12/income-inequality-in-the-u-s-is-rising-most-rapidly-among-asians/.

Kovats, R. S., D. H. Campbell-Lendrum, A. J. McMichel, A. Woodward, and J. St. H. Cox. "Early effects of climate change: Do they include changes in vector-borne disease?" *Philosophical Transactions of the Royal Society of London. Series B: Biological Sciences* 356, no. 1411 (2001): 1057–1068.

Kraut-Becher, Julie R., Thomas L. Gift, Anne C. Haddix, Kathleen L. Irwin, and Robert B. Greifinger. "Cost-effectiveness of universal screening for chlamydia and gonorrhea in US jails." *Journal of Urban Health* 81, no. 3 (2004): 453–471.

Kreston, Rebecca. "Blood money: Hookworm economics in the Postbellum South." *Discover Magazine*. Published April 25, 2011. https://www.discovermagazine.com/health/blood-money-hookworm-economics-in-the-postbellum-south.

Kromm, Chris. "The South's economic crisis." *Facing South*. Published October 18, 2011. https://www.facingsouth.org/2011/10/the-souths-economic-crisis.html.

Laiño, M. A., M. V. Cardinal, G. F. Enriquez, A. Alvedro, M. S. Gaspe, and R. E. Gürtler. "An oral dose of Fluralaner administered to dogs kills pyrethroid-resistant and susceptible Chagas disease vectors for at least four months." *Veterinary Parasitology* 268 (2019): 98–104.

Lamberton, Poppy H., and Peter M. Jourdan. "Human ascariasis: Diagnostics update." *Current Tropical Medicine Reports* 2, no. 4 (2015): 189–200.

Lavelle, Kristen, and Joe Feagin. "Hurricane Katrina: The race and class debate." *Monthly Review* 58, no. 3 (2006): 52.

Leaning, Jennifer, and Debarati Guha-Sapir. "Natural disasters, armed conflict, and public health." *New England Journal of Medicine* 369, no. 19 (2013): 1836–1842.

Lee, Bruce Y., Kristina M. Bacon, Maria Elena Bottazzi, and Peter J. Hotez. "Global economic burden of Chagas disease: A computational simulation model." *The Lancet Infectious Diseases* 13, no. 4 (2013): 342–348.

Lee, Harper. *To Kill a Mockingbird.* New York: Grand Central Publishing, 1960.

Lee, Rachel M., Laura B. Moore, Maria Elena Bottazzi, and Peter J. Hotez. "Toxocariasis in North America: A systematic review." *PLoS Neglected Tropical Diseases* 8, no. 8 (2014): e3116.

Lee, Su Hyun, Kwang Woo Nam, Ji Yeon Jeong, Seung Jin Yoo, Young-Sang Koh, Seogjae Lee, Sang Taek Heo, Seung-Yong Seong, and Keun Hwa Lee. "The effects of climate change and globalization on mosquito vectors: Evidence from Jeju Island, South Korea on the potential for Asian tiger mosquito (Aedes albopictus) influxes and survival from Vietnam rather than Japan." *PLoS One* 8, no. 7 (2013): e68512.

Lee, Sung-jin, Kathleen R. Parrott, and Mira Ahn. "Exploring housing challenges of low-income minority populations in the Southern United States." *Cityscape* 14, no. 1 (2012): 73–98.

Lei, Serena. "An unwaged war on deep poverty." *The Urban Institute*. Published December 15, 2013. https://www.urban.org/features/unwaged-war-deep-poverty.

Lenk, Edeltraud J., William K. Redekop, Marianne Luyendijk, Christopher Fitzpatrick, Louis Niessen, Wilma A. Stolk, Fabrizio Tediosi, et al. "Socioeconomic benefit to individuals of achieving 2020 targets for four neglected tropical diseases controlled/eliminated by innovative and intensified disease management: Human African trypanosomiasis, leprosy, visceral leishmaniasis, Chagas disease." *PLoS Neglected Tropical Diseases* 12, no. 3 (2018): e0006250.

Leuchtenburg, William E. "The origins of Franklin D. Roosevelt's "court-packing" plan." *The Supreme Court Review* (1966).

———. "When Franklin Roosevelt clashed with the supreme court—And lost." *Smithsonian Magazine*. Published May 2005. https://www.smithsonianmag.com/history/when-franklin-roosevelt-clashed-with-the-supreme-court-and-lost-78497994/.

Levernier, William. "An analysis of poverty in the American South: How are metropolitan areas different from nonmetropolitan areas?" *Contemporary Economic Policy* 21, no. 3 (2003): 372–382.

Levey, Linda M., James P. Curry, and Samuel Levey. "Rural-urban differences in access to Iowa child health services." *The Journal of Rural Health* 4, no. 2 (1988): 59–72.

Li, Quan-yue, Dong-hai Zhao, Hai-yan Qu, and Chuan-nong Zhou. "Life-threatening complications of ascariasis in trauma patients: A review of the literature." *World Journal of Emergency Medicine* 5, no. 3 (2014): 165–170.

Lishner, Denise M., Mary Richardson, Phyllis Levine, and Donald Patrick. "Access to primary health care among persons with disabilities in rural areas: A summary of the literature." *The Journal of Rural Health* 12, no. 1 (1996): 45–53.

Liu, Eugene W., Kimberly A. Workowski, Laura H. Taouk, Jay Schulkin, William E. Secor, and Jeffrey L. Jones. "Survey of obstetrician-gynecologists in the United States about trichomoniasis, 2016." *Sexually Transmitted Diseases* 46, no. 1 (2019): 9.

Loftus, John, Elizabeth M. Allen, Kathleen Thiede Call, and Susan A. Everson-Rose. "Rural-urban differences in access to preventive health care among publicly insured Minnesotans." *The Journal of Rural Health* 34 (2018): s48–s55.

Lora, Jessika. "Ascariasis." Last modified December 2004. https://web.stanford.edu/group/parasites/ParaSites2005/Ascaris/JLora_ParaSite.htm.

Ludlam, Joel A. "Prevalence of trachoma among Navajo Indian children." *American Journal of Optometry and Physiological Optics* 55, no. 2 (1978): 116–118.

Ma, Guangxu, Celia V. Holland, Tao Wang, Andreas Hofmann, Chia-Kwung Fan, Rick M. Maizels, Peter J. Hotez, and Robin B. Gasser. "Human toxocariasis." *The Lancet Infectious Diseases* 18, no. 1 (2018): e14–e24.

Mabaso, M. L. H., C. C. Appleton, J. C. Hughes, and E. Gouws. "The effect of soil type and climate on hookworm (Necator americanus) distribution in KwaZulu-Natal, South Africa." *Tropical Medicine & International Health* 8, no. 8 (2003): 722–727.

Mack, Elizabeth A., and Sarah Wrase. "A burgeoning crisis? A nationwide assessment of the geography of water affordability in the United States." *PLoS One* 12, no. 1 (2017): e0169488.

Mackey, Tim K., Bryan A. Liang, Raphael Cuomo, Ryan Hafen, Kimberly C. Brouwer, and Daniel E. Lee. "Emerging and reemerging neglected tropical diseases: A review of key characteristics, risk factors, and the policy and innovation environment." *Clinical Microbiology Reviews* 27, no. 4 (2014): 949–979.

Madrigal, Alexis. "Why the Gulf Coast is uniquely vulnerable to disasters." *The Atlantic.* Published August 29, 2017. https://www.theatlantic.com/technology/archive/2017/08/why-the-gulf-coast-is-uniquely-vulnerable-to-disasters-hurricane-harvey/538374/.

Mammen, Sheila, Jean W. Bauer, and Leslie Richards. "Understanding persistent food insecurity: A paradox of place and circumstance." *Social Indicators Research* 92, no. 1 (2009): 151.

Mann, Joshua R., Suzanne McDermott, Timothy L. Barnes, James Hardin, Haikun Bao, and Li Zhou. "Trichomoniasis in pregnancy and mental retardation in children." *Annals of Epidemiology* 19, no. 12 (2009): 891–899.

Manne-Goehler, Jennifer, Michael R. Reich, and Veronika J. Wirtz. "Access to care for Chagas disease in the United States: A health systems analysis." *The American Journal of Tropical Medicine and Hygiene* 93, no. 1 (2015): 108–113.

Marchildon, Jackie. "Neglected tropical diseases: The most dangerous diseases you've never heard of." *Global Citizen*. Published January 18, 2018. https://www.globalcitizen.org/en/content/neglected-tropical-diseases/

Markovits, Daniel. *The Meritocracy Trap: How America's Foundational Myth Feed Inequality, Dismantles the Middle Class, and Devours the Elite*. New York: Penguin Press, 2019.

Marmot, Michael. "The influence of income on health: Views of an epidemiologist." *Health Affairs* 21, no. 2 (2002): 31–46.

Marmot, Michael G., Stephen Stansfeld, Chandra Patel, Fiona North, Jenny Head, Ian White, Eric Brunner, Amanda Feeney, and G. Davey Smith. "Health inequalities among British civil servants: The Whitehall II study." *The Lancet* 337, no. 8754 (1991): 1387–1393.

Martínez, Deyanira Nevárez, María G. Rendón, and Diego Arroyo. "Los Olvidados/The forgotten: Reconceptualizing colonias as viable communities." *Progress in Planning* 133 (2019): 100450.

Marx, C., J. Lin, M. R. Masruha, M. G. Rodrigues, A. J. Da Rocha, L. C. P. Vilanova, and Alberto Alain Gabbai. "Toxocariasis of the CNS simulating acute disseminated encephalomyelitis." *Neurology* 69, no. 8 (2007): 806–807.

Marx, Jerry D. "American social policy in the great depression and World War II." Accessed October 21, 2019. https://socialwelfare.library.vcu.edu/eras/great-depression/american-social-policy-in-the-great-depression-and-wwii/.

Masozera, Michel, Melissa Bailey, and Charles Kerchner. "Distribution of impacts of natural disasters across income groups: A case study of New Orleans." *Ecological Economics* 63, no. 2–3 (2007): 299–306.

Massara, Cristiano Lara, and Martin Johannes Enk. "Treatment options in the management of Ascaris lumbricoides." *Expert Opinion on Pharmacotherapy* 5, no. 3 (2004): 529–539.

McCarrier, Kelly P., Frederick J. Zimmerman, James D. Ralston, and Diane P. Martin. "Associations between minimum wage policy and access to health care: Evidence from the Behavioral Risk Factor Surveillance System, 1996–2007." *American Journal of Public Health* 101, no. 2 (2011): 359–367.

McGreal, Chris. "America's poorest border town: No immigration papers, no American dream." *The Guardian*. Published November 19, 2015. https://www.theguardian.com/us-news/2015/nov/19/americas-poorest-border-town-no-immigration-papers-no-american-dream.

———. "America's poorest white town: Abandoned by coal, swallowed by drugs." *The Guardian*. Published November 12, 2015. https://www.theguardian.com/us-news/2015/nov/12/beattyville-kentucky-and-americas-poorest-towns.

———. "Where even Walmart won't go: How dollar general took over rural America." *The Guardian*. Published August 13, 2018. https://www.theguardian.com/business/2018/aug/13/dollar-general-walmart-buhler-haven-kansas.

McIntyre, Mary. "Notice: Environmental study in Lowndes County, Alabama, fails to prove hookworm infection." *Alabama State Department of Health*. Published April 9, 2018. http://www.alabamapublichealth.gov/infectiousdiseases/assets/hookworm-notice.pdf.

McKenna, Megan L., Shannon McAtee, Patricia E. Bryan, Rebecca Jeun, Tabitha Ward, Jacob Kraus, Maria E. Bottazzi, Peter J. Hotez, Catherine C. Flowers, and Rojelio Mejia. "Human intestinal parasite burden and poor sanitation in rural Alabama." *The American Journal of Tropical Medicine and Hygiene* 97, no. 5 (2017): 1623–1628.

McNeil, Donald J. "Rare infection threatens to spread in blood supply." *The New York Times*. Published November 18, 2003. https://www.nytimes.com/2003/11/18/science/rare-infection-threatens-to-spread-in-blood-supply.html.

Meyer, Bruce D., and James X. Sullivan. "Winning the war: Poverty from the great society to the great recession." *No. w18718*. National Bureau of Economic Research, 2013. https://www.nber.org/papers/w18718.pdf.

Meyers, Alyssa C., Marvin Meinders, and Sarah A. Hamer. "Widespread Trypanosoma cruzi infection in government working dogs along the Texas-Mexico border: Discordant serology, parasite genotyping and associated vectors." *PLoS Neglected Tropical Diseases* 11, no. 8 (2017): e0005819.

Meza, Emily. "Examining wastewater treatment struggles in Lowndes County, AL." *Duke University Library*. Published April 27, 2018.

Micks, Don W., and William B. Moon. "Aedes aegypti in a Texas coastal county as an index of dengue fever receptivity and control." *The American Journal of Tropical Medicine and Hygiene* 29, no. 6 (1980): 1382–1388.

Miller Center. "January 8, 1964: State of the Union." *University of Virginia*. Accessed December 2, 2019. https://millercenter.org/the-presidency/presidential-speeches/january-8-1964-state-union.

Miller, Daniel P. "Accessibility of summer meals and the food insecurity of low-income households with children." *Public Health Nutrition* 19, no. 11 (2016): 2079–2089.

Miller, Keith, Kristina Costa, and Donna Cooper. *How to Upgrade and Maintain Our Nation's Wastewater and Drinking-Water Infrastructure*. Washington, D.C.: Center for American Progress, 2012.

Miller, Leigh Ann, Kate Colby, Susan E. Manning, Donald Hoenig, Elizabeth McEvoy, Susan Montgomery, Blaine Mathison, et al. "Ascariasis in humans and pigs on small-scale farms, Maine, USA, 2010–2013." *Emerging Infectious Diseases* 21, no. 2 (2015): 332.

Miller, William C., Heidi Swygard, Marcia M. Hobbs, Carol A. Ford, Mark S. Handcock, Martina Morris, John L. Schmitz, Myron S. Cohen, Kathleen Mullan Harris, and J. Richard Udry. "The prevalence of trichomoniasis in young adults in the United States." *Sexually Transmitted Diseases* 32, no. 10 (2005): 593–598.

Milman, Oliver. "'We're not a dump'—Poor Alabama towns struggle under the stench of toxic landfills." *The Guardian*. Published April 15, 2019. https://www.theguardian.com/us-news/2019/apr/15/were-not-a-dump-poor-alabama-towns-struggle-under-the-stench-of-toxic-landfills.

Mnif, Wissem, Aziza Ibn Hadj Hassine, Aicha Bouaziz, Aghleb Bartegi, Olivier Thomas, and Benoit Roig. "Effect of endocrine disruptor pesticides: A review." *International Journal of Environmental Research and Public Health* 8, no. 6 (2011): 2265–2303.

Molina, I., F. Salvador, A. Sánchez-Montalvá, B. Treviño, N. Serre, A. Sao Avilés, and B. Almirante. "Toxic profile of benznidazole in patients with chronic Chagas disease: Risk factors and comparison of the product from two different manufacturers." *Antimicrobial Agents and Chemotherapy* 59, no. 10 (2015): 6125–6131.

Montgomery, Susan P., Monica E. Parise, Ellen M. Dotson, and Stephanie R. Bialek. "What do we know about Chagas disease in the United States?" *The American Journal of Tropical Medicine and Hygiene* 95, no. 6 (2016): 1225–1227.

Morillo, Carlos A., Jose Antonio Marin-Neto, Alvaro Avezum, Sergio Sosa-Estani, Anis Rassi, Jr., Fernando Rosas, Erick Villena, et al. "Randomized trial of benznidazole for chronic Chagas' cardiomyopathy." *New England Journal of Medicine* 373, no. 14 (2015): 1295–1306.

Mostafalou, Sara, and Mohammad Abdollahi. "Pesticides and human chronic diseases: Evidences, mechanisms, and perspectives." *Toxicology and Applied Pharmacology* 268, no. 2 (2013): 157–177.

Mubarak, Mohammad Yousuf, Abram L. Wagner, Bradley F. Carlson, and Matthew L. Boulton. "Hygienic behaviors and risks for ascariasis among college students in Kabul, Afghanistan." *The American Journal of Tropical Medicine and Hygiene* 97, no. 2 (2017): 563–566.

Munson, Erik, Timothy Kramme, Maureen Napierala, Kimber L. Munson, Cheryl Miller, and Jeanne E. Hryciuk. "Female epidemiology of transcription-mediated amplification-based Trichomonas vaginalis detection in a metropolitan setting with a high prevalence of sexually transmitted infection." *Journal of Clinical Microbiology* 50, no. 12 (2012): 3927–3931.

Murphy, J. Michael, Cheryl A. Wehler, Maria E. Pagano, Michelle Little, Ronald E. Kleinman, and Michael S. Jellinek. "Relationship between hunger and psychosocial functioning in low-income American children." *Journal of the American Academy of Child & Adolescent Psychiatry* 37, no. 2 (1998): 163–170.

Murray, Christopher J. L., Theo Vos, Rafael Lozano, Mohsen Naghavi, Abraham D. Flaxman, Catherine Michaud, Majid Ezzati, et al. "Disability-adjusted life years (DALYs) for 291 diseases and injuries in 21 regions, 1990–2010: A systematic analysis for the Global Burden of Disease Study 2010." *The Lancet* 380, no. 9859 (2012): 2197–2223.

National Alliance to End Homelessness. "Racial disparities in homelessness in the United States." Published June 6, 2018. https://endhomelessness.org/resource/racial-disparities-homelessness-united-states/.

———. "State of homelessness." Accessed December 1, 2019. https://endhomelessness.org/homelessness-in-america/homelessness-statistics/state-of-homelessness-report/.

National Collaborating Centre for Acute Care (UK). *Nutrition Support for Adults: Oral Nutrition Support, Enteral Tube Feeding and Parenteral Nutrition*, no. 32. London: National Collaborating Centre for Acute Care, 2006. https://www.ncbi.nlm.nih.gov/books/NBK49258/.

National Council on Aging. "Economic security for seniors facts." Last modified 2016. https://www.ncoa.org/news/resources-for-reporters/get-the-facts/economic-security-facts/.

National Health Service. "Trichomoniasis—Prevention." Last modified October 23, 2018. https://www.nhs.uk/conditions/trichomoniasis/prevention/.

National Housing Law Project. "Fair housing & housing for people with disabilities." Accessed November 1, 2019. https://www.nhlp.org/initiatives/fair-housing-housing-for-people-with-disabilities/.

National Rural Health Association. "About rural health care." Accessed December 2019. https://www.ruralhealthweb.org/about-nrha/about-rural-health-care.

Nejsum, Peter, E. Davis Parker, Jane Frydenberg, Allan Roepstorff, Jaap Boes, Rashidul Haque, Ingrid Astrup, Jørgen Prag, and Uffe B. Skov Sørensen. "Ascariasis is a zoonosis in Denmark." *Journal of Clinical Microbiology* 43, no. 3 (2005): 1142–1148.

Nellis, Ashley. "The color of justice: Racial and ethnic disparity in state prisons." *The Sentencing Project*. Published June 14, 2016. https://www.sentencingproject.org/publications/color-of-justice-racial-and-ethnic-disparity-in-state-prisons/.

Nelson, Suchitra, Tom Greene, and Claire B. Ernhart. "Toxocara canis infection in preschool age children: Risk factors and the cognitive development of preschool children." *Neurotoxicology and Teratology* 18, no. 2 (1996): 167–174.

Neumann, Todd C., Price V. Fishback, and Shawn Kantor. "The dynamics of relief spending and the private urban labor market during the new deal." *The Journal of Economic History* 70, no. 1 (2010): 195–220.

Neumayer, Eric, and Thomas Plümper. "Inequalities of income and inequalities of longevity: A cross-country study." *American Journal of Public Health* 106, no. 1 (2016): 160–165.

Nicolopoulou-Stamati, Polyxeni, Sotirios Maipas, Chrysanthi Kotampasi, Panagiotis Stamatis, and Luc Hens. "Chemical pesticides and human health: The urgent need for a new concept in agriculture." *Frontiers in Public Health* 4 (2016): 148.

NIH: National Institute of Allergy and Infectious Diseases. "Neglected tropical diseases." Last modified July 11, 2016. https://www.niaid.nih.gov/research/neglected-tropical-diseases.

Nijhawan, Ank E., Alison K. DeLong, David D. Celentano, Robert S. Klein, Jack D. Sobel, Denise J. Jamieson, and Susan Cu-Uvin. "The association between Trichomonas infection and incarceration in HIV-seropositive and at-risk HIV-seronegative women." *Sexually Transmitted Diseases* 38, no. 12 (2011): 1094.

Nord, Mark, and Kathleen Romig. "Hunger in the summer: Seasonal food insecurity and the National School Lunch and Summer Food Service programs." *Journal of Children and Poverty* 12, no. 2 (2006): 141–158.

Norris, Jeremiah, Carol Adelman, Yulya Spantchak, and Kacie Marano. "Social and economic impact review on neglected tropical diseases." *Economic Policy/Briefing Paper*. Washington, D.C.: Hudson Institute, 2012.

Nunes, Maria Carmo Pereira, Andrea Beaton, Harry Acquatella, Caryn Bern, Ann F. Bolger, Luis E. Echeverria, Walderez O. Dutra, et al. "Chagas cardiomyopathy: An update of current clinical knowledge and management: A scientific statement from the American Heart Association." *Circulation* 138, no. 12 (2018): e169–e209.

Nuwer, Rachel. "How a worm gave the south a bad name." *PBS*. Published April 27, 2016. https://www.pbs.org/wgbh/nova/article/how-a-worm-gave-the-south-a-bad-name/.

O'Connell, Heather A. "The impact of slavery on racial inequality in poverty in the contemporary US South." *Social Forces* 90, no. 3 (2012): 713–734.

OECD Wealth Distribution Database. "Income inequality." Last modified 2020. https://data.oecd.org/inequality/income-inequality.htm.

———. "Wealth." Last modified January 2018. https://stats.oecd.org/Index.aspx?DataSetCode=WEALTH.

O'lorcain, P., and C. V. Holland. "The public health importance of Ascaris lumbricoides." *Parasitology* 121, no. S1 (2000): S51–S71.

Ong, Samuel, David A. Talan, Gregory J. Moran, William Mower, Michael Newdow, Victor C. W. Tsang, and Robert W. Pinner. "Neurocysticercosis in radiographically imaged seizure patients in US emergency departments." *Emerging Infectious Diseases* 8, no. 6 (2002): 608.

Orrenius, Pia M., Madeline Zavodny, and Leslie Lukens. "Why stop there?: Mexican migration to the US border region." *No. 0803*. Federal Reserve Bank of Dallas, 2008.

Ortiz, Larry, Lydia Arizmendi, and Llewellyn J. Cornelius. "Access to health care among Latinos of Mexican descent in colonias in two Texas counties." *The Journal of Rural Health* 20, no. 3 (2004): 246–252.

Osman, K. A., and M. Stoytcheva. *Pesticides in the Modern World–Effects of Pesticides Exposure*, London: IntechOpen Limited, 2011.

Owusu-Edusei, Jr., Kwame, Harrell W. Chesson, Thomas L. Gift, Guoyu Tao, Reena Mahajan, Marie Cheryl Bañez Ocfemia, and Charlotte K. Kent. "The estimated direct medical cost of selected sexually transmitted infections in the United States, 2008." *Sexually Transmitted Diseases* 40, no. 3 (2013): 197–201.

Pace, Paola. "Migration and the right to health: A review of international law." *International Organization for Migration*. Published 2009. https://publications.iom.int/system/files/pdf/iml_19.pdf.

Pack, Robert P., Ralph J. Diclemente, Edward W. Hook, III, and M. Kim Oh. "High prevalence of asymptomatic STDs in incarcerated minority male youth: A case for screening." *Sexually Transmitted Diseases* 27, no. 3 (2000): 175–177.

Packchanian, Ardzroonv. "Infectivity of the Texas strain of Trypanosoma cruzi to man." *The American Journal of Tropical Medicine and Hygiene* 1, no. 3 (1943): 309–314.

———. "Natural infection of Triatoma gerstakeri with Trypanosoma cruzi in Texas." *Public Health Reports (1896–1970)* 54 (1939): 1547–1554.

———. "The problem of Chagas' disease in Texas." *Texas State Journal of Medicine* 43, no. 3 (1947): 179–183.

Parsons, Jim C. "Ascarid infections of cats and dogs." *Veterinary Clinics of North America: Small Animal Practice* 17, no. 6 (1987): 1307–1339.

Pathak, Dipali. "Hookworms, poverty, poor sanitation linked in rural Alabama." *Baylor College of Medicine*. Published September 6, 2017. https://www.bcm.edu/news/school-of-tropical-medicine/hookworm-poverty-sanitation-alabama.

Patrick, Kayla. "National snapshot: Poverty among women and families, 2016." *National Women's Law Center*. Published September 2017. https://nwlc.org/wp-content/uploads/2017/09/Poverty-Snapshot-Factsheet-2017.pdf.

Pega, Frank, Sze Yan Liu, Stefan Walter, Roman Pabayo, Ruhi Saith, and Stefan K. Lhachimi. "Unconditional cash transfers for reducing poverty and vulnerabilities: Effect on use of health services and health outcomes in low-and middle-income countries." *Cochrane Database of Systematic Reviews* 11 (2017).

Pet Leadership Council. "2015–2016 APPA national pet owners survey—Generational report." Accessed August 19, 2019. https://www.google.com/url?rct=j&sa=t&url=http://www.americanpetproducts.org/pubs_generationalreport.asp&ct=ga&cd=CAIyGjMyOWZlN2U4NmFkZjU2M2E6Y29tOmVuOlVT&usg=AFQjCNGzc1w9n3jhBk5rW-wRiuk6JFhh8Q.

Peters, Louk W. H., Gerjo Kok, Geert T. M. Ten Dam, Goof J. Buijs, and Theo G. W. M. Paulussen. "Effective elements of school health promotion across behavioral domains: A systematic review of reviews." *BMC Public Health* 9, no. 1 (2009): 182.

Petkova, Elisaveta P., Kristie L. Ebi, Derrin Culp, and Irwin Redlener. "Climate change and health on the US Gulf Coast: Public health adaptation is needed to address future risks." *International Journal of Environmental Research and Public Health* 12, no. 8 (2015): 9342–9356.

Petrin, Dino, Kiera Delgaty, Renuka Bhatt, and Gary Garber. "Clinical and microbiological aspects of Trichomonas vaginalis." *Clinical Microbiology Reviews* 11, no. 2 (1998): 300–317.

Pettus, Emily. "Entrenched poverty tough to shake in the Mississippi Delta." *Clarion Ledger*. Last modified August 8, 2017. https://www.clarionledger.com/story/news/2017/08/07/mississippi-delta-poverty/544601001/#:~:targetText=Although%20opportunities%20have%20improved%20in,it's%2030%20to%2040%20percent.

Philip, Phinse Mappalakayil, Srinivasan Kannan, and Neetu Ambali Parambil. "Community-based interventions for health promotion and disease prevention in noncommunicable diseases: A narrative review." *Journal of Education and Health Promotion* 7 (2018).

Philips, Matthew. "What's the best way to measure poverty: Income or consumption?" *Freakonomics*. Published September 14, 2011. http://freakonomics.com/2011/09/14/whats-the-best-way-to-measure-poverty-income-or-consumption/.

Pickett, Kate E., and Michelle Pearl. "Multilevel analyses of neighbourhood socioeconomic context and health outcomes: A critical review." *Journal of Epidemiology & Community Health* 55, no. 2 (2001): 111–122.

Pimpare, Stephen. *A People's History of Poverty in America*. New York: The New Press, 2008.

Pink, Ross. "Child rights, right to water and sanitation, and human security." *Health and Human Rights* 14 (2012): E78–E87.

Piontak, Joy Rayanne, and Michael D. Schulman. "Food insecurity in rural America." *Contexts* 13, no. 3 (2014): 75–77.

Plaster, Ashley N., Julia E. Painter, Dylan H. Tjersland, and Kathryn H. Jacobsen. "University students' knowledge, attitudes, and sources of information about Zika virus." *Journal of Community Health* 43, no. 4 (2018): 647–655.

Polson, Jim. "More Americans are getting their electricity cut off." *Bloomberg.com* . Published October 13, 2017. https://www.bloomberg.com/news/articles/2017-10-13/in-great-american-blackout-millions-go-dark-due-to-unpaid-bills.

Posey, Drew L., Brian G. Blackburn, Michelle Weinberg, Elaine W. Flagg, Luis Ortega, Marianna W. Wilson, Evan Secor, Kolby Sanders-Lewis, Kimberly Won, and James H. Maguire. "High prevalence and presumptive treatment of schistosomiasis and strongyloidiasis among African refugees." *Clinical Infectious Diseases* 45, no. 10 (2007): 1310–1315.

Primary Care Progress. "The case of primary care." Accessed September 14, 2018. https://www.primarycareprogress.org/primary-care-case/.

Pugh, Tony. "Shift from infectious diseases has left the U.S. more vulnerable." *McClatchy DC Bureau.* Published May 25, 2007. https://www.mcclatchydc.com/latest-news/article24452836.html.

Radke, Elizabeth G., Christopher J. Gregory, Kristina W. Kintziger, Erin K. Sauber-Schatz, Elizabeth A. Hunsperger, Glen R. Gallagher, Jean M. Barber, et al. "Dengue outbreak in key west, Florida, USA, 2009." *Emerging Infectious Diseases* 18, no. 1 (2012): 135–137.

Raju, Sarath, Corinne A. Keet, Laura M. Paulin, Elizabeth C. Matsui, Roger D. Peng, Nadia N. Hansel, and Meredith C. McCormack. "Rural residence and poverty are independent risk factors for chronic obstructive pulmonary disease in the United States." *American Journal of Respiratory and Critical Care Medicine* 199, no. 8 (2019): 961–969.

Raphael, Steven, and Eugene Smolensky. "Immigration and poverty in the United States." *American Economic Review* 99, no. 2 (2009): 41–44.

Raphelson, Samantha. No "easy answer" to growing number of stray dogs in the US, advocate says." *KPBS Public Media.* Published December 29, 2017. https://www.kpbs.org/news/2017/dec/29/no-easy-answer-to-growing-number-of-stray-dogs-in/.

Rasberry, Catherine N., Sarah M. Lee, Leah Robin, B. A. Laris, Lisa A. Russell, Karin K. Coyle, and Allison J. Nihiser. "The association between school-based physical activity, including physical education, and academic performance: A systematic review of the literature." *Preventive Medicine* 52 (2011): S10–S20.

Ratcliffe, Michael, Charlynn Burd, Kelly Holder, and Alison Fields. "Defining rural at the US Census Bureau." *American Community Survey and Geography Brief* 1, no. 8 (2016).

Reardon, Sean F., Joseph P. Robinson, and Ericka S. Weathers. "Patterns and trends in racial/ethnic and socioeconomic academic achievement gaps." In *Handbook of Research in Education Finance and Policy*, pp. 497–516. Chandler, AZ: AEFP, 2008.

Rearwin, David T., J. H. Tang, and James W. Hughes. "Causes of blindness among Navajo Indians: An update." *Journal of the American Optometric Association* 68, no. 8 (1997): 511–517.

Redekop, William K., Edeltraud J. Lenk, Marianne Luyendijk, Christopher Fitzpatrick, Louis Niessen, Wilma A. Stolk, Fabrizio Tediosi, et al. "The socioeconomic benefit to individuals of achieving the 2020 targets for five preventive chemotherapy neglected tropical diseases." *PLoS Neglected Tropical Diseases* 11, no. 1 (2017): e0005289.

Reed, Sharon L., and James H. McKerrow. "Why funding for neglected tropical diseases should be a global priority." *Clinical Infectious Diseases* 67, no. 3 (2018): 323–326.

Reilly, John J., J. Kelly, and D. C. Wilson. "Accuracy of simple clinical and epidemiological definitions of childhood obesity: Systematic review and evidence appraisal." *Obesity Reviews* 11, no. 9 (2010): 645–655.

Riggs, E., J. Hughes, D. Irvin, and K. Leopard. *An Overview of Clean Water Access Challenges in the United States*. Chapel Hill, NC: Global Water Challenge and the Environmental Finance Center, School of Government, University of North Carolina, 2017.

Rockefeller Foundation. "Rockefeller Sanitary Commission (RSC)." Accessed January 26, 2019. https://rockfound.rockarch.org/rockefeller-sanitary-commission.

Roeleveld, Nel, and Reini Bretveld. "The impact of pesticides on male fertility." *Current Opinion in Obstetrics and Gynecology* 20, no. 3 (2008): 229–233.

Rogan, Joe, Producer. "Joe Rogan experience." *Peter Hotez on Vaccines and Tropical Diseases* [Podcast audio]. Published March 23, 2019. https://podcastnotes.org/2019/03/23/hotez/.

Rollins, Brad. "A sprawling slum in San Marcos' shadow." *San Marcos Mercury*. Published November 14, 2011. http://smmercury.com/2011/11/14/a-sprawling-slum-in-san-marcos-shadow/.

Romo, Matthew L. "Need for pharmacist awareness of Chagas disease." *American Journal of Health-System Pharmacy* 71, no. 13 (2014): 1069–1070.

Rosenbaum, Janet, Jonathan Zenilman, Eve Rose, Gina Wingood, and Ralph DiClemente. "Cash, cars, and condoms: Economic factors in disadvantaged adolescent women's condom use." *Journal of Adolescent Health* 51, no. 3 (2012): 233–241.

Ross, Catherine E., and Chia-ling Wu. "The links between education and health." *American Sociological Review* 60, no. 5 (1995): 719–745.

Rostrup, Morten. "The role of nongovernmental organizations in providing health care." Text delivered at the Annual *World Bank Conference on Development Economics*, p. 6, 2001.

Roy, Priti Kumar, Shubhankar Saha, and Fahad Al Basir. "Effect of awareness programs in controlling the disease HIV/AIDS: An optimal control theoretic approach." *Advances in Difference Equations* 217, no. 1 (2015): 1–18.

Rude, Emelyn. "The American South is still eating white dirt." *Vice*. Published June 5, 2015. https://www.vice.com/en_us/article/pgxwvk/the-american-south-is-still-eating-white-dirt.

Rueckert, Phineas. "Millions of poor Americans are contracting these 'diseases of poverty'—But can't afford pills to cure them." *Global Citizen*. Published December 11, 2017. https://www.globalcitizen.org/en/content/hookworm-drug-prices-poverty-alabama/.

Rush, Benjamin. "An account of the bilious remitting fever: As it appeared in Philadelphia, in the summer and autumn of the year 1780." *The American Journal of Medicine* 11, no. 5 (1951): 546–550.

Rysavy, Tracy. "What does sewage have to do with it?" *Green America*. Accessed September 20, 2019. https://greenamerica.org/drinking-water-risk/what-does-sewage-have-do-it.

Salameh, Pascale, Mirna Waked, Isabelle Baldi, Patrick Brochard, and Bernadette Abi Saleh. "Respiratory diseases and pesticide exposure: A case-control study in Lebanon." *Journal of Epidemiology & Community Health* 60, no. 3 (2006): 256–261.

Sanborn, Margaret, K. J. Kerr, L. H. Sanin, D. C. Cole, K. L. Bassil, and C. Vakil. "Non-cancer health effects of pesticides: Systematic review and implications for family doctors." *Canadian Family Physician* 53, no. 10 (2007): 1712–1720.

Satterwhite, Catherine Lindsey, Elizabeth Torrone, Elissa Meites, Eileen F. Dunne, Reena Mahajan, M. Cheryl Bañez Ocfemia, John Su, Fujie Xu, and Hillard Weinstock. "Sexually transmitted infections among US women and men: Prevalence and incidence estimates, 2008." *Sexually Transmitted Diseases* 40, no. 3 (2013): 187–193.

Schantz, P. M., C. F. Von Reyn, T. Welty, F. L. Andersen, M. G. Schultz, and I. G. Kagan. "Epidemiologic investigation of echinococcosis in American Indians living in Arizona and New Mexico." *The American Journal of Tropical Medicine and Hygiene* 26, no. 1 (1977): 121–126.

Schiller, Jeannine S., Jacqueline W. Lucas, and Jennifer A. Peregoy. "Summary health statistics for US adults: National health interview survey, 2011." (2012).

Schwebke, Jane R., and Renee A. Desmond. "A randomized controlled trial of partner notification methods for prevention of trichomoniasis in women." *Sexually Transmitted Diseases* 37, no. 6 (2010): 392–396.

Scott, J. Allen. "The prevalence and distribution of hookworm infection in Egypt." *American Journal of Epidemiology* 26, no. 3 (1937): 455–505.

Scott, Janny, and David Leonhardt. "Shadowy lines that still divide." *The New York Times*. Published 2005. https://www.nytimes.com/2005/05/15/us/class/shadowy-lines-that-still-divide.html.

Scott, Logan. Interview with corresponding author, unpublished, 2009.

Scott, Robert. "The manufacturing footprint and the importance of U.S. manufacturing jobs." *Economic Policy Institute*. Published January 22, 2015. https://www.epi.org/publication/the-manufacturing-footprint-and-the-importance-of-u-s-manufacturing-jobs/.

Semchuk, Karen M., Edgar J. Love, and Robert G. Lee. "Parkinson's disease and exposure to agricultural work and pesticide chemicals." *Neurology* 42, no. 7 (1992): 1328.

Semenza, Jan C., Jonathan E. Suk, Virginia Estevez, Kristie L. Ebi, and Elisabet Lindgren. "Mapping climate change vulnerabilities to infectious diseases in Europe." *Environmental Health Perspectives* 120, no. 3 (2012): 385–392.

Semuels, Alana. "Good school, rich school; bad school, poor school." *The Atlantic*. Published August 25, 2016. https://www.theatlantic.com/business/archive/2016/08/property-taxes-and-unequal-schools/497333/.

———. "The American neighborhoods without water, sewers, or building codes." *The Atlantic*. Published March 3, 2016. https://www.theatlantic.com/business/archive/2016/03/the-americans-without-running-water/471909/.

Séralini, Gilles-Eric, Emilie Clair, Robin Mesnage, Steeve Gress, Nicolas Defarge, Manuela Malatesta, Didier Hennequin, and Joël Spiroux de Vendômois. "Republished study: Long-term toxicity of a roundup herbicide and a roundup-tolerantgenetically modified maize." *Environmental Sciences Europe* 26, no. 1 (2014): 14.

Sethia, Babulal, and Parveen Kumar, eds. *Essentials of Global Health*, Amsterdam: Elsevier Health Sciences, 2019.

Shah, Jamil, and Abul Shahidullah. "Ascaris lumbricoides: A startling discovery during screening colonoscopy." *Case Reports in Gastroenterology* 12, no. 2 (2018): 224–229.

Shariatpanahi, Seyed Peyman, Afshin Jafari, Maryam Sadeghipour, Nasibeh Azadeh-Fard, Keivan Majidzadeh-A, Leila Farahmand, and Alireza Madjid Ansari. "Assessing the effectiveness of disease awareness programs: Evidence from Google Trends data for the world awareness dates." *Telematics and Informatics* 34, no. 7 (2017): 904–913.

Shariff, Azim F., Dylan Wiwad, and Lara B. Aknin. "Income mobility breeds tolerance for income inequality: Cross-national and experimental evidence." *Perspectives on Psychological Science* 11, no. 3 (2016): 373–380.

Sherman, Irwin W. *Twelve Diseases That Changed the World*. Washington, D.C.: ASM Press, 2007.

Shi, Leiyu, and Barbara Starfield. "Primary care, income inequality, and self-rated health in the United States: A mixed-level analysis." *International Journal of Health Services* 30, no. 3 (2000): 541–555.

Shipler, David K. *The Working Poor: Invisible in America*. New York: Borzoi Book, 2004.

Simile, Catherine, and Kristen S. Miller. "They could see stars from their beds: The plight of the rural poor in the aftermath of Hurricane Hugo." (1992).

Singh, Gopal K., Gem P. Daus, Michelle Allender, Christine T. Ramey, Elijah K. Martin, Chrisp Perry, Andrew A. De Los Reyes, and Ivy P. Vedamuthu. "Social determinants of health in the United States: Addressing major health inequality trends for the nation, 1935–2016." *International Journal of MCH and AIDS* 6, no. 2 (2017): 139–164.

Skwarecki, Beth. *Outbreak!: 50 Tales of Epidemics That Terrorized the World*. Avon, MA: Adams Media, 2016.

Smeeding, Timothy. "Poor people in rich nations: The United States in comparative perspective." *Journal of Economic Perspectives* 20, no. 1 (2006): 69–90.

Smith, Catharine. "Why the U.S., one of the world's richest countries, struggles with diseases of poverty." *Huffington Post*. Last modified March 2, 2018. https://www.huffingtonpost.com/entry/america-diseases-of-poverty_us_5a69f610e4b0dc592a0fe66a.

Smith, Dawn. "The HIV epidemiology research study, HIV out-patient study, and the spectrum of disease studies." *JAIDS Journal of Acquired Immune Deficiency Syndromes* 17 (1998): S17–S19.

Smith, Neil. "There's no such thing as a natural disaster: Understanding Katrina." *SSRC Perspectives from the Social Sciences* (2006).

Somers, Margaret R., and Fred Block. "From poverty to perversity: Ideas, markets, and institutions over 200 years of welfare debate." *American Sociological Review* 70, no. 2 (2005): 260–287.

Sorvillo, Frank, Lisa Smith, Peter Kerndt, and Lawrence Ash. "Trichomonas vaginalis, HIV, and African-Americans." *Emerging Infectious Diseases* 7, no. 6 (2001): 927.

Spach, David H., Andrew S. Kanter, Molly J. Dougherty, Ann M. Larson, Marie B. Coyle, Don J. Brenner, Bala Swaminathan, et al. "Bartonella (Rochalimaea) quintana bacteremia in inner-city patients with chronic alcoholism." *New England Journal of Medicine* 332, no. 7 (1995): 424–428.

Sparks, S. D. "New student majority in south and west: Poor children." *Education Week* 33, no. 9 (2013): 6.

Spatig-Amerikaner, Ary. "Unequal education: Federal loophole enables lower spending on students of color." *Center for American Progress* (2012).

Stanford University. "History of discovery." Accessed August 2019. https://web.stanford.edu/group/parasites/ParaSites2002/trichomoniasis/History.html.

State Health Access Data Assistance Center. "Study of the impact of the ACA implementation in Kentucky." *Foundation for a Healthy Kentucky*. Published 2016. http://files.constantcontact.com/1b4946a6001/7cc9e76b-04fa-45d3-8ac3-6ef33d321d13.pdf.

Steele, Jennifer L. "Whatever it takes: Geoffrey Canada's quest to change Harlem and America." *Harvard Educational Review* 79, no. 3 (2009).

Stillwaggon, Eileen. "The ecology of poverty: Nutrition, parasites, and vulnerability to HIV/AIDS." In *AIDS, Poverty and Hunger: Challenges and Responses*, pp. 167–180. Washington, D.C.: International Food Policy Research Institute, 2006.

Stimpert, Kelly K., and Susan P. Montgomery. "Physician awareness of Chagas disease, USA." *Emerging Infectious Diseases* 16, no. 5 (2010): 871.

Stivers, Camilla. ""'So poor and so black": Hurricane Katrina, public administration, and the issue of race." *Public Administration Review* 67 (2007): 48–56.

Stone, Judy. "Chagas: An emerging infectious disease threat in the U.S." *Forbes*. Published October 1, 2015. https://www.forbes.com/sites/judystone/2015/10/01/chagas-an-emerging-infectious-disease-threat-in-u-s/#155348876530.

———. "Hurricanes, poverty, and neglected infections." *Scientific American Blog Network*. Published August 30, 2012. https://blogs.scientificamerican.com/molecules-to-medicine/hurricane-katrina-poverty-and-neglected-infections/.

Stoner, Amanda. "Regulatory deficiencies in wastewater infrastructure in rural Appalachia." *Sustainable Development Law & Policy* 18 (2017): 30.

Suro, Roberto, Jill H. Wilson, and Audrey Singer. "Immigration and poverty in America's suburbs." *Metropolitan Opportunity Series at Brookings Institute* (2011).

Sutton, Madeline, Maya Sternberg, Emilia H. Koumans, Geraldine McQuillan, Stuart Berman, and Lauri Markowitz. "The prevalence of Trichomonas vaginalis infection among reproductive-age women in the United States, 2001–2004." *Clinical Infectious Diseases* 45, no. 10 (2007): 1319–1326.

Swaby, Andrielle N., Mark D. Lucas, and Robert M. Ross. *The Teacher-Friendly Guide to the Earth Science of the Southeastern US*, 2nd ed. Ithaca, NY: Paleontological Research Institution, 2016.

Swanson, Kelby. "WRITE TEAM: Rethinking crime and punishment." *The Times*. Published September 25, 2019. https://www.mywebtimes.com/2019/09/24/write-team-rethinking-crime-and-punishment/ax0k4kt/.

Swinny, B. "Abstract of discussion: Severe reactions from insect stings." *Texas State Journal of Medicine* 46, no. 8 (1950): 640.

Swygard, H., A. C. Sena, M. M. Hobbs, and M. S. Cohen. "Trichomoniasis: Clinical manifestations, diagnosis and management." *Sexually Transmitted Infections* 80, no. 2 (2004): 91–95.

Tavernise, Sabrina. "A toilet, but no proper plumbing: A reality in 500,000 U.S. homes." *The New York Times*. Published September 27, 2016. https://www.nytimes.com/2016/09/27/health/plumbing-united-states-poverty.html.

Tenney, Trevor D., Rachel Curtis-Robles, Karen F. Snowden, and Sarah A. Hamer. "Shelter dogs as sentinels for Trypanosoma cruzi transmission across Texas." *Emerging Infectious Diseases* 20, no. 8 (2014): 1323–1326.

Tessum, Christopher W., Joshua S. Apte, Andrew L. Goodkind, Nicholas Z. Muller, Kimberley A. Mullins, David A. Paolella, Stephen Polasky, et al. "Inequity in consumption of goods and services adds to racial–ethnic disparities in air pollution exposure." *Proceedings of the National Academy of Sciences* 116, no. 13 (2019): 6001–6006.

Texas A&M University Colonias Program. "Who we are." Accessed September 12, 2019. https://colonias.arch.tamu.edu/about/who-we-are/index.html.

Texas Archive of the Moving Image. "The poverty tours (1964)." Accessed August 1, 2018. https://texasarchive.org/2010_00054.

Texas Department of Health and Human Services. "Data: Dengue fever & dengue hemorrhagic fever (DHF)." Last modified April 3, 2019. https://www.dshs.texas.gov/IDCU/disease/dengue/Data.aspx.

Texas State University. "Chagas disease: A silent killer with a cure." *Infection Control Today*. Published April 18, 2019. https://www.infectioncontroltoday.com/infectious-diseases-conditions/chagas-disease-silent-killer-cure.

Thakur, Darshana Sudip, Rajashree Khot, P. P. Joshi, Madhuri Pandharipande, and Keshav Nagpure. "Glyphosate poisoning with acute pulmonary edema." *Toxicology International* 21, no. 3 (2014): 328.

The Alabama Department of Environmental Management. "State revolving fund (SRF)." Last modified 2019. http://www.adem.state.al.us/programs/water/srf.cnt.

The END Fund. "Annual report 2012." Published 2013. https://end.org/cms/assets/uploads/2018/01/2012-Annual-Report.pdf.

The United Nations Human Rights Office of the High Commissioner. "Fact sheet on the right to adequate housing toolkit." Accessed November 1, 2019. https://www.ohchr.org/EN/Issues/Housing/toolkit/Pages/RighttoAdequateHousingToolkit.aspx.

———. "United Nations millennium declaration general assembly resolution 55/2." Published September 8, 2000. https://www.ohchr.org/EN/ProfessionalInterest/Pages/Millennium.aspx.

The Urban Institute. "Katrina: Demographics of a disaster." Published September 9, 2005. https://www.urban.org/sites/default/files/publication/52091/900835-katrina-demographics-of-a-disaster_0.pdf.

Thiede, Brian C., Daniel T. Lichter, and Tim Slack. "Working, but poor: The good life in rural America?" *Journal of Rural Studies* 59 (2018): 183–193.

Thiermann, A. B., and R. R. Frank. "Human leptospirosis in Detroit and the role of rats as chronic carriers." *International Journal of Zoonoses* 7, no. 1 (1980): 62–72.

Thornthwaite, Charles Warren. "An approach toward a rational classification of climate." *Geographical Review* 38, no. 1 (1948): 55–94.

Torstensson, David. "Beyond the city: Lyndon Johnson's war on poverty in rural America." *Journal of Policy History* 25, no. 4 (2013): 587–613.

Traub, Rebecca J., Ian D. Robertson, Peter Irwin, Norbert Mencke, and R. C. Andrew Thompson. "The prevalence, intensities and risk factors associated with geohelminth infection in tea-growing communities of Assam, India." *Tropical Medicine & International Health* 9, no. 6 (2004): 688–701.

Tsai, Tyjen, and Paola Scommegna. "U.S. has world's highest incarceration rate." *Population Reference Bureau*. Published August 10, 2012. https://www.prb.org/us-incarceration/.

Tulin, Leah J. "Poverty and chronic conditions during natural disasters: A glimpse at health, healing, and Hurricane Katrina." *Georgetown Journal on Poverty Law and Policy* 14 (2007): 115.

U.S. Department of Education. "Equity of opportunity." Accessed October 15, 2019. https://www.ed.gov/equity.

U.S. Department of Health and Human Services Office of Minority Health. "Profile: Black/African Americans." Accessed December 2019. https://minorityhealth.hhs.gov/omh/browse.aspx?lvl=3&lvlid=61.

Umetsu, Shuichiro, Tsuyoshi Sogo, Kentaro Iwasawa, Takeo Kondo, Tomoyuki Tsunoda, Manari Oikawa-Kawamoto, Haruki Komatsu, Ayano Inui, and Tomoo Fujisawa. "Intestinal ascariasis at pediatric emergency room in a developed country." *World Journal of Gastroenterology: WJG* 20, no. 38 (2014): 14058.

UN Water. "World toilet day 2019." Accessed October 15, 2019. https://www.worldtoiletday.info/.

United Nations General Assembly. "Sixty-ninth session of the United National General Assembly: Draft outcome document of the United Nations summit for the adoption of the post-2015 development agenda." Published August 12, 2015. http://www.un.org/ga/search/view_doc.asp?symbol=A/69/L.85&Lang=E.

United Nations Sustainable Development Goals. "Water and sanitation." Accessed August 15, 2019. https://www.un.org/sustainabledevelopment/water-and-sanitation/.

United Way. "Measure of society." Last modified 2016. https://www.unitedway.org/our-impact/stories/ar-measure-of-a-society.

Upshur, Ross. "Ethics and infectious disease." *Bulletin of the World Health Organization* 86 (2008): 654.

Ura, Alexa, and Elbert Wang. "Poverty in Texas drops to lowest levels in more than a decade." *Texas Tribune*. Published September 13, 2018. https://www.texastribune.org/2018/09/13/texas-poverty-census-2017-lowest-levels-decade/#targetT ext=And%20families%20living%20in%20the,that's%20double%20the%20state%20figure.&targetText=The%20latest%20estimates%20released%20Thursday,of%2018.5%20percent%20in%202011.

Urlacher, Samuel S., Peter T. Ellison, Lawrence S. Sugiyama, Herman Pontzer, Geeta Eick, Melissa A. Liebert, Tara J. Cepon-Robins, Theresa E. Gildner, and J. Josh Snodgrass. "Tradeoffs between immune function and childhood growth among Amazonian forager-horticulturalists." *Proceedings of the National Academy of Sciences* 115, no. 17 (2018): e3914–e3921.

US Census Bureau. "How the Census Bureau measures poverty." Accessed December 1, 2019. https://www.census.gov/topics/income-poverty/poverty/guidance/poverty-measures.html.

US Department of Health and Human Services. "LIHEAP home energy notebook for fiscal year 2011." (2014).

US Department of Housing and Urban Development. *Strategic Plan FY2000–FY2006*. Washington, D.C., 2000.

USAID and RTI International. "Neglected tropical disease control program final report." Published 2012, 9. http://www.ntdenvision.org/sites/default/files/docs/ntdcp_report_lo_update.pdf.

———. "The envision impact final report." Published December 31, 2019. https://www.ntdenvision.org/sites/default/files/docs/PA00WB3N.pdf.

USAID Neglected Tropical Disease Program. "Mass drug administration." Published 2019. https://www.neglecteddiseases.gov/about/what-we-do/mass-drug-administration.

Vaitla, Bapu, Stephen Devereux, and Samuel Hauenstein Swan. "Seasonal hunger: A neglected problem with proven solutions." *PLoS Medicine* 6, no. 6 (2009): e1000101.

Vazquez-Prokopec, Gonzalo M., Audrey Lenhart, and Pablo Manrique-Saide. "Housing improvement: A novel paradigm for urban vector-borne disease control?" *Transactions of the Royal Society of Tropical Medicine and Hygiene* 110, no. 10 (2016): 567–569.

Vermeer, Donald E., and Dennis A. Frate. "Geophagy in a Mississippi county." *Annals of the Association of American Geographers* 65, no. 3 (1975): 414–424.

Victora, Cesar G., Fernando C. Barros, Rosângela C. Lima, Dominique P. Behague, Helen Gonçalves, Bernardo L. Horta, Denise P. Gigante, and J. Patrick Vaughan. "The Pelotas birth cohort study, Rio Grande do Sul, Brazil, 1982–2001." *Cadernos de saude publica* 19, no. 5 (2003): 1241–1256.

Vinetz, Joseph M., Gregory E. Glass, Charles E. Flexner, Paul Mueller, and David C. Kaslow. "Sporadic urban leptospirosis." *Annals of Internal Medicine* 125, no. 10 (1996): 794–798.

Vock, Daniel. "People are literally being poisoned: How sewage problems in Alabama got so bad—And why other states should worry." *Governing*. Published July 17, 2018. https://www.governing.com/topics/transportation-infrastructure/gov-alabama-hookworm-sewage.html.

Wagstaff, Adam. "Poverty and health sector inequalities." *Bulletin of the World Health Organization* 80 (2002): 97–105.

Waide, R. B., M. R. Willig, C. F. Steiner, G. Mittelbach, L. Gough, S. I. Dodson, G. P. Juday, and R. Parmenter. "The relationship between productivity and species richness." *Annual Review of Ecology and Systematics* 30, no. 1 (1999): 257–300.

Wallace, P. *Eat White Dirt*. Directed by Forrester A. United States: Public Broadcasting Service, 2015.

Walsh, Michael G., and M. A. Haseeb. "Reduced cognitive function in children with toxocariasis in a nationally representative sample of the United States." *International Journal for Parasitology* 42, no. 13–14 (2012): 1159–1163.

Wayland, III, Robert H., and E. T. Oppelt. "Onsite wastewater treatment systems manual." United States: Environmental Protection Agency, 2002.

Weaver, Haylee J., John M. Hawdon, and Eric P. Hoberg. "Soil-transmitted helminthiases: Implications of climate change and human behavior." *Trends in Parasitology* 26, no. 12 (2010): 574–581.

Webster, Joanne P., David H. Molyneux, P. J. Hotez, and Alan Fenwick. "The contribution of mass drug administration to global health: Past, present and future." *Philosophical Transactions of the Royal Society B: Biological Sciences* 369, no. 1645 (2014): 20130434.

Weiman, David F. "Imagining a world without the new deal." *The Washington Post*. Published August 12, 2011. https://www.washingtonpost.com/opinions/imagining-a-world-without-the-new-deal/2011/08/03/gIQAtJoBBJ_story.html.

Weinthal, Erika, Elizabeth Albright, Catherine C. Flowers, and Emily Stewart. "Solution-centered collaborative research in rural Alabama." *Social Science Research Council*. Published March 6, 2018. https://items.ssrc.org/insights/solution-centered-collaborative-research-in-rural-alabama/.

Weisenburger, Dennis D. "Human health effects of agrichemical use." *Human Pathology* 24, no. 6 (1993): 571–576.

Wesseling, Catharina, Rob McConnell, Timo Partanen, and Christer Hogstedt. "Agricultural pesticide use in developing countries: Health effects and research needs." *International Journal of Health Services* 27, no. 2 (1997): 273–308.

Whitehead, Nadia. "The U.S. thought it was rid of hookworm. Wrong." *NPR.org*. Published September 12, 2017. https://www.npr.org/sections/goatsandsoda/2017/09/12/550387650/the-u-s-thought-it-was-rid-of-hookworm-wrong.

Wilemon, Tom. "TN, KY are miles apart on Medicaid." *The Tennessean*. Published July 22, 2013. https://passportmedia.wordpress.com/2013/07/22/tn-ky-are-miles-apart-on-medicaid/.

Willers, Denise M., Jeffrey F. Peipert, Jenifer E. Allsworth, Michael D. Stein, Jennifer S. Rose, and Jennifer G. Clarke. "Prevalence and predictors of sexually transmitted infection among newly incarcerated females." *Sexually Transmitted Diseases* 35, no. 1 (2008): 68–72.

Williams, Brian. ""That we may live": Pesticides, plantations, and environmental racism in the United States South." *Environment and Planning E: Nature and Space* 1, no. 1–2 (2018): 243–267.

Wills, John, Louis Garrison, and Itzhak Jacoby. *Report of the Graduate Medical Education National Advisory Committee to the Secretary, Department of Health and Human Services: Modeling, Research, and Data Technical Panel*. Washington,

D.C.: US Department of Health and Human Services, Public Health Service, Health Resources Administration, Office of Graduate Medical Education, 1981.

Wølner-Hanssen, Pål, John N. Krieger, Claire E. Stevens, Nancy B. Kiviat, Laura Koutsky, Cathy Critchlow, Timothy DeRouen, Sharon Hillier, and King K. Holmes. "Clinical manifestations of vaginal trichomoniasis." *JAMA* 261, no. 4 (1989): 571–576.

Wood, David. "Effect of child and family poverty on child health in the United States." *Pediatrics* 112, no. 3 (2003): 707–711.

Wood, Sherwin F. "New localities for Trypannosoma cruzi Chagas in southwestern United States." *American Journal of Epidemiology* 34, no. 1 (1941): 1–13.

Woodhall, Dana M., Mark L. Eberhard, and Monica E. Parise. "Neglected parasitic infections in the United States: Toxocariasis." *The American Journal of Tropical Medicine and Hygiene* 90, no. 5 (2014): 810–813.

Woody, Norman C., and Hannah B. Woody. "American trypanosomiasis (Chagas' disease); first indigenous case in the United States." *Journal of the American Medical Association* 159, no. 7 (1955): 676–677.

Woody, Norman C., Noel DeDianous, and Hannah B. Woody. "American Trypanosomiasis. II. Current serologie studies in Chagas' disease." *Journal of Pediatrics* 58, no. 5 (1961): 738–745.

Workowski, Kimberly A., and Stuart M. Berman. "Sexually transmitted diseases treatment guidelines, 2015." *MMWR. Morbidity and Mortality Weekly Report: Recommendations and Reports*. Published 2010. https://www.cdc.gov/mmwr/preview/mmwrhtml/rr5912a1.htm.

World Health Organization. "Accelerating work to overcome the global impact of neglected tropical diseases: A roadmap for implementation." Published 2012. https://unitingtocombatntds.org/wp-content/uploads/2017/11/who_ntd_roadmap.pdf.

———. "Keeping the vector out: Housing improvements for vector control and sustainable development." Published 2017. https://www.who.int/social_determinants/publications/keeping-the-vector-out/en/.

———. "Neglected Tropical diseases." Accessed March 15, 2019. http://www.who.int/neglected_diseases/diseases/en/.

———. "Probability of dying per 1000 live births: Data by country." Last modified October 14, 2019. http://apps.who.int/gho/data/node.main.525?lang=en.

———. *Public Health Impact of Pesticides Used in Agriculture*, 1990.

———. "Sanitation." Accessed October 15, 2019. http://www.who.int/topics/sanitation/en/.

———. "Yellow fever." Published May 7, 2019. https://www.who.int/en/news-room/fact-sheets/detail/yellow-fever.

———. "Yellow fever: Questions and answers." Published March 2, 2017. https://www.who.int/features/qa/yellow-fever/en/.

World Health Organization Department of Control of Neglected Tropical Diseases. *Sustaining the Drive to Overcome the Global Impact of Neglected Tropical Diseases: Second WHO Report on Neglected Diseases*. Geneva: World Health Organization, 2013. https://www.who.int/neglected_diseases/9789241564540/en/

Yale Law School. "Inaugural address of George W. Bush; January 20, 2001." Published 2008. https://avalon.law.yale.edu/21st_century/gbush1.asp.

Yan, Wudan. "Grappling with the health consequences of floods: Hurricanes, monsoons, and heavy rains have researchers studying how to prevent the diseases that often follow." *IEEE Pulse* 9, no. 2 (2018): 26–30.

Young, Maria-Elena De Trinidad, Gabriela León-Pérez, Christine R. Wells, and Steven P. Wallace. "More inclusive states, less poverty among immigrants? An examination of poverty, citizenship stratification, and state immigrant policies." *Population Research and Policy Review* 37, no. 2 (2018): 205–228.

Zekeri, Andrew A. "The causes of enduring poverty in Alabama's Black Belt." In *In the Shadows of Poverty: Strengthening the Rural Poverty Research Capacity of the South*. Mississippi State, MS: Mississippi State University, Rural Policy Research Institute's Rural Poverty Research Center, 2004.

Zera, Anthony J., and Lawrence G. Harshman. "The physiology of life history trade-offs in animals." *Annual Review of Ecology and Systematics* 32, no. 1 (2001): 95–126.

Zhan, Bin, Coreen M. Beaumier, Neima Briggs, Kathryn M. Jones, Brian P. Keegan, Maria Elena Bottazzi, and Peter J. Hotez. "Advancing a multivalent 'Pan-anthelmintic' vaccine against soil-transmitted nematode infections." *Expert Review of Vaccines* 13, no. 3 (2014): 321–331.

Zhang, Ping, Guoyu Tao, and Lynda A. Anderson. "Differences in access to health care services among adults in rural America by rural classification categories and age." *Australian Journal of Rural Health* 11, no. 2 (2003): 64–72.

Zhou, Xiao-Nong, Li-Ying Wang, Ming-Gang Chen, Tian-Ping Wang, Jia-Gang Guo, Xiao-Hua Wu, Qing-Wu Jiang, Jiang Zheng, and Xian-Yi Chen. "An economic evaluation of the national schistosomiasis control programme in China from 1992 to 2000." *Acta Tropica* 96, no. 2–3 (2005): 255–265.

Ziliak, J. "Modernizing SNAP benefits." *The Hamilton Project, Policy Proposal 2016–06*. https://www.hamiltonproject.org/assets/files/ziliak_modernizing_snap_benefits.pdf.

Zimmerman, Seth D. "Elite colleges and upward mobility to top jobs and top incomes." *American Economic Review* 109, no. 1 (2019): 1–47.

Zong, Jie, Jeanne Batalova, and Jeffrey Hallock. "Frequently requested statistics on immigrants and immigration in the United States." *Migration Policy Institute* 26 (2015): 1–18.

Zuckerman, Stephen, and Teresa Coughlin. "Initial health policy responses to hurricane Katrina and possible next steps." Washington D.C.: The Urban Institute, 2006.

Index

About the Authors

Dr. Christine Crudo Blackburn is an assistant research scientist and deputy director of the Pandemic and Biosecurity Policy Program with the Scowcroft Institute for International Affairs in the Bush School of Government & Public Service and an adjunct faculty member at in the Department of Health Promotion and Community Health Sciences in the School for Public Health at Texas A&M University. In these roles she conducts research on issues related to pandemics, zoonotic diseases, and health of vulnerable populations. Dr. Blackburn teaches course on infectious disease in low-income countries, refugee health, the social and political impacts of pandemics, and bioterrorism.

Prior to her position at the Scowcroft Institute she worked as a postdoctoral researcher in the Field Disease Investigation Unit in the College of Veterinary Medicine at Washington State University. Dr. Blackburn received her PhD in 2015 from Washington State University as part of the Individual Interdisciplinary Doctoral Program, a degree program that requires three major fields of study. Dr. Blackburn's doctoral fields were Political Science, Communication, and Veterinary Clinical Sciences.

Ms. Macey T. Lively received her Master of International Affairs degree from the Bush School of Government and Service at Texas A&M University. There, she studied American Homeland Security and courses offered by faculty of the Scowcroft Institute of International Affairs Pandemic and Biosecurity Policy Program. As a student, she has participated in research involving the economic impact of epidemics and improving business continuity in the Congo, the impact of health on violent extremism, and NTDs in the United States. Ms. Lively is currently a Master of Public Health student at the School of Public Health at Texas A&M University studying epidemiology while completing an internship with the Western Gulf Center of Excellence for Vector-Borne Diseases.

www.ingramcontent.com/pod-product-compliance
Lightning Source LLC
LaVergne TN
LVHW091533200926
848483LV00002B/387